T0339617

The Innate Immune Response to Noninfectious Stressors

Human and Animal Models

The Innate Immune Response to Noninfectious Stressors

Human and Animal Models

Edited by

Massimo Amadori

Laboratory of Cellular Immunology,
Istituto Zooprofilattico Sperimentale della
Lombardia e dell'Emilia-Romagna,
Brescia, Italy

AMSTERDAM • BOSTON • HEIDELBERG • LONDON
NEW YORK • OXFORD • PARIS • SAN DIEGO
SAN FRANCISCO • SINGAPORE • SYDNEY • TOKYO

Academic Press is an Imprint of Elsevier

Academic Press is an imprint of Elsevier
125 London Wall, London EC2Y 5AS, UK
525 B Street, Suite 1800, San Diego, CA 92101-4495, USA
50 Hampshire Street, 5th Floor, Cambridge, MA 02139, USA
The Boulevard, Langford Lane, Kidlington, Oxford OX5 1GB, UK

British Library Cataloguing-in-Publication Data
A catalogue record for this book is available from the British Library

Library of Congress Cataloging-in-Publication Data
A catalog record for this book is available from the Library of Congress

ISBN: 978-0-12-801968-9

For information on all Academic Press publications
visit our website at http://store.elsevier.com/

Publisher: Sara Tenney
Acquisition Editor: Linda Versteeg-Buschman
Editorial Project Manager: Halima Williams
Production Project Manager: Chris Wortley
Designer: Mark Rogers

Typeset by Thomson Digital
Printed and bound in the United States of America

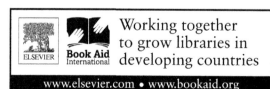

This book is dedicated to school teachers, colleagues, and friends who prompted me to doubt and question established dogmas, and deterred me from accepting easy and accessible truths for the sake of short-term community recognition.

Contents

7. Innate Immune Response and Psychotic Disorders

Jaana Suvisaari, Outi Mantere

8. Modulation of the Interferon Response by Environmental, Noninfectious Stressors

Elisabetta Razzuoli, Cinzia Zanotti, Massimo Amadori

9. **Disease-Predicting and Prognostic Potential of Innate Immune Responses to Noninfectious Stressors: Human and Animal Models**

Erminio Trevisi, Livia Moscati, Massimo Amadori

Contributors

Massimo Amadori Laboratory of Cellular Immunology, Istituto Zooprofilattico Sperimentale della Lombardia e dell'Emilia-Romagna, Brescia, Italy

Ryutaro Fukui Division of Infectious Genetics, Institute of Medical Science, Tokyo, Japan

Stefania Gallucci Department of Microbiology and Immunology, Laboratory of Dendritic Cell Biology, Temple University, School of Medicine, Philadelphia, PA, USA

Segundo González Departamento de Inmunología, Hospital Universitario Central de Asturias, Oviedo, Asturias, Spain

Nicola Lacetera Department of Agriculture, Forests, Nature and Energy, University of Tuscia, Viterbo, Italy

Carlos López-Larrea Departamento de Biología Funcional, Inmunología, Universidad de Oviedo, Instituto Universitario de Oncología del Principado de Asturias, Asturias, Spain

Alejandro López-Soto Departamento de Inmunología, Hospital Universitario Central de Asturias, Oviedo; Departamento de Biología Funcional, Inmunología, Universidad de Oviedo, Instituto Universitario de Oncología del Principado de Asturias, Asturias, Spain

Outi Mantere Department of Health, Mental Health Unit, National Institute for Health and Welfare, Helsinki, Finland

Yoshiro Maru Department of Pharmacology, Tokyo Women's Medical University, Shinjuku-ku, Tokyo, Japan

Kensuke Miyake Division of Infectious Genetics, Institute of Medical Science, Tokyo, Japan

Livia Moscati Laboratory of Clinical Sciences, Istituto Zooprofilattico Sperimentale Umbria e Marche, Perugia, Italy

Elisabetta Razzuoli Laboratory of Diagnostics, S.S. Genova, Istituto Zooprofilattico Sperimentale del Piemonte, Liguria e Valle d'Aosta, Piazza Borgo Pila, Genova, Italy

Elena Riboldi Department of Pharmaceutical Sciences, Università del Piemonte Orientale "Amedeo Avogadro," Novara, Italy

Antonio Sica Department of Pharmaceutical Sciences, Università del Piemonte Orientale "Amedeo Avogadro," Novara; Department of Inflammation and Immunology, Humanitas Clinical and Research Center, Rozzano, Italy

Jaana Suvisaari Department of Health, Mental Health Unit, National Institute for Health and Welfare, Helsinki, Finland

Erminio Trevisi Faculty of Agriculture, Food and Environmental Sciences, Istituto di Zootecnica, Università Cattolica del Sacro Cuore, Piacenza, Italy

Cinzia Zanotti Laboratory of Cellular Immunology, Istituto Zooprofilattico Sperimentale della Lombardia e dell'Emilia-Romagna, Brescia, Italy

Preface

The concept of innate immune response to noninfectious stressors needs a definition of its foundation and of relevant underlying tenets. This way, the reader can be confronted with a coherent, unitary conceptual framework, in which diverse biological features of such a response can be adequately grasped and traced back to common cause/effect mechanisms.

Individuals are prompted to adapt in order to improve and optimize the interaction with their environment. In this respect, animals usually adopt a "feed forward" strategy – animals mount a corrective action to potentially noxious stimuli before whichever problem becomes substantial.[1] This process is affected by animal needs, which may refer to vital resources or to particular actions underlying the access to vital resources. Adaptation implies a stepwise corrective action, whereby activity and energy expense are proportional to the perceived threat. In this scenario, inflammation should be interpreted as a protective attempt to restore a homeostatic state of the host. Threats are caused by stressors, meant as whatever biological, or physico-chemical entities, real or unreal (psychotic) conditions affecting or potentially affecting the established levels of homeostasis, according to the host's perception. Adaptation to environmental stressors can be measured by different procedures, including the evaluation of physiological parameters. These indicate the onset of a biological defense action,[2] characterized by:

1. An early, biological response (neuro-endocrine and behavioral);
2. A later change of biological functions in different organs and apparata.

As for phase 2, immune functions represent a crucial reporter system of the adaptation process because of the strict functional and anatomical connections between brain and lymphoid organs; the brain itself is the main regulatory organ of the immune system. As highlighted in a previous review paper,[3] the two main circuits, "psycho-sensitive stimuli/behavioral response" and "antigenic stimuli/immune response," are indeed subsystems of a unitary integrated complex aimed at providing optimal conditions for the host's survival and adaptation (see Fig. P.1). In this conceptual framework, immune responses, stress, and inflammation should be considered an ancestral, overlapping set of responses aimed at the neutralization of stimuli perturbing body homeostasis.[4]

Within the immune system, innate immunity is the first line of defense against a plethora of *noxae* perturbing the host's homeostatic balance. It is based

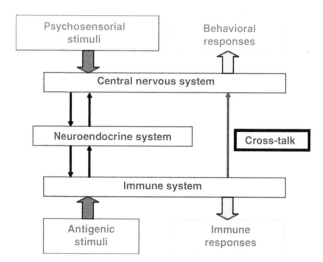

FIGURE P.1   The central nervous and immune systems are part of a unitary integrated complex.

on complex pathways of recognition and signaling for pathogen-associated molecular patterns (PAMPs) and damage-associated molecular patterns (DAMPs), as well as on diverse humoral and cell-mediated effector functions. Microbial components are recognized by means of pattern-recognition receptors (PRRs) including Toll-like and NOD-like receptors (TLRs and NLRs).[5] The activation of PRRs results in the expression of proinflammatory cytokines, chemokines, and antimicrobial peptides, initiating and regulating the immune response. The possible recognition of PAMPs and DAMPs implies that the innate immune system can detect (1) infectious microbial pathogens and (2) cellular stress caused by a plethora of noninfectious physico-chemical agents, or by the very response to microbial agents.[5] Both infectious and noninfectious agents can deliver in fact "danger" signals,[6] which are processed for subsequent humoral and cell-mediated responses. Danger signals may be soluble (DAMPs) or cell-associated (stress antigens) for a recognition by natural killer and some γδ T cell populations, in the framework of the "lymphoid stress surveillance system."[7]

The innate immune system may also have a profound impact on concomitant behavioral adaptation responses, as exemplified by the role of proinflammatory cytokines in the induction of sickness behavior (lethargy, anorexia, and curtailing of social and reproductive activities) that is a clearly defined motivational status.[8] Thus, the innate immune system reshuffles behavioral priorities toward a well-organized, integrated response to microbial infections; interestingly, behavioral depression was shown to provide an important adaptive advantage to sick animals, anorexia being thus associated to a better chance for survival under such conditions.[9]

The relationship between stress, inflammation, and immune functions deserves a few comments. Usually, transient acute stresses are not noxious for healthy individuals, and they may be associated with better immune responses. These events are even thought of as nature's adjuvant under field conditions.[10] On the whole, the consequences of stress on immune functions are generally adaptive in the short term, whereas they can be damaging when stress is chronic, including predisposition to disease occurrence.

If innate immune functions represent a crucial reporter system of effective versus noneffective adaptation to infectious and noninfectious stressors, it goes without saying that a sound panel of clinical immunology tests may reveal subjects at risk for disease occurrence, as a result of poor environmental adaptation. Predisposition to disease occurrence after exposure to chronic stress may have two faces in the same coin:

1. Reduced clearance of common environmental pathogens.
2. Poor homeostatic control of the inflammatory response.

In general, a defective innate immune response forces the host to a wider use of the adaptive immune response (antibody and cytotoxic T lymphocytes), which is demanding in terms of energy expense.[11]

The innate immune response must be regulated to enable efficient pathogen killing but also to limit detrimental tissue pathology.[12] This is the reason why a complex of sensing receptors and signaling pathways developed along the phylogenetic evolution to allow the coordinated expression of proinflammatory and anti-inflammatory cytokines in response to environmental stress. In particular, the signaling pathway consisting of phosphoinositide 3 (Pi3)-kinase, Akt, and mechanistic target of rapamycin (mTor) is a key regulator of innate immune responses to environmental stress.[13] Among mitogen-activated protein kinases, p38 plays a crucial role in the regulation of mTor activity. p38 can be activated by TLR ligands, cytokines, and most importantly, by diverse physicochemical, noninfectious stress signals.[14] p38- and Pi3-driven signals coordinately act on mTor to regulate the expression of IL-12 and IL-10 in myeloid immune cells.[12]

Therefore, the innate immune system can finely tune pro- and anti-inflammatory responses in tissues after exposure to both infectious and noninfectious stressors.

Innate immune responses to both infectious and noninfectious stressors are finely modulated by the host's microbiota, meant as the ensemble of microorganisms that resides in an established environment. There are clusters of bacteria in different parts of the body, such as the gut, skin, mouth, vagina, and so on. Gut microbiota corresponds to the huge microbial population living in the intestine, containing trillions of microorganisms with some 1000 different species, most of them specific to each subject. The recognition of commensal microorganisms is essential for the development and function of the immune system in the mucosal and peripheral districts.[15] The activities of the innate immune system are finely tuned by commensal bacteria. These can, for example, inhibit NF-κB activation by disrupting the host cell control over ubiquitination and degradation,[16] thus exerting an anti-inflammatory control action. Also,

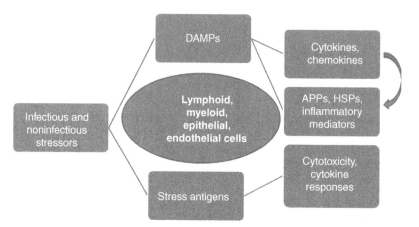

FIGURE P.2 **Common features of infectious and noninfectious stressors.** APPs, acute-phase proteins; HSPs, heat-shock proteins.

commensal bacteria can release metabolites of complex digested polysaccharides, which may induce the expression of anti-inflammatory cytokines such as IL-10.[17] Several aspects of innate immunity are stimulated by specific bacterial strains, whereas the whole microbiota exerts a substantial inflammatory control of the gut ecosystem and of pathogen susceptibility, in the framework of a continuous "cross-talk" with the mucosal immune system.[18] This interaction is critical; the microbiota is required for proper development and function of innate immune cells. In turn, these provide effector functions that maintain a stable microbiota, in the framework of interdependency and feedback mechanisms aimed at mutual homeostasis.[19]

The effective recognition of PAMPs and DAMPs and the related signaling pathways imply that *sensing, signaling, and effector mechanisms of the innate immune system are remarkably similar for both infectious and noninfectious stimuli, albeit differently modulated (Fig. P.2). This is the central tenet and subject of this book*, which deals with different kinds of noninfectious stressors in preclinical and clinical studies in both human and veterinary medicine.

Innate immune responses to noninfectious stressors can be best grasped by a few examples, in the light of consolidated research models:

- As illustrated in a previous review article,[3] a proinflammatory cytokine of the innate immune system like IL-1 induces activation of the hypothalamo-pituitary-adrenocortical axis as well as stimulation of cerebral noradrenaline; the effects of IL-1 are remarkably similar to those observed following either LPS administration (reminiscent of infectious stress) or acute, noninfectious stressing events in laboratory animals, such as electric shock or restraint.[20] Likewise, the brain produces interferon (IFN)-α in response to noninflammatory as well as inflammatory stress; the intracerebral injection of this cytokine may alter the brain activity to exert a feedback effect on the immune system.[21]

- Pigs mount an IFN-α response to early weaning, which also affect the usual pattern of constitutive expression of type I IFN genes.[22] Early weaning is associated with the expression of inflammatory cytokine genes in the proximal and distal parts of the small intestine.[23] Calves also mount IFN-α responses to long-distance road journeys in trucks (M. Amadori, unpublished results). In the mentioned studies, both pigs and cattle did not show evidence of concomitant viral infections.

- Abnormal inflammatory responses and activation of the innate immune system (cytokines, acute phase responses) can be detected in high-yielding dairy cows submitted to the metabolic stress of lactation onset.[24]

- Heat stress can induce innate immune responses in cattle, as shown by Peli et al. in a field survey in one beef and one veal farm located in Northern Italy.[25] The survey was carried out during a meteoalarm issued in July 2009 by the Italian environmental control authorities. Blood samples were collected from 10 head/farm 1–2 days before the announced heat wave and 3–4 days after, a heat wave being defined as average daily temperature humidity index (THI) ≥ 73. In both farms, this threshold value was overstepped as a result of sudden THI increase (+6.5 points). A significant increase of white blood cell (WBC) counts took place in cattle, showing no correlation with hematocrit values. Cattle showed increases of serum IL-4 ($P < 0.01$), IL-6, and TNF-α, as well as a significant decrease of serum IFN-γ levels ($P < 0.01$) over the heat stress period. In general, the impact of the heat stress was more serious in steers than in calves. These data are fully in agreement with previous findings in humans after traumatic and burn injuries, which confirm a major downregulation of the TH1 response and an upregulation of the TH2 response.[26] These findings should be offset against the current figures of high mortality rates of farm animals in hot summer periods,[27] which are of concern in terms of both animal health and welfare.

- The innate immune response to endocrine disruptors is a fascinating issue, largely investigated in fish models. Thus, there is evidence that the fish immune system is a potential target for environmental endocrine disruptors.[28] Oxidative stress (an imbalance between production and depletion of reactive oxygen species, ROS) is the first response to environmental stressors,[29] as shown, for example, in a zebrafish model of exposure to atrazine.[30] ROS are associated with cell injury or death, lipid peroxidation, and membrane damage. Therefore, they cause the release of DAMPs and relevant innate immune responses. Thus, in another zebrafish model, the exposure to phthalate esters caused a significant increase of mRNA levels of interferon (IFN)-gamma, interleukin (IL)-1 beta, Mx protein, lysozyme and complement factor C3B genes.[31]

- Widespread toxic compounds in forages and milk like mycotoxins also induce responses of the innate immune system. Mycotoxins are secondary metabolites of fungi, which may contaminate food and feeds. The same mold can produce different mycotoxins, but the presence of a particular mold does not always indicate that a certain mycotoxin is released; moreover, different fungi can contaminate the feed in different production phases (plant growth, harvest, and storage). In particular, mycotoxins can cause oxidative stress[32] and modulate the immune response, resulting in different forms of immunosuppression (depressed T- or B-lymphocyte activity, suppressed antibody production, and impaired macrophage/neutrophil-effector functions), and a release of proinflammatory cytokines (IL-1β, IL-6, and TNF-α), and acute phase proteins like haptoglobin and serum amyloid A.[33,34] Therefore, mycotoxins exert a two-sided interaction with the host, underlying (1) classical immunotoxic activities giving rise to different forms of immunosuppression[34] and (2) cellular stress causing innate immune responses. These two features may obviously overlap and act synergically in the host. Thus, increased susceptibility to human and animal infectious diseases can be observed after exposure to mycotoxins.[35] Because of their worldwide distribution and toxic effects mycotoxins are considered an important risk for human health.[36] Many studies demonstrated the immunotoxic and/or immunomodulatory effects of single mycotoxins, even though there are no clear data about the effects of a combined exposure to different mycotoxins.

- The systemic inflammatory response syndrome is an extremely serious innate immune response to tissue damages. This may be observed, for example, in some human patients with fractures, who develop high fever and shock after a couple of days. The traditional hypothesis of a reduced posttraumatic blood flow in the gut underlying increased intestinal permeability and bacteremia was discounted, since portal blood of these patients is sterile.[37] Instead, the plasma has a high concentration of mitochondrial DNA (a noninfectious stressor) as a result of cellular disruption by trauma. These mitochondrial DAMPs with evolutionarily conserved similarities to bacterial PAMPs can then signal through identical innate immune pathways to create a sepsis-like state.[37]

- As previously stated, one of the likely associations between noninfectious stress and innate immunity can be traced back to the lymphoid stress-surveillance system, that is, to the network of lymphocyte populations (mainly γδ T cells), which recognize neo-antigens like MIC on stressed cells,[7] that is, cells exposed to events as diverse as heat shock, infections, DNA damage, and so on. MIC and other proteins are ligands for the activating NK cell receptor NKG2D, expressed on NK cells, CD8+ αβ T cells and γδ T cells, also sustaining an IFN-γ response.[38] The response to stress antigens aims to control the negative consequences for the host in terms of tissue damage and biological fitness. This tenet is probably relevant to the impact of psychotic stressors, too. Thus, in murine models, the ability to control the consequences of mental stress is dependent on peripheral immunity. T cells specific to abundantly expressed CNS antigens are responsible for brain tissue homeostasis and help the individual to cope with stressful life episodes, their activity being checked by regulatory CD4+ CD25+ T cells.[39] Animals with immune deficiency show a reduced ability to check the consequences of stress in terms of anxiety and startle response.[40] Interestingly, a short exposure to a psychotic stressor can enhance T-cell infiltration to the brain, associated with increased ICAM-1 expression by choroid plexus cells. The mental stress response can be reduced by immunization with a CNS-related myelin peptide.[40] This is an interesting example of "protective autoimmunity," in which a primary stress response gives rise to a protective adaptive immune response to self-tissue antigens.

- Psychologically stressful states may underlie inflammation in the visceral fat and vasculature of patients with cardiovascular disease.[41] Also, a psychological stress condition induces a shift in the type-1/type-2 cytokine balance toward a type-2 response, which may play a role in the course of hepatitis B virus infection.[42]
- Nutrient overload (obesity model of metabolic stress) promotes inflammation, sustained by inflammatory cytokines.[43] Obesity is characterized by chronic low-grade inflammation with permanently increased oxidative stress, which damages cellular structures, and leads to the development of obesity-related complications.[44]

Regardless of the triggering cause, the findings mentioned indicate that the innate immune and inflammatory response is triggered in the host to achieve a better ability to deal with both infectious and noninfectious stress.[5] At the same time, this response needs to be accurately controlled to avoid tissue damage and waste of metabolic energy.

In this conceptual framework, the book aims to illustrate the aforementioned concepts in established models of response to noninfectious, physical, chemical, metabolic, and psychotic stressors in both animals and humans. The reader will be presented with updated contributions on these subjects and given ideas and perspectives of leading edge research activities in these and other related fields of investigation.

The book is opened by an overview of the innate immune response by Stefania Gallucci. This overview is mainly focused on a detailed description of the sensors implied in the recognition of noninfectious stressors, their main categories, and signaling pathways. This way the reader can be aware of the strategies adopted by the host to check these stressors and prevent unwanted consequences in terms of homeostatic balance.

The above chapter is strictly correlated with the contribution by Kensuke Miyake on "homeostatic inflammation." DAMPs are produced not only by damaged cells in disease, but also by undamaged cells. This leads in turn to the new fascinating concept of autoimmune disease as an outcome of an excessive response of innate immune sensors to their endogenous ligands. This implies that the host steadily exerts a fine tuning of low-grade, physiological inflammatory responses, aimed at optimizing homeostatic balance and major physiological functions. Homeostatic inflammation is therefore a foundation of successful environmental adaptation. Failure of either induction or control of these crucial circuits can give rise to serious clinical repercussions.

Lopèz-Soto et al. deals with the molecular basis of the immune response to stressed cells. The reader is confronted with the mechanisms controlling the expression of molecules (stress antigens) with key roles in immunity. The subsequent activation of dendritic cells and T-cell-mediated responses outlines an interesting model, whereby a primary signal of the innate immune system (stress antigens) gives rise to an effector innate response (NK cells), or to adaptive T cell responses. This is actually reminiscent of "protective autoimmunity" by the host's T cells, following exposure to the aforementioned psychotic stress. Since the response to stress antigens frequently takes place in the host, the prevalence of reactive NK and T cells may be high, which may have important consequences on diagnostic assays of cell-mediated immunity. These can be biased whenever responder lymphocytes are confronted *in vitro* with both Ag-specific and stress antigens, expressed, for example, in established cell lines.[45] Also, it would be worth investigating in the future the possible evolution of NK cell responses to self-stress antigens, in line with recent evidence of a "maturation" of NK responses to viral infections – NK cells can acquire in fact some form of immunological memory, and enhanced NK functions can be displayed during secondary, compared to primary exposure to virus infections.[46]

One of the major stressors involved in the generation of DAMPs is hypoxia, as illustrated in the contribution by Elena Riboldi and Antonio Sica. Hypoxia is linked to the production of reactive oxygen species (ROS), which underlies the generation of inflammasomes and the release of inflammatory cytokines like IL-1 and IL-18.[47] On the whole, hypoxia and inflammatory signals share selected transcriptional events, including the activation of members of both the hypoxia-inducible factor (HIF) and nuclear factor κB (NF-κB) families. These concepts are of paramount importance in the pathophysiology of human diseases ranging from cancer, to infections, to chronic inflammation. This is also relevant to an important large animal model, the pig. The percentage weight of the heart muscle has decreased from 0.38% in wild boars to 0.21% in modern Landrace pigs.[48] Such pigs show an accentuated mean capillary-to-fiber distance in larger (type II) muscle fibers, which hampers an effective removal of toxic metabolites and favors lactic acid accumulation.[49] The resulting tissue hypoxia induces conditions of persistent oxidative stress response, which paves the way to serious clinical conditions such as Mulberry Heart Disease, Porcine Stress Syndrome, and Osteochondrosis. Disease predisposition as a result of genetic selection of pigs is also highlighted in the chapter by Erminio Trevisi, Livia Moscati, and Massimo Amadori. In agreement with the preceding statements, lean muscle pigs show in fact abnormally high serum concentrations of reactive oxygen metabolites (ROMs), as opposed to rural swine.[48]

The concept of metabolic stress and its recognition by the innate immune system is highlighted in the chapter by Nicola Lacetera in another large animal model – the high-yielding dairy cow. In this chapter, fundamental features of a major metabolic stress (energy deficit and oxidative stress after lactation onset) are analyzed with respect to heat-shock protein (HSP) responses. HSPs can act as signaling intermediates and regulate innate and adaptive immune responses. The outcome of these regulatory actions may dictate the inflammatory profile of the immune response during infections and diseases. *De facto*, the prevalence of diverse disease cases and culling rates are high in the early lactation phase of high-yielding dairy cows.[50,51] These findings are also commented in the chapter by Erminio Trevisi, Livia Moscati, and Massimo Amadori.

The chapter by Yoshiro Maru deals with the role of innate immune responses in cancer metastasis. These are substantially different from those observed in primary tumor tissues, in that they can alter microenvironments, whether physically and functionally, in the organs that are distant from the primary site. This remote control cultivates the so-called "soil" before the actual arrival of tumor cells as "seed" from the primary site. It can be argued that fundamental components of the innate immune system, mainly Toll-like receptors and inflammasomes, play a fundamental role in effective metastatization of primary tumor cells. In this model, the innate immune response to a noninfectious, tumor stressor may turn detrimental to the host and give rise to serious clinical repercussions.

The correlation between innate immune responses and generation of psychotic disorders in humans is the topic of the chapter by Jaana Suvisaari and Outi Mantere. The authors outline fundamentals of psychoneuroimmunology (PNEI), as a comprehensive conceptual framework in which complex laboratory and clinical findings can be correctly grasped and evaluated. In practice, the canonical boundaries between immune and neuroendocrine control systems can be no longer recognized in a continuum of homeostatic circuits, in which a single recognized effector function is part of a wider strategy for better survival and adaptation. Such a strategy is based upon networks of multidirectional signaling and feedback regulations effected by neuroendocrine- and immunocyte-derived mediators.[52] In this scenario, the reader can understand why proinflammatory activation of the innate immune system and T-cells of the adaptive immune system underlie first-episode psychosis and chronic psychotic disorders. Whereas such alterations are most pronounced in the acute clinical phase, chronic psychotic disorders and chronic inflammation proceed together, and they are often accompanied by metabolic comorbidities such as obesity, type 2 diabetes, and dyslipidemias. In the framework of PNEI, Suvisaari and Mantere outline psychotic disorders as neurodevelopmental diseases. In this scenario, they review scientific data about alterations in innate immune response during neonatal period and data on childhood exposures that could be linked to psychotic disorders via inflammatory mechanisms. Also, they discuss animal and genetic studies on schizophrenia supporting the role of immunological factors for disease occurrence.

The modulation of the IFN system by environmental, noninfectious stressors is illustrated in the chapter by Elisabetta Razzuoli, Cinzia Zanotti, and Massimo Amadori. Most data reviewed by the authors refer to Type I interferons, that is, a heterogeneous group including several distinct families (IFN-α, IFN-β, IFN-ϵ, IFN-ω, IFN-κ, IFN-δ, and IFN-τ), with some of them (like IFN-α) consisting of different subtypes.[53] Although type I IFNs were discovered as a potent antiviral substance accumulated in chick chorioallantoic membranes more than 50 years ago,[54] these cytokines were subsequently shown to exert a plethora of regulatory functions under both health and disease conditions: activation of immune effector cells, induction of Th1 responses, modulation of MHC expression, adrenocortical-stimulating, opioid-like and pyrectic properties, and induction of behavioral (psychotic) responses, to cite a few.[55] On the whole, type I IFNs have been highlighted as physiological modulators, with only one of their functions being the ability to hinder viral replication intracellularly. In this scenario, the authors review the accumulated evidence of an important role of Type I IFNs as homeostatic agents in the inflammatory response. As such, these cytokines can be detected following exposure to diverse environmental, noninfectious stressors inducing an inflammatory response in the host. IFN responses can be thus detected in large animal models of commingling, truck transportation, early weaning, as well as in human and animal models of psychotic stress and autoimmune diseases. The authors also discuss the constitutive expression of IFNs in tissues of healthy individuals, in view of its possible role and functions in the response to infectious and noninfectious stressors. Constitutive expression and a prevalent posttranscriptional control of expression outline a peculiar response system, dealt with by the authors on the basis of accumulated evidence in clinical and preclinical studies.

Clinical repercussions of altered innate immune responses to environmental stressors are illustrated in the final chapter by Erminio Trevisi, Livia Moscati, and Massimo Amadori. Cattle and pig models are illustrated in terms of timecourse of a few clinical immunology and chemistry parameters, depicting the process of environmental adaptation in critical phases of the farming activities, in agreement with the contents of Lacetera's chapter. In particular, the authors illustrate the disease-predicting and prognostic potential of some laboratory parameters of innate immune responses to noninfectious stressors. The chapter is mainly focused on large animal models, that is, dairy cows and pigs, for which strong evidence has been accumulated of a timely prediction of disease risks on the basis of laboratory parameters of innate immunity. These large animal models are compared with human models of innate immune responses and their predictive and prognostic value for disease occurrence. The authors also discuss the diagnostic and prognostic potential of common parameters of immunosuppression in man and animals like the plasma concentrations of widespread opportunistic viruses (Anelloviridae and the like).

On the whole, the chapters of this book provide a robust, comprehensive view of the critical interactions between environmental, noninfectious stressors, and the host's innate immune system, in a unitary and coherent conceptual framework. The "One Health" approach of this book aims to reconcile apparently diverging findings in different animal species with common interpretative views, and to provide a convenient framework to complex biological phenomena. In particular, the choice of large animal models stems from a critical reappraisal of current preclinical investigation strategies, whereby the need for an improved conceptual framework is both diverse and substantial. Large animal models are founded on animal species like pig, more closely related to humans than mice in terms of phylogenetic evolution, and showing anatomical and physiologic characters comparable to humans. Most importantly, moving beyond the mouse into large animal models should allow for better translation into clinical research.[56] In this scenario, the book can be conducive to fruitful links between preclinical and clinical research centers and to a relevant, positive impact on diagnostic, prophylactic, and therapeutic schemes for animal and human diseases.

REFERENCES

1. Broom DM. Adaptation. *Berl Munch Tierarztl Wochenschr* 2006;**119**:1–6.
2. Moberg GP. Biological response to stress: key to assessment of animal well-being? In: Moberg GP, editor. *Animal Stress*. Bethesda, Maryland: American Physiological Society; 1985. p. 27–49.
3. Amadori M, Stefanon B, Sgorlon S, Farinacci M. Immune system response to stress factors. *Ital J Anim Sci* 2009;**8**:287–99.
4. Ottaviani E, Franceschi C. A new theory on the common evolutionary origin of natural immunity, inflammation and stress response: the invertebrate phagocytic immunocyte as an eye-witness. *Domest Anim Endocrinol* 1998;**15**:291–6.
5. Gallo PM, Gallucci S. The dendritic cell response to classic, emerging, and homeostatic danger signals. Implications for autoimmunity. *Front Immunol* 2013;**4**:138.
6. Matzinger P. An innate sense of danger. *Ann NY Acad Sci* 2002;**961**:341–2.
7. Hayday AC. γδ T cells and the lymphoid stress-surveillance response. *Immunity* 2009;**31**:184–96.
8. Kelley KW, Bluthe RM, Dantzer R, Zhou JH, Shen WH, Johnson RW, et al. Cytokine-induced sickness behavior. *Brain Behav Immun* 2003;**17**(Suppl 1):S112–8.
9. Dantzer R, Kelley KW. Twenty years of research on cytokine-induced sickness behavior. *Brain Behav Immun* 2007;**21**:153–60.
10. Dhabhar FS, Viswanathan K. Short-term stress experienced at time of immunization induces a long-lasting increase in immunologic memory. *Am J Physiol Regul Integr Comp Physiol* 2005;**289**:R738–44.
11. Martin 2nd LB, Navara KJ, Weil ZM, Nelson RJ. Immunological memory is compromised by food restriction in deer mice *Peromyscus maniculatus*. *Am J Physiol Regul Integr Comp Physiol* 2007;**292**:R316–20.
12. Katholnig K, Kaltenecker CC, Hayakawa H, Rosner M, Lassnig C, Zlabinger GJ, et al. P38α senses environmental stress to control innate immune responses via mechanistic target of rapamycin. *J Immunol* 2013;**190**:1519–27.

13. Powell JD, Pollizzi KN, Heikamp EB, Horton MR. Regulation of immune responses by mTOR. *Annu Rev Immunol* 2012;**30**:39–68.

14. Coulthard LR, White DE, Jones DL, McDermott MF, Burchill SA. p38 (MAPK): stress responses from molecular mechanisms to therapeutics. *Trends Mol Med* 2009;**15**:369–79.

15. Macpherson AJ, Harris NL. Interactions between commensal intestinal bacteria and the immune system. *Nat Rev Immunol* 2004;**4**:478–85.

16. Neish AS, Gewirtz AT, Zeng H, Young AN, Hobert ME, Karmali V, et al. Prokaryotic regulation of epithelial responses by inhibition of IκB-α ubiquitination. *Science* 2000;**289**:1560–3.

17. Saemann MD, Bohmig GA, Osterreicher CH, Burtscher H, Parolini O, Diakos C, et al. Anti-inflammatory effects of sodium butyrate on human monocytes: potent inhibition of IL-12 and up-regulation of IL-10 production. *FASEB J* 2000;**14**:2380–2.

18. Tellez G. Prokaryotes versus eukaryotes: who is hosting whom? *Front Vet Med* 2014;**1**. http://journal.frontiersin.org/article/10.3389/fvets.2014.00003/full).

19. Thaiss CA, Levy M, Suez J, Elinav E. The interplay between the innate immune system and the microbiota. *Curr Opin Immunol* 2014;**26**:41–8.

20. Dunn AJ, Wang J, Ando T. Effects of cytokines on cerebral neurotransmission. Comparison with the effects of stress. *Adv Exp Med Biol* 1999;**461**:117–27.

21. Hori T, Katafuchi T, Take S, Shimizu N. Neuroimmunomodulatory actions of hypothalamic interferon-alpha. *Neuroimmunomodulation* 1998;**5**:172–7.

22. Razzuoli E, Villa R, Sossi E, Amadori M. Characterization of the interferon-alpha response of pigs to the weaning stress. *J Interf Cytokine Res* 2011;**31**:237–47.

23. Pie S, Lalles JP, Blazy F, Laffitte J, Seve B, Oswald IP. Weaning is associated with an upregulation of expression of inflammatory cytokines in the intestine of piglets. *J Nutr* 2004;**134**:641–7.

24. Trevisi E, Amadori M, Cogrossi S, Razzuoli E, Bertoni G. Metabolic stress and inflammatory response in high-yielding, periparturient dairy cows. *Res Vet Sci* 2012;**93**:695–704.

25. Peli A, Scagliarini L, Famigli Bergamini P, Prosperi A, Bernardini D, Pietra M. Effetto dello stress da caldo sull'immunità del bovino da carne. *Large Ani Rev* 2013;**19**:215–8 [in Italian].

26. Miller AC, Rashid RM, Elamin EM. The "T" in trauma: the helper T-cell response and the role of immunomodulation in trauma and burn patients. *J Trauma* 2007;**63**:1407–17.

27. Vitali A, Lana E, Amadori M, Bernabucci U, Nardone A, Lacetera N. Analysis of factors associated with mortality of heavy slaughter pigs during transport and lairage. *J Anim Sci* 2014;**92**:5134–41.

28. Ahmed SA. The immune system as a potential target for environmental estrogens (endocrine disruptors): a new emerging field. *Toxicology* 2000;**150**:191–206.

29. Livingstone DR. Contaminant-stimulated reactive oxygen species production and oxidative damage in aquatic organisms. *Mar Pollut Bull* 2001;**42**:656–66.

30. Jin Y, Zhang X, Shu L, Chen L, Sun L, Qian H, et al. Oxidative stress response and gene expression with atrazine exposure in adult female zebrafish (*Danio rerio*). *Chemosphere* 2010;**78**:846–52.

31. Xu H, Yang M, Qiu W, Pan C, Wu M. The impact of endocrine-disrupting chemicals on oxidative stress and innate immune response in zebrafish embryos. *Env Toxicol Chem* 2013;**32**:1793–9.

32. Schaaf GJ, Nijmeijer SM, Maas RF, Roestenberg P, de Groene EM, Fink-Gremmels J. The role of oxidative stress in the ochratoxin A-mediated toxicity in proximal tubular cells. *Biochim Biophys Acta* 2002;**1588**:149–58.

33. Mikami O, Kubo M, Murata H, Muneta Y, Nakajima Y, Miyazaki S, et al. The effects of acute exposure to deoxynivalenol on some inflammatory parameters in miniature pigs. *J Vet Med Sci* 2011;**73**:665–71.

34. Oswald IP, Marin DE, Bouhet S, Pinton P, Taranu I, Accensi F. Immunotoxicological risk of mycotoxins for domestic animals. *Food Addit Contam* 2005;**22**:354–60.

35. Antonissen G, Martel A, Pasmans F, Ducatelle R, Verbrugghe E, Vandenbroucke V, et al. The impact of *Fusarium* mycotoxins on human and animal host susceptibility to infectious diseases. *Toxins (Basel)* 2014;**6**:430–52.

36. Massart F, Saggese G. Oestrogenic mycotoxin exposures and precocious pubertal development. *Int J Androl* 2010;**33**:369–76.

37. Zhang Q, Raoof M, Chen Y, Sumi Y, Sursal T, Junger W, et al. Circulating mitochondrial DAMPs cause inflammatory responses to injury. *Nature* 2010;**464**:104–7.

38. Guzman E, Birch JR, Ellis SA. Cattle MIC is a ligand for the activating NK cell receptor NKG2D. *Vet Immunol Immunopathol* 2010;**136**:227–34.

39. Cohen H, Ziv Y, Cardon M, Kaplan Z, Matar MA, Gidron Y, et al. Maladaptation to mental stress mitigated by the adaptive immune system via depletion of naturally occurring regulatory CD4+ CD25+ cells. *J Neurobiol* 2006;**66**:552–63.

40. Lewitus GM, Cohen H, Schwartz M. Reducing post-traumatic anxiety by immunization. *Brain Behav Immun* 2008;**22**:1108–14.

41. Black PH. The inflammatory consequences of psychologic stress: relationship to insulin resistance, obesity, atherosclerosis and diabetes mellitus, type II. *Med Hypotheses* 2006;**67**:879–91.

42. He Y, Gao H, Li X, Zhao Y. Psychological stress exerts effects on pathogenesis of hepatitis B via type-1/type-2 cytokines shift toward type-2 cytokine response. *PLoS ONE* 2014;**9**:e105530.

43. Febbraio MA. Role of interleukins in obesity: implications for metabolic disease. *Trends Endocrinol Metab* 2014;**25**:312–9.

44. Marseglia L, Manti S, D'Angelo G, Nicotera A, Parisi E, Di Rosa G, et al. Oxidative stress in obesity: a critical component in human diseases. *Int J Mol Sci* 2014;**16**:378–400.

45. Tran PD, Christiansen D, Winterhalter A, Brooks A, Gorrell M, Lilienfeld BG, et al. Porcine cells express more than one functional ligand for the human lymphocyte activating receptor NKG2D. *Xenotransplantation* 2008;**15**:321–32.

46. Horowitz A, Stegmann KA, Riley EM. Activation of natural killer cells during microbial infections. *Front Immunol* 2012;**2**:88.

47. Martinon F, Mayor A, Tschopp J. The inflammasomes: guardians of the body. *Annu Rev Immunol* 2009;**27**:229–65.

48. Brambilla G, Civitareale C, Ballerini A, Fiori M, Amadori M, Archetti LI, et al. Response to oxidative stress as a welfare parameter in swine. *Redox Rep* 2002;**7**:159–63.

49. Dämmrich K. Organ change and damage during stress-morphological diagnosis. In: Viepkema PR, van Adrichem PWM, editors. *Biology of stress in farm animals: an integrated approach.* Dordrecht, The Netherlands: Martinus Nijhoff; 1987. p. 71–8.

50. Drackley JK. ADSA Foundation Scholar Award. Biology of dairy cows during the transition period: the final frontier? *J Dairy Sci* 1999;**82**:2259–73.

51. Mulligan FJ, Doherty ML. Production diseases of the transition cow. *Vet J* 2008;**176**:3–9.

52. Plytycz B, Seljelid R. Stress and immunity: mini review. *Folia Biol-Krakow* 2002;**50**:181–9.

53. Soos JM, Szente BE. Type I interferons. In: Thomson AW, Lotze MT, editors. *The cytokine handbook.* London: Academic Press; 2003. p. 549–66.

54. Isaacs A, Lindenmann I. Virus interference. I. The interferon. *Proc R Soc (London) Ser B* 1957;**147**:258–73.

55. Amadori M. The role of IFN-alpha as homeostatic agent in the inflammatory response: a balance between danger and response? *J Interferon Cytokine Res* 2007;**27**:181–9.

56. Meurens F, Summerfield A, Nauwynck H, Saif L, Gerdts V. The pig: a model for human infectious diseases. *Trends Microbiol* 2012;**20**:50–7.

Chapter 1

An Overview of the Innate Immune Response to Infectious and Noninfectious Stressors

Stefania Gallucci

Department of Microbiology and Immunology, Laboratory of Dendritic Cell Biology, Temple University, School of Medicine, Philadelphia, PA, USA

INTRODUCTION

The immune system is a complex network of cells and molecules, whose main function is to protect the body from the invasion of harmful microorganisms – the pathogens.[1]

In most vertebrates, including human and mammals in general, the immune system is composed of two branches, the *innate* and *adaptive* immune systems, which collaborate in fighting infections. The innate system activates first and then it stimulates the adaptive immunity. The innate immune system, as the name suggests, is already operational at birth and it gets started fast in a few hours because it is mediated by cascades of molecules that activate in a matter of minutes. These cascades include the complement, antimicrobial peptides, and cytokines such as type I interferons. The innate immunity is also mediated by cells like the phagocytes (granulocytes, dendritic cells (DCs), and macrophages) and the natural killer cells, which activate in a few hours. The adaptive immunity (also called acquired immunity), on the other hand, is mediated by T and B lymphocytes, which become fully operational only after birth, and requires days to be ready to face the pathogens.[1]

In order to efficiently fight infections without harming the body, cells of the innate immune system perform four main functions: first, they recognize presence and "dangerousness" of an infection (*recognition*); second, they fuel the inflammatory process and fight the infection, through phagocytosis and cytotoxicity, these events occur during the first days from the encounter with a pathogen, that is new to the immune system, when the adaptive immunity is not ready yet (*effector phase*); third, they activate the adaptive immune response by presenting the antigen (Ag) to T cells and they determine the kind of adaptive immune response to be activated by secreting specific cytokines (*Ag presentation and T helper (Th) class regulation*); finally, cells of the innate immune system participate in repairing the tissues damaged either by the pathogen, or by the immune response triggered by the pathogen, and in maintaining the homeostasis of tissues and organs of our body (*tissue repair and homeostasis*).[1]

This chapter will focus on the rules and molecular players, ligands, and receptors for the function of recognition by the innate immune system.

RECOGNITION

One of the main questions in the history of immunology is how the immune system recognizes if it is appropriate to mount an immune response (i.e., against a pathogen) or if it is more useful to become tolerant (i.e., to self Ags). When lymphocytes encounter their Ag, the molecule that they are specific for, they can either mount an immune response or be tolerized; this decision depends on the state of activation of the cells that are presenting the Ag to them, the Ag-presenting cells (APCs).[2] The most important APCs are DCs, but macrophages and B cells can also present Ags, and initiate adaptive immune responses. The DCs[3,4] reside in all the tissues and organs of the body in a resting state and, as sentinels, they monitor the environment waiting for an activation signal. At this stage, the dendritic cells do not present Ags, rather they sample their environment through the processes of macropinocytosis and phagocytosis.[5] Once the dendritic cells receive signals of activation, they migrate to the draining lymph nodes and are able to stimulate T lymphocytes by processing the uptaken Ags, and display them on the cell surface in association with MHC class I and II molecules (signal 1), upregulating costimulatory molecules, such as CD80 and CD86 (signal 2), and secreting proinflammatory cytokines (signal 3), in order to start an immune response.[6]

Until the 1970s, immunologists thought that lymphocytes were designed to activate in the mere presence of the Ag. The immune system was considered incapable of mounting an immune response against the Ags of its own body (self-Ags) because the autoreactive lymphocytes were all physically eliminated during development. Experimental evidence indicates that autoreactive lymphocytes are present in healthy individuals, so that explanation was not sufficient.

The first idea that the innate immune system and not the lymphocytes discriminates what is self from what is nonself came from Charlie Janeway Jr, who wrote in 1989[7] that the innate immunity, and now we know the dendritic cells, sense the infectious foreign agent, through an array of pattern recognition receptors (PRRs). These receptors bind conserved features of molecules shared by families of evolutionary distant organisms like bacteria, and he called these molecules pathogen-associated molecular patterns (PAMPs). These PAMPs have to be essential for the survival or pathogenicity of microorganisms, otherwise the microbes would lose them in order to escape from the immune system. And they cannot be expressed by host organisms otherwise they would trigger autoreactivity.[8]

This theoretical model of immune recognition provided a new molecular basis to support the classic self–nonself model of immunity that had been widely accepted by immunologists for 50 years. But it could not explain the occurrence of important immune responses in the absence of any pathogen: clinical situations such as the rejection of transplants, chronic inflammatory diseases, tumor immunity, trauma-induced systemic inflammatory response syndrome, and other inflammatory conditions like atherosclerosis or ischemia – reperfusion injury – are mediated by a "sterile inflammation," in which the innate immune system is activated by signals that do not come from an infectious agent.[9]

In 1994, Polly Matzinger proposed an alternative model, the Danger Model, that says that the dendritic cells sense danger.[10] She theorized that the dendritic cells are activated by endogenous molecules, secreted by cells undergoing stress, or released during tissue damage or by necrotic cells. A similar "injury hypothesis," was also proposed by W.G. Land, inspired by his experience in transplantation.[11] Seong and Matzinger subsequently called these endogenous danger signals damage-associated molecular patterns (DAMPs),[12] using the same nomenclature of Janeway. In the beginning the two models were seen as mutually exclusive, but two decades of experimental evidence now indicate that the innate immune system is indeed activated through PRRs that are triggered by PAMPs and also by DAMPs, and many scientists call PAMPs and DAMPs as the "danger signals,"[9,13,14] using an inclusive nomenclature that suggests that PRRs recognize the molecular features of a pathologic status that can be the result of pathogens and trauma/stress.

To summarize, the innate immune cells have *specificity* for a limited number of molecules, namely the PAMPs and DAMPs, which signal infectious nonself and damaged self as danger or alarm. PAMPs are molecular structures conserved in large families of bacteria, viruses, or other microorganisms, and they are usually considered associated with pathogens; since PAMPs are also expressed by the normal flora of the mammalian mucosa, they are also called microbial-associated molecular patterns (MAMPs).[15] DAMPs are endogenous molecules that are actively secreted by cells undergoing stress, or are passively released by necrotic cells or liberated upon tissue damage. The innate immune cells express a limited *diversity* of receptors, called PRRs, that are germ-line encoded, which means they are transcribed from a limited number of genes that remain the same throughout the life of an individual as most of the genes do. These receptors survey the extracellular and intracellular space for conserved danger signals that serve as indicators of infection and tissue damage.

PRRs AND PAMPs

PRRs are presently divided into several main families of receptors, which have been increasing in number in the last few years, thanks to the continuous discovery of novel pathways. The best-known families so far are the toll-like receptors (TLRs), the C-type lectin receptors (CLRs), the nucleotide-binding domain, leucine-rich repeat (LRR) containing (or NOD-like) receptors (NLRs), the RIG-I-like receptors (RLRs), the cGAS-STING, and the AIM2-like receptors (ALRs) (Table 1.1).[14,16] Furthermore, some PRRs belong to other families of receptors, like the immunoglobulin superfamily. Most PRRs are expressed by DCs and other APCs, and they are involved in recognizing PAMPs and DAMPs during infections by viruses, bacteria, and fungi, and during tissue damage and sterile inflammation, stimulating APC activation and inflammatory processes. Cytokine receptors, like the interleukin-1 receptor and the type I interferon receptor, also activate similar functions. Moreover, PRRs can be expressed also by T cells and by nonimmune cells, influencing the class of the adaptive immune response, through the production of specific cytokines.

In the following sections, the families of PRRs will be described together with the main PAMPs that they recognize, while the DAMPs will be described in independent sections in the second part of the chapter, in order to provide to the mediators of noninfectious stressors the space and the details appropriate to the focus of this book.

TABLE 1.1 The DAMPs

DAMP	Source	Receptor	Activating the inflammasome
Extracellular nucleic acids	Dead cells, NETs, damaged mitochondria	TLR7, TLR9	No
Intracellular/retroviral DNA	Cytoplasmic EVE or mtDNA	cGAS-STING, RLRs, ALRs	Yes
ATP	Dead cells, damaged mitochondria	P2Z/P2X$_7$, NLRs	Yes
Uric acid, alum, CPPD crystals	Nucleic acid breakdown, dead cells	TLRs, NLRs	Yes
Heat-shock proteins	Dead cells	TLRs, CD91, CLRs	n.d.
HMGB1	Dead cells, activated immune cells	TLRs, RAGE, CXCR4	No
EMC degradation products	ECM	TLRs, P2X, NLRs	Yes
Homeostatic perturbations	Changes in cellular environment	mTOR, ?	Yes

Toll-Like Receptors

TLRs were the first family of PRRs discovered and still the most studied. Ruslan Medzhitov, while working in the lab of CA Janeway, Jr., cloned the first mammalian receptor that activates the transcription factor central to the immune activation, NFκB, predicting it would be an analog of the toll protein.[17] Toll had been previously shown to control the dorsal–ventral patterning during early embryonic development in *Drosophila melanogaster* and was also known to stimulate the production of antimicrobial proteins and trigger antifungal immune responses in adult *Drosophila*.[18] Beutler et al. then showed that TLR4 recognizes the most known PAMP, the lipopolysaccharide (LPS) from Gram-negative bacteria.[19] The importance of the discovery of TLRs for our understanding of the initiation and regulation of the immune response has been recognized in 2011 by the Nobel Prize[20] to J.A. Hoffmann for the studies in *Drosophila*,[18] to B. Beutler for the mammalian studies,[19] and to R. Steinman for initiating[21] and driving the research on the dendritic cells.[2,3] The TLR family presently includes 13 members in mice and 10 in humans that have in common homology of structure and signaling adaptors.[14] TLRs are transmembrane glycoproteins characterized by an extracellular domain that is responsible for ligand recognition through variable LRR modules.[22] TLRs form homo- or heterodimers and some are localized on the cell surface (TLR1, 2, 4, 5, and 6), where they recognize a variety of molecules conserved in extracellular bacteria and fungi; for example, the main PAMP that triggers TLR4 is LPS from Gram-negative bacteria, but TLR4 can also recognize fusion proteins from the respiratory syncytial virus, mouse mammary tumor virus envelope proteins, and the pneumolysin from *Streptococcus pneumoniae.* TLR2, forming heterodimers with TLR1 and TLR6, recognizes a wide range of PAMPs derived from bacteria, fungi, parasites, and viruses,[23] such as lipopeptides from Gram-positive bacteria and mycoplasma, peptidoglycan, and lipoteichoic acid from Gram-positive bacteria, zymosan from fungi, lipoarabinomannan from mycobacteria, tGPI-mucin from *Trypanosoma cruzi,* and the hemagglutinin protein from measles virus. TLR5 is triggered by flagellin from flagellated bacteria. TLRs are also expressed in the endosomal compartment (TLR 3, 7, 8, and 9) and recognize mostly nucleic acids. TLR3 recognizes double-stranded (ds) RNA, TLR7-8 recognizes single-stranded (ss) RNA, and TLR9 recognizes unmethylated 2′-deoxyribo-cytidine-phosphateguanosine (CpG) DNA motifs that can come from intracellular pathogens like viruses or DNA endocytosed from the extracellular space.[14,23] The triggering of TLRs often requires accessory molecules that strengthen the binding with the ligand and also provide qualitative difference in the signaling pathways activated downstream of the receptor. As an example, MD-2 is an accessory molecule associated with TLR4 and required for its activation, and indeed MD-2 deficient cells do not respond to LPS.[24] Moreover, CD14 also associates with TLR4 and affects how TLR4 binds to its ligands: it has been suggested that CD14 preferentially increases the binding of DAMPs.[22]

Signaling

The intracellular tail of TLRs is associated to adaptor molecules that are responsible for triggering the signaling pathways leading to the initiation of the innate immune response, from transcription of costimulatory molecules, proinflammatory cytokine and type I interferons (I-IFNs), to upregulation of phagocytosis, autophagy, cell metabolism, and in some case cell death. The two main signaling pathways downstream TLRs are (1) the pathway mediated by the adaptor MyD88 that leads, through a cascade of signaling events, to NFκB activation, translocation to the nucleus and NFκB-mediated transcription; (2) the pathway mediated by the adaptor TRIF that leads, through the activation of IRFs (interferon regulatory factors), to the transcription of type I IFN alpha/beta; the response to the autocrine production of type I IFNs induces the expression of interferon stimulated genes (ISGs), generating an interferon positive feedback loop.[25] The master regulator of the production of type I IFNs is IRF7, which is highly expressed in dendritic cells and especially in plasmacytoid dendritic cells, the major producers of type I IFNs, and it is strongly upregulated upon stimulation with type I IFN, directing the amplification of the interferon positive feedback loop.[26] Both pathways also activate the pathway of the MAP kinases, that is, Erk, p38, and JNK, which leads to the activation of the transcription factor AP-1 and the expression of proinflammatory cytokines.[14] Most TLRs utilize the MyD88-mediated pathway; TLR3 utilizes only the TRIF pathway, while TLR4 utilizes both pathways, with implications for the quality and strength of the downstream response. The autocrine production of type I interferons is necessary to mediate the full activation of APCs, and APCs, both dendritic cells and macrophages, which do not respond to type I interferons, either because they do not express the type I interferon receptor (IFNAR) or the pivotal signal transducers downstream of IFNAR, STAT1, and STAT2, are deficient in the upregulation of the costimulatory molecules and proinflammatory cytokines that are characteristic of full innate cell activation.[27–29]

C-Type Lectin Receptors

CLRs are a family of receptors important in the immunity against bacteria, viruses, and fungi. They contain at least one C-type lectin-like domain (CTLD), a conserved motif that has evolved to adapt to a variety of ligands, either of microbial origin or released by damaged host cells.[30] CTLDs were originally named because they can bind carbohydrates in a calcium-dependent manner, but many can also bind glycans, proteins, or lipids in a calcium-independent manner. CLRs are expressed on the cell surface of DCs, macrophages, and other myeloid cells, and also on epithelial cells. Dectin-1/CARD9,* Dectin-2/Mincle, DC-SIGN, and mannose receptor are examples of CLRs that, once they recognize microbes, induce phagocytosis and microbicidal activities to degrade

---

* Many of these receptors have a complex nomenclature, with two or more names indicating the same molecule.

them or shuttle them to Ag presentation.[31] Moreover, many CLRs also recognize damaged and dead cells and they can distinguish between cells dying by apoptosis, considered anti-inflammatory (recognized by receptors like Mgl-1/Clec10a), from those dying by necrosis/necroptosis, types of death considered proinflammatory (recognized by receptors like Mincle/CLEC4E and DNGR-1/CLEC9A).[32] Therefore, CLRs expressed in myeloid cells can regulate their endocytic traffic, signaling pathways, and gene transcription in order to initiate immunity or tolerance for the Ags coming from necrotic or apoptotic cells, respectively. DNGR-1 is expressed mostly in CD8α dendritic cells and it recognizes necrotic cells by binding the protein F-actin, a cytosolic component of the cytoskeleton that is exposed to the extracellular space by necrotic cells. DNGR-1 binding marks the phagocytosed dead cell as necrotic and shuttles it to the class I pathway for cross-presentation.[33] Another proinflammatory CLR is LOX-1, (lectin-like oxidized low-density lipoprotein), the primary receptor for oxidized low-density lipoprotein (ox-LDL) in endothelial cells, which can recognize other DAMPs, such as heat-shock proteins,[30] and it is involved in the pathogenesis of atherosclerosis.[34]

Signaling

Some CLRs, like Dectin-1 and DNGR-1, activate the signaling molecule Syk through an ITAM-like motif. This signaling pathway leads to DC and macrophage activation, via NFκB and MAP kinase, downstream of Dectin but not of DNGR-1. Indeed, DNGR-1 has not been shown to trigger DC activation but rather to promote cross-priming, that is, the presentation of extracellular Ags with MHC class I molecules, in DCs already activated by other PRRs.[30]

The RIG-I-Like Receptors

The recognition of viral infections and host defense in invertebrates and plants is mostly carried out by RNA interference and the Dicer nuclease family of host immune receptors.[35] In the vertebrates and mammals in particular, the immune system relies on the production of type I[25] and III interferons[36] and ISGs, which are produced upon recognition of intracellular RNA and DNA by the PRR families of RLRs and ALRs.[14,37] The RLRs retinoic acid-inducible gene I (RIG-I) and melanoma differentiation factor 5 (MDA5) are cytoplasmic PRRs, which belong to the larger family of helicases.[38] They are expressed not only by APCs or immune cells, but also by most cells of our body, and are pivotal in antiviral responses by recognizing RNAs in the cytosol. They contain three important domains: (1) a C-terminal repressor domain (RD) embedded within the C-terminal domain (CTD); (2) a central ATPase containing DExD/H-box helicase domain, which binds the RNAs; and (3) two amino-terminal caspase recruiting domains (CARD) that mediate downstream signaling.[38] RIG-I binds the terminal 5′ triphosphate and the blunt-end base pair at the 5′-end of ss- and dsRNA; MDA5 binds the internal duplex segments of consensus dsRNAs.[39]

Using poly (I:C) as a synthetic dsRNA mimic, studies have shown that MDA5 binds long, but not short, dsRNA.

Signaling

The binding of the RNA ligands induces a conformational change in the RLRs, releasing the CARD, which then can start the activation of the downstream signaling pathway by associating, via CARD–CARD interactions, with the membrane-associated adaptor mitochondrial antiviral signaling (MAVS, also known as IPS-1, VISA, and Cardif).[40] Once activated, MAVS starts to aggregate and activate in a prion-like manner other MAVS molecules,[40] amplifying the activation of the downstream events, which include activation of TBK1, MAPKs, NFκB, and IRFs, leading to production of inflammatory cytokines and interferons, as most PRRs do.[14]

NLRs and the Inflammasome

Nucleotide-binding domain, LRR-containing (or NOD-like) receptors (NLRs) are involved in responses to a wide range of microbial pathogens, in inflammatory diseases, cancer, and metabolic and autoimmune disorders.[16] Although results from genetically deficient cells and mice support an important role for NLRs in immunity against infections, no direct binding of NLRs to PAMPs has been found so far,[16] suggesting that NLRs may be pure PRRs for DAMPs released or generated upon intracellular damage. A number of mechanisms have been proposed to trigger NLR activation, including potassium efflux, an increase in intracellular calcium and a decrease in cellular cyclic AMP, pore-forming actions driven by the host or bacteria, phagolysosomal destabilization, changes in cell volume and mitochondrial-derived reactive oxygen species (ROS), and oxidized mitochondrial DNA (mtDNA).[41] NLRs are cytoplasmic receptors that can be divided in two subfamilies: (1) the NOD subfamily, characterized by the presence of one or more CARD domains, and (2) the LRR and pyrin domain (PYD) -containing proteins (NLRP), characterized by the presence of a pyrin domain. Once activated, several NLRs, like NLRP1b, NLRP3, and NLRC4, associate with the adaptor protein ASC (apoptosis-associated speck-like protein containing a CARD), which forms a platform that recruits the procaspase-1 to form the multiprotein complex "inflammasome."[42]

Signaling

The multimeric complex of proteins of the inflammasome assembles in the cytoplasm of macrophages and dendritic cells, by reorganizing the cytoplasmic ASC into a single "speck" of 0.8–1 μm, which is considered a hallmark of inflammasome assembly. This speck is crucial for the recruitment of caspase-1 and the amplification of the events downstream of the inflammasome, which are the cleavage by caspase 1 of pro-IL-1β and pro-IL-18 into biologically active cytokines, ready to be secreted outside the cells. The production of these procytokines occurs prior to the activation of the inflammasome and is induced by the triggering of other PRRs, such as TLRs. Moreover, the inflammasome triggers the proinflammatory cell death "pyroptosis," again through the activation of caspase 1 and 11.[41]

A noncanonical pathway to activate the inflammasome is initiated by intracytosolic LPS that directly activates caspase 11 in an ASC-independent manner, upon priming by autocrine type I interferons. This scenario possibly occurs when LPS gains access to the cytosol thanks to bacterial secretion systems. Moreover, the inflammasome can also be activated by some CLRs like Dectin-1, by forming a noncanonical complex with caspase 8 and ASC that can cleave pro-IL-1b.[43]

AIM2-Like Receptors

ALRs[44] are intracellular sensors of dsDNA derived from bacteria, viruses, and autoinflammatory sterile conditions. They comprise members of the PYHIN family, that is, human AIM2 (absent in melanoma 2) and interferon-inducible protein 16(IFI16). The PYHIN family of proteins is defined by an N-terminal PYD, involved in homotypic protein–protein interactions, and one or two C-terminal DNA-binding HIN domains (HIN hematopoietic interferon-inducible nuclear Ag). AIM2 is expressed in the cytoplasm, while IFI16 is mostly nuclear and it can translocate to the cytoplasm during cellular stress, such as upon UV irradiation. Most cells, like fibroblasts, epithelial cells, macrophages, dendritic cells, and T cells express ALRs, with differences in distribution and functions of the different members. AIM2 recognizes DNA in a nonsequence specific manner via electrostatic attraction between the positively charged HIN domain and the negatively charged dsDNA sugar-phosphate backbone.[44] The positive charge of the HIN domain also plays an important role in the regulation of AIM2. In AIM2, the HIN domain is normally bound to the negatively charged PYD, maintaining AIM2 in an autoinhibited state prior to the binding to dsDNA. In the presence of dsDNA, the domain HIN will bind to the DNA, releasing the negatively charged PYD that is able to bind ASC, activate the inflammasome, and the downstream cleavage of pro-IL1β and pro-IL18, to the bioactive cytokines.[45] Moreover, dsDNA also generates a platform to recruit more AIM2 molecules, further amplifying a process that is already autocatalytic.

Similarly to AIM2, IFI16 recognizes dsDNA in a GC and sequence-independent manner, but it shows specificity for length, binding preferably fragments of dsDNA, which are around 150 base pairs long. This length requirement may explain why IFI16, although localized in the nucleus, is not constantly activated by the host DNA, which normally exposes linker dsDNA between nucleosomes that are 10–20 bp long, and therefore too short to activate IFI-16.[46,47]

Signaling

Activated IFI16 assembles a multimeric complex, similar to AIM2, which is translocated to the cytoplasm, where it can trigger the activation of the inflammasome, but it can also bind and activate the endoplasmic resident adaptor protein stimulator of interferon genes (STING), inducing the production of type I interferons (described further).[44]

C-GAS and Other DNA Sensors

Besides the ALRs, other cytosolic DNA sensors have been recently discovered to participate in the initiation of antiviral responses. These sensors include DNA-dependent activator (DAI) of IFN-regulatory factors; DEAD (aspartate-glutamate-alanine-aspartate)-box polypeptide 41 (DDX41); DNA-dependent protein kinase (DNA-PK);[44] and cGAMP synthetase (cGAS).[48] The latter is involved in sensing viral DNA in host defense as well as self-DNA in autoimmunity. Indeed, cGAS has been shown to recognize dsDNA and upon activation, generate the endogenous cyclic dinucleotide GMP–AMP (cGAMP). cGAS directly binds dsDNA in a sequence-independent manner through electrostatic and hydrogen bond interactions with the sugar–phosphate backbone of DNA; this binding induces a conformational change in cGAS and allows ATP and GTP to reach the catalytic pocket in cGAS that synthesizes the cGAMP.[48]

Signaling

In a similar manner to the bacterial cyclic dinucleotides (CDNs), cGAMP then activates STING, which subsequently activates the transcription factors NFκB and IRF3, through the kinases IKK and TBK1, respectively, leading to the production of type I interferon and proinflammatory cytokines, and maturation of APCs.[48]

RAGE

The receptor for advanced glycosylation end products (RAGE) is an important receptor of DAMPs. Initially discovered to bind advanced glycosylation end products (AGE), RAGE is a transmembrane receptor of the immunoglobulin superfamily, containing an extracellular region that binds DAMPs through its V domain, and a cytoplasmic region mediating the downstream signaling. RAGE can also become soluble, upon alternate splicing or protease processing, and acts as a decoy receptor by preventing DAMPs from triggering transmembrane RAGE. The expression of RAGE is upregulated by the presence of its ligands, creating a positive feedback loop that amplifies its activation. RAGE and TLRs share common ligands and signaling pathways, suggesting a cooperative interaction in stimulating the immune response. Indeed, RAGE binding triggers the activation of NFκB, cell proliferation, and TGF-β production.[49] RAGE has been mostly studied for its role in inflammation and tissue damage, but it can also bind PAMPs, such as bacterial or viral DNA that are chaperoned by HMGB1 (see the next section).

Soluble PRRs

A special class of PRRs consists of soluble molecules that recognize pathogens and modified self. The collectins and ficolins recognize microorganisms and can trigger the lectin pathway of complement, leading to the activation of the complement cascade and the initiation of complement-dependent inflammation, phagocytosis, and cell lysis. The family of pentraxins comprises of short pentraxins, that is, the C-reactive protein (CRP) and the serum amyloid P (SAP), which are acute phase proteins, mainly secreted by the hepatocytes during inflammation in response to IL-6 and IL-1, and the long pentraxins such as PTX3. PTX3 is expressed by dendritic cells and monocytes/macrophages, but also by endothelial and epithelial cells, and it is induced by TLR triggering and proinflammatory cytokines; furthermore, PTX3 is also stored in preformed granules in the neutrophils, ready to be secreted in the presence of pathogens or upon TLR triggering. PTX3 can bind bacteria, viruses, and fungi, as well as dead cells, and promote their complement-mediated lysis and phagocytosis.[50]

PRR LOCALIZATION

The immune system can mount different types of immune responses, humoral or cell mediated, that are promoted by distinct subsets of Th cells: Th1 T cells help the CD8 T cells to become cytotoxic T cells (CTL), pivotal in host defense against viruses and intracellular parasites; Th1 T cells also activate macrophages to increase their ability to kill and digest the pathogens that they have phagocytosed or the intracellular pathogens that have infected them; Th2 cells participate in the host defense against extracellular parasites and also promote allergy. Follicular Th cells help B cells to mature and produce antibodies (Abs); Th17 cells contribute to the clearance of extracellular bacteria and fungi by recruiting neutrophils and macrophages in the site of infection.[1] These different subsets of Th cells mediate their functions through the secretion of cytokines. Last but not the least, there are the CD4 regulatory T cells (Treg) that are characterized by the expression of CD25 and of the transcription regulator FOXP-3. Tregs suppress the immune response, as a part of the maintenance of peripheral tolerance. The immune system deploys these different types of immune strategies depending on the kind of pathogens it is facing, the microenvironment in which the infection is taking place, intracellular or extracellular, and also depending on the tissues involved; responses in the gut can be very different from the ones in the skin or in the eye. These differentiations are dictated by the encounter of different PAMPs triggering specific PRRs. Moreover, the simultaneous exposure to specific DAMPs can further affect the activation pattern of the APCs, influencing the cocktail of cytokines that they will produce, and therefore the type of adaptive immune response that they can initiate.

TLRs, CLRs, and RAGE are expressed on the cell surface or in the endosomal compartment, and their localization is important to detect the presence of PAMPs and DAMPs, directly exposed in the extracellular space or that require processing upon phagocytosis in the endosomal compartment, respectively. On the contrary, NLRs, RIG-Is, ALRs, and other nucleic acid sensors are localized in the cytoplasm and detect pathogens that penetrate into the cells and DAMPs produced directly by the stressed cells. Depending on their localization, PRRs can provide information about the whereabouts of the pathogen/stress, and therefore direct the most appropriate immune strategy to deal with it: extracellular strategies such as antibody production, complement activation, Th17 or Th2 types of adaptive responses are deployed for an extracellular pathogen/stress, while CTL killers and the macrophages inducing the delayed type IV hypersensitivity (DTH) are activated in the presence of intracellular pathogens. The PRR compartmentalization is also an important strategy to avoid inappropriate exposure of PRRs to DAMPs in the absence of tissue damage.[13,16,22,51] Indeed, DAMPs are normally sequestered from PRRs through the compartmentalization of PRRs. For example, PRRs recognizing nucleic acids are associated to the endosomes and therefore, are not exposed to the DNA present in the nucleus or the RNA present in the cytoplasm, but to extracellular nucleic acids that are released during major surgery, trauma, or cancer, clinical situations, in which necrotic cell death is occurring.[52]

DAMPs

The DAMPs can be defined as primary endogenous danger signals, as they originate directly from the damaged cells or tissues[53–55] (Table 1.1). A second category of endogenous danger signals consists of secondary danger signals, which are cytokines produced by activated immune cells that behave as danger signals, activating dendritic cells and initiating innate immunity[55] (see the next section dedicated to the secondary danger signals). DAMPs are very heterogeneous in structure, physical, chemical, and biological properties, but they have in common the property to be normally sequestered from the PRRs and become exposed to them upon cellular and tissue damage.[9,13] In the late 1990s, the labs of Janeway and Beutler were showing that the immune system is activated by pathogens through the activation of TLR by PAMPs,[8,17,19] Matzinger and coworkers showed that necrotic cells and a prototypic endogenous danger signal, type I interferons, can stimulate the activation of dendritic cells into APCs, which are able to present Ags to T cells and initiate adaptive immune responses *in vivo* (e.g., DTH and CTLs) in the absence of any pathogen, therefore acting as endogenous adjuvants.[54,56–58] These discoveries opened the new field of the endogenous danger signals as immune stimulators.[55] Since then, a large number of literature has been detailing the molecular players that trigger and sustain sterile inflammation (Table 1.1).

Nucleic Acids

Nucleic acids are potent PAMPs, important in initiating immune responses in host defense against viral and also bacterial infections, and they are also

DAMPs, involved in autoimmunity and antitumor immunity. Endogenous DNA is normally sequestered in the nucleus, hidden from TLRs and cytoplasmic DNA sensors. During the programmed cell death apoptosis, the maintenance of membrane integrity and activation of DNAse prevent the release of endogenous DNA in the extracellular compartment.[59] Such a careful elimination does not occur during necrosis and other forms of proinflammatory cell death, such as necroptosis, the RIP-3-dependent programmed necrotic cell death;[60] in these kinds of necrotic cell death, DNA and RNA are released into the extracellular milieu, becoming available to be uptaken by APCs and trigger endosomal TLRs.[52] This process is considered an important pathogenic step in autoimmunity and especially in systemic lupus erythematosus (SLE), in which nucleic acids, possibly coming from necrotic cells,[61] play the double role of autoadjuvants, triggering TLR7 and TLR9, and of Ags, eliciting specific and diagnostic auto-Abs.[62] DNA is also actively extruded by neutrophils as a strategy to trap and kill bacteria in the phenomenon called "neutrophil extracellular traps (NETs)";[63] this extracellular DNA can activate innate immunity and production of type I IFNs, and it has been suggested to participate in the pathogenesis of autoimmunity.[64]

The cytosol can also be a source of DNA as DAMPs. This fact was made evident by the discovery that there is a constitutive activation of DNA sensors dependent on STING, with subsequent production of type I interferons and autoimmunity, in human and murine models of TREX1 deficiency, a $3'5'$-exonuclease present in the cytosol. It has been proposed that TREX1, also called DNAse III, normally degrades DNA produced by endogenous viral elements (EVE) like integrated retroviruses.[65–67] In the absence of TREX1, such endogenous viral DNA accumulates in the cytoplasm above the threshold of sensitivity of the DNA sensors, thus triggering the IFN response. In this case, this EVE DNA can be considered a PAMP, because of its viral origin, and a DAMP, because it is derived from sequences integrated in the mammalian genome during evolution.

Moreover, it has been recently proposed that DNA derived from tumor cells can stimulate APCs to produce type I interferons in a TLR-independent manner. This tumor-derived host DNA has been shown to activate cytosolic PRRs that trigger the signaling pathways mediated by STING, although it remains to be understood how phagocytosed DNA can exit the endosomal compartment and access the cytosol of APCs.[68]

ATP

The concept of DAMP compartmentalization is highlighted by the single nucleotide ATP, which is normally present in the cytosol without immunological consequences, but when it is secreted in the extracellular milieu at high concentration, it can activate DCs by triggering the purinergic receptors P2Z/P2X$_7$ present on the cell surface.[69,70] ATP is one of the most ancient and conserved DAMP, conserved in evolution from prokaryotes, to plants and mammals.[71] In collaboration with TLRs, ATP is a mediator of the activation of NLRP3 and the inflammasome, leading to the activation of caspase 1 and the production of mature IL-1β. Extracellular ATP is one of the mediators of the sterile inflammation induced by necrotic cells, for example, during the massive death of tumor cells induced by chemotherapy.[68] The immunological role of ATP is rather complex and the concentration of extracellular ATP is tightly regulated through hydrolysis by the ectonucleotidases CD39 and CD73; the adenosine generated from ATP degradation were shown to have immunosuppressive effects that can promote tumor growth and resistance to immunosurveillance *in vivo*.[68] Moreover, low concentrations of ATP do not induce DC maturation but rather the migration of phagocytes, and it has been proposed that ATP at low concentrations functions as a "find-me signal" released by apoptotic cells to recruit phagocytes and increase apoptotic body clearance.[9,72] These complex results suggest that extracellular ATP plays an important role in defining the response of innate immune cells to dead cells, either apoptotic or necrotic, or tissue damage, and therefore controlling ATP concentrations is of paramount importance in the global regulation of the immune response.

Uric Acid

One of the first DAMPs to be shown to act as an adjuvant *in vivo*, and induce CTL responses important in immunotherapy of tumors, is uric acid.[57,58] Uric acid is a small molecule that is present in the extracellular milieu at low concentration with no immunological effects. When it is released at high concentrations, it precipitates and forms insoluble crystals of monosodium urate (MSU), which are highly inflammatory. It has been very well known for a long time that uric acid, the end product of purine nucleotide catabolism, can accumulate as MSUs and induce inflammation in the joints of patients with gout. Recently, it has been shown that MSU triggers DC activation upon release by dead cells, that is, during chemotherapy. Several mechanisms may underline the proinflammatory effects of MSU. These involve the activation of the inflammasome, which MSU stimulates together with the increased concentrations of extracellular ATP derived from damaged mitochondria, which are released by dead cells. In turn, MSU causes the stimulation of IL-1β production and, possibly, of pyroptosis.[16] The induction of inflammasome-dependent pyroptosis in the macrophages, which respond to necrotic cells, seems to establish a positive feedback loop. The induction of ROS further amplifies the inflammatory process.[73]

Alum is highly utilized as a safe adjuvant in the preparations of vaccines for the human population. In analogy to MSU and to calcium pyrophosphate dehydrate (CPPD), Alum has been shown to form crystals, accumulate at the site of injection and induce inflammasome activation. It has been proposed that when phagocytes uptake MSU or other crystals, the physical rigidity of the crystals damage the phagolysosomes, and this leads to the leakage of proinflammatory mediators into the cytosol, triggering the activation of the inflammasome.[74]

More generally, Davis et al. proposed in 2011[16] that the inflammasome can recognize host-derived crystalline or polymer moieties associated to a special ability to recognize "mislocalization of these endogenous molecules." Indeed, to quote their words "ATP, MSU, and CPPD are normally cytosolic constituents; however, if they are sensed in the extracellular environment, an inflammatory response is initiated (inside out). Likewise, if extracellular cholesterol crystals, hyaluronan, or amyloid β are internalized (outside in), a similar response is initiated."[16]

Heat-Shock Proteins

Heat-shock proteins are highly abundant molecules, normally expressed intracellularly, that act as chaperones and play a vital role in the protein synthesis machinery by maintaining proteins in their correct folding. Their names have been derived by the fact that the expression of important members of this large family of proteins is upregulated by several noninfectious stressors, such as elevated temperature, osmotic shock, and cytotoxic agents.[75] Srivastava and coworkers first showed that HSPs are released by necrotic cells, they act as danger signals that activate dendritic cells and induce Ag presentation, and initiate immune responses.[76] HSPs such as HSP70, HSP90, calreticulin, and GP96, have been involved in antitumor immunity, where they act as DAMPs. Moreover, as chaperones, HSPs can also participate in Ag processing, delivering Ags, and possibly autoantigens to APCs.[9,77] In particular, calreticulin, normally present in the ER lumen, upon cellular stress caused, for example, by chemotherapy, can translocate to the plasma membrane, where it interacts with the HSP receptor CD91 on phagocytes, promoting the phagocytosis of dead tumor cells. Several HSPs, like calreticulin and GP96, trigger CD91 on APCs and induce APC activation, production of proinflammatory cytokines, and T cell polarization toward the Th17 phenotype, which contributes to antitumor immunity. Indeed, high expression of calreticulin in tumors has been associated with favorable prognosis.[68]

Mitochondrial Danger Signals

Mitochondria are pivotal players in the activation of the innate immune response. Indeed, they are important sources of danger signals, PAMPs and DAMPs, and are required for the appropriate activation of the immune cells. Mitochondria are ancient symbionts that express molecules of bacterial origin that can be considered PAMPs, such as the mtDNA,[78] which contains CpG motifs capable of stimulating TLR9, and N-formyl peptides, analogs to bacterial peptides.[9] During cellular stress, mitochondria are damaged and released by necrotic cells in the extracellular milieu, where their danger signals participate in the activation of the innate immune cells. In fact, major traumatic injury causes elevated serum levels of mtDNA, which contributes to the severity of the sterile shock.[78] Mitochondria also contribute to the execution of cell death program and the shift from apoptosis to necrosis/necroptosis, participating in the qualification of cell death as pro- or anti-inflammatory.[79] Finally, mitochondria are major stations of production of energy and recent evidence shows that the modulation of their ability to increase production of ATP, as a source of energy in this case, not as a DAMP, strongly affect the strength of the innate and adaptive immune response.[80]

HMGB1

High Mobility Group Box protein 1 (HMGB1) is a nonhistonic DNA-binding protein, which is normally localized in the nucleus as part of the chromatin, where it contributes to the stabilization of the nucleosomal structure, and to the regulation of gene transcription.[81] HMGB1 is highly conserved in evolution and it is a member of a family of four chromatin proteins, HMG1, 2, 14, and 17. HMGB1 binds to DNA, thanks to its high positive charge. Although it is well known as a DAMP, it is becoming clear that HMGB1 has several other functions, depending on the compartment, in which it resides, and the posttranslational modifications that it has received, such as oxidation and hyperacetylation (see the end of this section).[82]

DAMP

HMGB1 can be released by necrotic cells during tissue injury and activate dendritic cells by triggering TLR4, inducing activation of NFκB, and production of proinflammatory cytokines such as TNF-α. HMGB1 can also trigger other PRRs like TLR2 and RAGE, on the cell surface of APCs. The importance of HMGB1 as a major DAMP released by necrotic cells is supported by the observed decrease in stimulatory capacity of necrotic cells genetically lacking HMGB1, and by the ability of neutralizing Abs to ameliorate inflammation.[83,84] Moreover, high levels of HMGB1 have been found in the sera of patients upon brain and myocardial ischemia and during sepsis; furthermore, clinical studies and reports in animal models support a pathogenic role for HMGB1 in the late phase of septic shock.[83]

Chaperone

Since HMGB1 is released by necrotic cells still bound to DNA, it can act as a chaperone to shuttle nuclei acids into the endosomal compartment of APCs, and possibly facilitate the triggering of nucleic acid sensors such as TLR9. During apoptosis, HMBG1 has been shown to bind firmly to the chromatin and therefore to remain sequestered in the apoptotic bodies. Under normal circumstances, this strategy would keep HMGB1 hidden from the PRRs and bound to be degraded during clearance of apoptotic cells. In case of defects in the clearance of apoptotic cells, such as in autoimmune diseases,[85] late apoptotic cells could become necrotic and release HMGB1 chaperoning DNA. HMGB1 also has the ability to bind LPS, at the level of lipid A, possibly because of its electric charge, and it can chaperone it to the CD14-TLR4 MD2 complex, increasing the response of macrophages to the LPS.[86] Therefore, HMGB1 stimulates the innate immune response not only as a DAMP but also as a chaperone of PAMPs and coreceptor of PRRs.[13]

Secondary Danger Signal

HMGB1 can also act as a secondary danger signal, when it is actively secreted like a cytokine by innate immune cells, such as macrophages and dendritic cells, upon TLR stimulation or exposure to TNF-α. In this case, HMGB1 is hyper-acetylated and translocated to the cytoplasm, where it is then secreted in the ex-tracellular compartment through a noncanonical mechanism, independent from the Golgi system.[87] Furthermore, an autocrine secretion of HMGB1 has been proposed to mediate dendritic cell activation and the induction of Th1-polarized adaptive immune responses.[88]

Chemokine

HMGB1 can also be secreted in a chemical form that allows it to bind to the chemokine CXCL12 and form a heterodimer, which can trigger the chemokine receptor CXCR4, and recruit leukocytes at the site of inflammation. This che-moattractant effect also facilitates the migration of smooth muscle stem cells that promote the repair of the necrotic tissues.

Redox State

HMGB1 can act as a chromatin protein, chemokine, DAMP, chaperone, and also as a cytokine. These different functions depend on the redox state of HMGB1.[13] Indeed, intracellular *chromatin* HMGB1 has three cysteines that are in a reduced (all-thiol) state; when HMGB1 is secreted in the extracellu-lar environment still in the all-thiol state, it can bind to CXCL12 and act as a chemokine;[89] upon oxidation of two cysteines, and the formation of a disulfide bond, HMGB1 is able to bind TLRs and act as a DAMP. If all the cysteines are oxidized, HMGB1 loses all the proinflammatory activities.[90] The complex regulation of different functions of HMGB1 is justified by its important role in tolerance and immunity.

Degradation Products of the Extracellular Matrix

Another important family of DAMPs consists of molecules generated by the degradation of components of the extracellular matrix (ECM).[9] Indeed, both infectious and sterile tissue damages are associated with the disruption of ECM, leading to the production of low molecular weight-degradation products like the glycosaminoglycan heparin sulfate and hyaluronic acid (HA). These soluble

ECM fragments trigger multiple PRRs, mostly TLR2 and TLR4, to activate dendritic cells and promote inflammation. Proteoglycans (PGs), such as biglycan and decorin, are released during tissue damage by the proteolytic activity of the enzymes, such as bone morphogenetic protein (BMP)-1, matrix metalloproteinases (MMP)-2, -3, and -13, and granzyme B.[51] Many other glycoproteins, like the fibronectin extra domain A (EDA), extravascular fibrinogen, and tenascin C, can act as DAMPs binding to TLR4, while PGs can trigger TLR2 and TLR4, and biglycan can also activate the NLRP3 inflammasome through the purinergic receptor P2X, leading to IL-1β production. The glycoprotein tenascins are highly expressed during the embryonic development in vertebrates and then during tissue injury and tumor growth. Their levels are found increased in inflammatory situations, such as, in rheumatoid arthritis, and mice deficient in tenascin-C show rapid resolution of inflammation, confirming the role of these DAMPs as amplifiers of inflammation.[51] Further evidence indicates that ECM molecules act as initiators/amplifiers of the autoimmune process in autoimmune diseases like rheumatoid arthritis, and in antitumor immunity.[68] The fact that so many DAMPs activate the immune cells through TLR4, posed the problem of discriminating the real stimulatory effects of the tested endogenous danger signals from the possible contamination of reagents with LPS. *In vivo* evidence generated using mice deficient for specific DAMPs, together with special attention to minimize the levels of LPS in the preparations, dissolved the initial concerns.[51]

SECONDARY ENDOGENOUS DANGER SIGNALS

The secondary endogenous danger signals are cytokines, such as IL-1β, TNF-α, and the interferons, which are produced by activated immune cells upon PRR triggering and initiate and mediate the activation of innate and adaptive immunity.[55] Although they are not considered classic DAMPs because they are produced upon PRR triggering, they activate and sustain the signaling pathways and the effector functions of the classic PRRs, such as the activation of the transcription factor NFκB, and the induction of proinflammatory processes, respectively.

Interestingly, the same cytokines can also be classified as DAMPs when they are secreted by damaged or stressed cells.[55] This is the case of type I interferons, which are also secreted by virally infected cells to warn of a viral infection. A second example is the production of IL-1β by cells dying of pyroptosis, as a consequence of a stressor that activated the NLRP3 inflammasome.[68]

Emerging and Homeostatic Danger Signals

In addition to the classic danger signals, derived from infectious nonself or damaged self, there are growing numbers of novel danger signals that belong to a third category of stressors. These novel danger signals neither derive from microorganisms, nor from stressed or dead cells, rather they are made up of inorganic material that can induce tissue damage and therefore the release of DAMPs.[9] Previous paragraphs have described the ability of MSU crystals to stimulate the inflammasome. Similarly, crystals of silica and other inorganic matter, which do not normally form in our body but can be generated upon exposure to environmental pollutants, can induce damage of phagocytes, through the destabilization of the phagolysosomes.[51]

Novel materials are also introduced into our bodies as wonders of modern medicine. Indeed, nanoparticles, either of organic origin such as liposomes, or made up of gold or any other precious metal, or polymers used for prosthetics, are not immunologically neutral, and evidence suggests that they may initiate the activation of the innate immune response by generating stress, cell death, and eliciting DAMPs.[9] Moreover, inorganic particulate matter may have, in common with DAMPs, a property of hydrophobicity that Seong and Matzinger have described to be shared by PAMPs and DAMPs.[12]

Another category of danger signals, has been recently proposed, which does not include either organic or inorganic, self or nonself molecules, but rather perturbations in the steady state of the cells and the tissues, which alert the cells of the immune system of the occurrence of injury or infections. Gallo and Gallucci called these alarms "homeostatic danger signals."[9] Localized acidosis, changes in osmolarity, hypoxia, oxidative stress with increased levels of ROS, and other metabolic disturbances, are conditions often associated with inflammation, either sterile or directly caused by bacterial growth. APCs are capable of directly sensing some of these perturbations. For example, macrophages can directly activate the inflammasome in a hypotonic environment because of the efflux of potassium and chloride induced by the mechanism that acts to reestablish the correct intracellular volume in case of decreased extracellular osmolarity.[41] Moreover, the signaling molecule mTOR, has been suggested to be involved in the sensing of osmotic stress.[91] Instead other perturbations induce the release of classic DAMPs, like high temperature ($>40°C$) that induces the upregulation of HSP70 and the subsequent activation of dendritic cells.[9] These perturbations can trigger the activation of signaling pathways in common with the PRRs, such as the inflammasome, and they may also trigger novel mechanisms that have not been discovered yet.

CONCLUSIONS

The innate immune response has a powerful ability to recognize a pathologic status caused by pathogens and/or trauma/stress through a set of receptors, very conserved in evolution, the PRRs, which are triggered by a diversified group of danger signals. These signals can be infectious or noninfectious, organic or inorganic, self or nonself molecules, and even perturbations in the physical and chemical microenvironment of the extracellular and intracellular spaces. Although these molecules are very heterogeneous, they trigger a very limited number of PRRs, and even more limited signaling pathways, suggesting that the purpose of the diversification is to maximize the ability to recognize pathologic conditions, even in the face of changes in the molecular diversity, that infectious agents implement as evasion strategies. It remains to be understood how few PRRs and signal transduction pathways can tailor the most efficient immune response to ward off the stressor, and the least damaging response for the tissue, in which such a response is occurring. Future studies will clarify how this happens; it is important that such studies are conducted by focusing on the DAMPs rather than the PAMPs, because they are possibly the ones that can provide the correct flavor of the tissue, and suggest the best immune response.

REFERENCES

1. Murphy K. *Janeway's Immunobiology*. 8th ed. New York: Garland Science; 2011.
2. Steinman RM, Hawiger D, Nussenzweig MC. Tolerogenic dendritic cells. *Annu Rev Immunol* 2003;**21**:685–711.
3. Bancereau J, Steinman RM. Dendritic cells and the control of immunity. *Nature* 1998;**392**(6673):245–52.
4. Merad M, Sathe P, Helft J, Miller J, Mortha A. The dendritic cell lineage: ontogeny and function of dendritic cells and their subsets in the steady state and the inflamed setting. *Annu Rev Immunol* 2013;**31**:563–604.
5. Sallusto F, Cella M, Danieli C, Lanzavecchia A. Dendritic cells use macropinocytosis and the mannose receptor to concentrate macromolecules in the major histocompatibility complex class II compartment: downregulation by cytokines and bacterial products. *J Exp Med* 1995;**182**(2):389–400.
6. Banchereau J, Briere F, Caux C, Davoust J, Lebecque S, Liu YJ, et al. Immunobiology of dendritic cells. *Annu Rev Immunol* 2000;**18**:767–811.
7. Janeway Jr CA. Approaching the asymptote? Evolution and revolution in immunology. *Cold Spring Harb Symp Quant Biol* 1989;**54**:1–13 Pt 1.
8. Medzhitov R, Janeway Jr CA. Innate immunity: the virtues of a nonclonal system of recognition. *Cell* 1997;**91**(3):295–8.
9. Gallo PM, Gallucci S. The dendritic cell response to classic, emerging, and homeostatic danger signals. Implications for autoimmunity. *Front Immunol* 2013;**4**:138.
10. Matzinger P. Tolerance, danger, and the extended family. *Annu Rev Immunol* 1994;**12**: 991–1045.
11. Land W, Schneeberger H, Schleibner S, Illner WD, Abendroth D, Rutili G, et al. The beneficial effect of human recombinant superoxide dismutase on acute and chronic rejection events in recipients of cadaveric renal transplants. *Transplantation* 1994;**57**(2):211–7.
12. Seong SY, Matzinger P. Hydrophobicity: an ancient damage-associated molecular pattern that initiates innate immune responses. *Nat Rev Immunol* 2004;**4**(6):469–78.
13. Broggi A, Granucci F. Microbe- and danger-induced inflammation. *Mol Immunol* 2015;**63**(2):127–33.
14. Kawai T, Akira S. The role of pattern-recognition receptors in innate immunity: update on Toll-like receptors. *Nat Immunol* 2010;**11**(5):373–84.
15. Eberl G, Boneca IG. Bacteria and MAMP-induced morphogenesis of the immune system. *Curr Opin Immunol* 2010;**22**(4):448–54.

16. Davis BK, Wen H, Ting JP. The inflammasome NLRs in immunity, inflammation, and associated diseases. *Annu Rev Immunol* 2011;**29**:707–35.

17. Medzhitov R, Preston-Hurlburt P, Janeway Jr CA. A human homologue of the *Drosophila* Toll protein signals activation of adaptive immunity. *Nature* 1997;**388**(6640):394–7.

18. Lemaitre B, Nicolas E, Michaut L, Reichhart JM, Hoffmann JA. The dorsoventral regulatory gene cassette spatzle/Toll/cactus controls the potent antifungal response in *Drosophila* adults. *Cell* 1996;**86**(6):973–83.

19. Poltorak A, He X, Smirnova I, Liu MY, Van Huffel C, Du X, et al. Defective LPS signaling in C3H/HeJ and C57BL/10ScCr mice: mutations in *Tlr4* gene. *Science* 1998;**282**(5396):2085–8.

20. Immunology in the limelight. *Nat Immunol* 2011;**12**(12):1127.

21. Steinman RM, Cohn ZA. Identification of a novel cell type in peripheral lymphoid organs of mice. I. Morphology, quantitation, tissue distribution. *J Exp Med* 1973;**137**(5):1142–62.

22. Brubaker SW, Bonham KS, Zanoni I, Kagan JC. Innate immune pattern recognition: a cell biological perspective. *Annu Rev Immunol* 2015;**33**:257–90.

23. Akira S, Uematsu S, Takeuchi O. Pathogen recognition and innate immunity. *Cell* 2006;**124**(4):783–801.

24. Meng J, Gong M, Bjorkbacka H, Golenbock DT. Genome-wide expression profiling and muta-genesis studies reveal that lipopolysaccharide responsiveness appears to be absolutely depen-dent on TLR4 and MD-2 expression and is dependent upon intermolecular ionic interactions. *J Immunol* 2011;**187**(7):3683–93.

25. Theofilopoulos AN, Baccala R, Beutler B, Kono DH. Type I interferons (alpha/beta) in immu-nity and autoimmunity. *Annu Rev Immunol* 2005;**23**:307–36.

26. Ikushima H, Negishi H, Taniguchi T. The IRF family transcription factors at the interface of innate and adaptive immune responses. *Cold Spring Harb Symp Quant Biol* 2013;**78**:105–16.

27. Steen HC, Gamero AM. STAT2 phosphorylation and signaling. *JAKSTAT* 2013;**2**(4):e25790.

28. Xu J, Zoltick PW, Gamero AM, Gallucci S. TLR ligands up-regulate Trex1 expression in mu-rine conventional dendritic cells through type I Interferon and NF-κB-dependent signaling pathways. *J Leukoc Biol* 2014;**96**(1):93–103.

29. Hoebe K, Janssen EM, Kim SO, Alexopoulou L, Flavell RA, Han J, et al. Upregulation of costimulatory molecules induced by lipopolysaccharide and double-stranded RNA occurs by Trif-dependent and Trif-independent pathways. *Nat Immunol* 2003;**4**(12):1223–9.

30. Sancho D, Reis e Sousa C. Sensing of cell death by myeloid C-type lectin receptors. *Curr Opin Immunol* 2013;**25**(1):46–52.

31. Plato A, Hardison SE, Brown GD. Pattern recognition receptors in antifungal immunity. *Semin Immunopathol* 2015;**37**(2):97–106.

32. Miyake Y, Yamasaki S. Sensing necrotic cells. *Adv Exp Med Biol* 2012;**738**:144–52.

33. Ahrens S, Zelenay S, Sancho D, Hanc P, Kjaer S, Feest C, et al. F-actin is an evolutionarily conserved damage-associated molecular pattern recognized by DNGR-1, a receptor for dead cells. *Immunity* 2012;**36**(4):635–45.

34. Sawamura T, Kakino A, Fujita Y. LOX-1: a multiligand receptor at the crossroads of response to danger signals. *Curr Opin Lipidol* 2012;**23**(5):439–45.

35. Ding SW. RNA-based antiviral immunity. *Nat Rev Immunol* 2010;**10**(9):632–44.

36. Durbin RK, Kotenko SV, Durbin JE. Interferon induction and function at the mucosal surface. *Immunol Rev* 2013;**255**(1):25–39.

37. Beutler B, Eidenschenk C, Crozat K, Imler JL, Takeuchi O, Hoffmann JA, et al. Genetic analy-sis of resistance to viral infection. *Nat Rev Immunol* 2007;**7**(10):753–66.

38. Paro S, Imler JL, Meignin C. Sensing viral RNAs by Dicer/RIG-I like ATPases across species. *Curr Opin Immunol* 2015;**32**:106–13.

39. Vabret N, Blander JM. Sensing microbial RNA in the cytosol. *Front Immunol* 2013;**4**:468.
40. Chan YK, Gack MU. RIG-I-like receptor regulation in virus infection and immunity. *Curr Opin Virol* 2015;**12C**:7–14.
41. Man SM, Kanneganti TD. Regulation of inflammasome activation. *Immunol Rev* 2015;**265**(1):6–21.
42. Vanaja SK, Rathinam VA, Fitzgerald KA. Mechanisms of inflammasome activation: recent advances and novel insights. *Trends Cell Biol* 2015;**25**(5):308–15.
43. Gringhuis SI, Kaptein TM, Wevers BA, Theelen B, van der Vlist M, Boekhout T, et al. Dectin-1 is an extracellular pathogen sensor for the induction and processing of IL-1beta via a noncanonical caspase-8 inflammasome. *Nat Immunol* 2012;**13**(3):246–54.
44. Connolly DJ, Bowie AG. The emerging role of human PYHIN proteins in innate immunity: implications for health and disease. *Biochem Pharmacol* 2014;**92**(3):405–14.
45. Hornung V, Ablasser A, Charrel-Dennis M, Bauernfeind F, Horvath G, Caffrey DR, et al. AIM2 recognizes cytosolic dsDNA and forms a caspase-1-activating inflammasome with ASC. *Nature* 2009;**458**(7237):514–8.
46. Morrone SR, Wang T, Constantoulakis LM, Hooy RM, Delannoy MJ, Sohn J. Cooperative assembly of IFI16 filaments on dsDNA provides insights into host defense strategy. *Proc Natl Acad Sci USA* 2014;**111**(1):E62–71.
47. Unterholzner L, Keating SE, Baran M, Horan KA, Jensen SB, Sharma S, et al. IFI16 is an innate immune sensor for intracellular DNA. *Nat Immunol* 2010;**11**(11):997–1004.
48. Cai X, Chiu YH, Chen ZJ. The cGAS-cGAMP-STING pathway of cytosolic DNA sensing and signaling. *Mol Cell* 2014;**54**(2):289–96.
49. Lee EJ, Park JH. Receptor for advanced glycation endproducts (RAGE), its ligands, and soluble RAGE: potential biomarkers for diagnosis and therapeutic targets for human renal diseases. *Genomics Inform* 2013;**11**(4):224–9.
50. Jaillon S, Bonavita E, Gentile S, Rubino M, Laface I, Garlanda C, et al. The long pentraxin PTX3 as a key component of humoral innate immunity and a candidate diagnostic for inflammatory diseases. *Int Arch Allergy Immunol* 2014;**165**(3):165–78.
51. Schaefer L. Complexity of danger: the diverse nature of damage-associated molecular patterns. *J Biol Chem* 2014;**289**(51):35237–45.
52. Jiang N, Reich CF, 3rd, Pisetsky DS. Role of macrophages in the generation of circulating blood nucleosomes from dead and dying cells. *Blood* 2003;**102**(6):2243–50.
53. Matzinger P. The danger model: a renewed sense of self. *Science* 2002;**296**(5566):301–5.
54. Gallucci S, Lolkema M, Matzinger P. Natural adjuvants: endogenous activators of dendritic cells. *Nat Med* 1999;**5**(11):1249–55.
55. Gallucci S, Matzinger P. Danger signals: SOS to the immune system. *Curr Opin Immunol* 2001;**13**(1):114–9.
56. Sauter B, Albert ML, Francisco L, Larsson M, Somersan S, Bhardwaj N. Consequences of cell death: exposure to necrotic tumor cells, but not primary tissue cells or apoptotic cells, induces the maturation of immunostimulatory dendritic cells. *J Exp Med* 2000;**191**(3):423–34.
57. Shi Y, Zheng W, Rock KL. Cell injury releases endogenous adjuvants that stimulate cytotoxic T cell responses. *Proc Natl Acad Sci USA* 2000;**97**(26):14590–5.
58. Shi Y, Evans JE, Rock KL. Molecular identification of a danger signal that alerts the immune system to dying cells. *Nature* 2003;**425**(6957):516–21.
59. Erwig LP, Henson PM. Immunological consequences of apoptotic cell phagocytosis. *Am J Pathol* 2007;**171**(1):2–8.
60. Pasparakis M, Vandenabeele P. Necroptosis and its role in inflammation. *Nature* 2015;**517**(7534):311–20.

61. Eloranta ML, Lovgren T, Finke D, Mathsson L, Ronnelid J, Kastner B, et al. Regulation of the interferon-alpha production induced by RNA-containing immune complexes in plasmacytoid dendritic cells. *Arthritis Rheum* 2009;**60**(8):2418–27.

62. Marshak-Rothstein A, Rifkin IR. Immunologically active autoantigens: the role of toll-like receptors in the development of chronic inflammatory disease. *Annu Rev Immunol* 2007;**25**:419–41.

63. Brinkmann V, Reichard U, Goosmann C, Fauler B, Uhlemann Y, Weiss DS, et al. Neutrophil extracellular traps kill bacteria. *Science* 2004;**303**(5663):1532–5.

64. Garcia-Romo GS, Caielli S, Vega B, Connolly J, Allantaz F, Xu Z, et al. Netting neutrophils are major inducers of type I IFN production in pediatric systemic lupus erythematosus. *Sci Transl Med* 2011;**3**(73): P 73ra20.

65. Yang YG, Lindahl T, Barnes DE. Trex1 exonuclease degrades ssDNA to prevent chronic checkpoint activation and autoimmune disease. *Cell* 2007;**131**(5):873–86.

66. Stetson DB, Ko JS, Heidmann T, Medzhitov R. Trex1 prevents cell-intrinsic initiation of auto-immunity. *Cell* 2008;**134**(4):587–98.

67. Gall A, Treuting P, Elkon KB, Loo YM, Gale Jr M, Barber GN, et al. Autoimmunity initiates in nonhematopoietic cells and progresses via lymphocytes in an interferon-dependent autoimmune disease. *Immunity* 2012;**36**(1):120–31.

68. Woo SR, Corrales L, Gajewski TF. Innate immune recognition of cancer. *Annu Rev Immunol* 2015;**33**:445–74.

69. Krysko DV, Agostinis P, Krysko O, Garg AD, Bachert C, Lambrecht BN, et al. Emerging role of damage-associated molecular patterns derived from mitochondria in inflammation. *Trends Immunol* 2011;**32**(4):157–64.

70. Mutini C, Falzoni S, Ferrari D, Chiozzi P, Morelli A, Baricordi OR, et al. Mouse dendritic cells express the P2X7 purinergic receptor: characterization and possible participation in antigen presentation. *J Immunol* 1999;**163**(4):1958–65.

71. Heil M, Land WG. Danger signals – damaged-self recognition across the tree of life. *Front Plant Sci* 2014;**5**:578.

72. Ravichandran KS. Beginnings of a good apoptotic meal: the find-me and eat-me signaling pathways. *Immunity* 2011;**35**(4):445–55.

73. Rock KL, Kataoka H, Lai JJ. Uric acid as a danger signal in gout and its comorbidities. *Nat Rev Rheumatol* 2013;**9**(1):13–23.

74. Cassel SL, Eisenbarth SC, Iyer SS, Sadler JJ, Colegio OR, Tephly LA, et al. The Nalp3 inflam-masome is essential for the development of silicosis. *Proc Natl Acad Sci USA* 2008;**105**(26): 9035–40.

75. Srivastava P. Roles of heat-shock proteins in innate and adaptive immunity. *Nat Rev Immunol* 2002;**2**(3):185–94.

76. Basu S, Binder RJ, Suto R, Anderson KM, Srivastava PK. Necrotic but not apoptotic cell death releases heat shock proteins, which deliver a partial maturation signal to dendritic cells and activate the NF-κ B pathway. *Int Immunol* 2000;**12**(11):1539–46.

77. Biswas C, Sriram U, Ciric B, Ostrovsky O, Gallucci S, Argon Y. The N-terminal fragment of GRP94 is sufficient for peptide presentation via professional antigen-presenting cells. *Int Immunol* 2006;**18**(7):1147–57.

78. Zhang Q, Raoof M, Chen Y, Sumi Y, Sursal T, Junger W, et al. Circulating mitochondrial DAMPs cause inflammatory responses to injury. *Nature* 2010;**464**(7285):104–7.

79. Galluzzi L, Kepp O, Kroemer G. Mitochondria: master regulators of danger signalling. *Nat Rev Mol Cell Biol* 2012;**13**(12):780–8.

80. Everts B, Pearce EJ. Metabolic control of dendritic cell activation and function: recent advances and clinical implications. *Front Immunol* 2014;**5**:203.

81. Andersson U, Tracey KJ. HMGB1 is a therapeutic target for sterile inflammation and infection. *Annu Rev Immunol* 2011;**29**:139–62.

82. Harris HE, Andersson U, Pisetsky DS. HMGB1: a multifunctional alarmin driving autoimmune and inflammatory disease. *Nat Rev Rheumatol* 2012;**8**(4):195–202.

83. Bianchi ME. DAMPs, PAMPs and alarmins: all we need to know about danger. *J Leukoc Biol* 2007;**81**(1):1–5.

84. Bianchi ME, Manfredi AA. High-mobility group box 1 (HMGB1) protein at the crossroads between innate and adaptive immunity. *Immunol Rev* 2007;**220**:35–46.

85. Cohen PL, Caricchio R. Genetic models for the clearance of apoptotic cells. *Rheum Dis Clin North Am* 2004;**30**(3):473–86.

86. Youn JH, Oh YJ, Kim ES, Choi JE, Shin JS. High mobility group box 1 protein binding to lipopolysaccharide facilitates transfer of lipopolysaccharide to CD14 and enhances lipopolysaccharide-mediated TNF-alpha production in human monocytes. *J Immunol* 2008;**180**(7):5067–74.

87. Bonaldi T, Talamo F, Scaffidi P, Ferrera D, Porto A, Bachi A, et al. Monocytic cells hyperacetylate chromatin protein HMGB1 to redirect it towards secretion. *EMBO J* 2003;**22**(20):5551–60.

88. Dumitriu IE, Baruah P, Valentinis B, Voll RE, Herrmann M, Nawroth PP, et al. Release of high mobility group box 1 by dendritic cells controls T cell activation via the receptor for advanced glycation end products. *J Immunol* 2005;**174**(12):7506–15.

89. Schiraldi M, Raucci A, Munoz LM, Livoti E, Celona B, Venereau E, et al. HMGB1 promotes recruitment of inflammatory cells to damaged tissues by forming a complex with CXCL12 and signaling via CXCR4. *J Exp Med* 2012;**209**(3):551–63.

90. Yang H, Antoine DJ, Andersson U, Tracey KJ. The many faces of HMGB1: molecular structure-functional activity in inflammation, apoptosis, and chemotaxis. *J Leukoc Biol* 2013;**93**(6): 865–73.

91. Desai BN, Myers BR, Schreiber SL. FKBP12-rapamycin-associated protein associates with mitochondria and senses osmotic stress via mitochondrial dysfunction. *Proc Natl Acad Sci USA* 2002;**99**(7):4319–24.

Chapter 2

Homeostatic Inflammation as Environmental-Adaptation Strategy

Kensuke Miyake, Ryutaro Fukui

Division of Infectious Genetics, Institute of Medical Science, Tokyo, Japan

INTRODUCTION

Homeostatic inflammation is similar to chronic inflammation; moreover, this concept has wider implications than inflammation. "Does inflammation work as pathogenic or protective response?," is a continuously asked question that raises a very important discussion, because a number of diseases are based on inflammation. According to the concept of homeostatic inflammation, inflammation is a part of homeostasis.[1] For example, metabolites work as ligands for innate immune sensors and induce inflammation, but if the inflammation is reversible and not progressive to the stage of vicious circle, homeostatic inflammation even works to maintain a stable immune environment (Fig. 2.1).

In this chapter, we focus on three topics. The first one is modulation of inflammation by metabolites and recognition of metabolites by innate immune sensors. These processes are closely linked to the interaction between immunity and metabolism. The second topic is protective and pathogenic functions of homeostatic inflammation. Although homeostatic inflammation is a part of homeostasis, accumulation of damage caused by homeostatic inflammation is a risk of lethal inflammation. The third one is the strategy to control homeostatic inflammation. Control means both induction and suppression, which is a goal of homeostatic inflammation.

INNATE IMMUNE SENSORS RECOGNIZE VARIOUS ENDOGENOUS LIGANDS INCLUDING METABOLITES

Innate immune sensors recognize pathogen-associated molecular patterns (PAMPs) and induce immune responses to protect the host from pathogens.[2–5] PAMPs are not pathogen-specific and innate immune sensors would not recognize

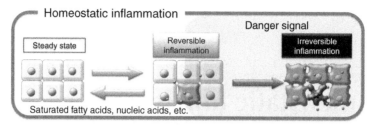

FIGURE 2.1   Concept of homeostatic inflammation. Danger signals underlie inflammation, which are induced by DAMPs released from damaged cells. In case of homeostatic inflammation, there is a spontaneous activation of innate immune sensors induced by endogenous ligands. If homeostatic inflammation is limited and reversible, it is a part of homeostasis. Collapse of control systems of homeostatic inflammation leads, of course, to pathogenic and irreversible inflammation and diseases.

self-derived molecular patterns under normal conditions, however, self-derived molecules sharing the construct with pathogens are also recognized as endogenous ligands by innate immune sensors.[6,7]

Some of the well-known host-derived molecules are called damage-associated molecular patterns (DAMPs). DAMPs are released from damaged cells and recognized by innate immune sensors to induce inflammation and facilitate clearance of damaged cells by phagocytes.[8,9] Digested cells no longer release DAMPs, thus originally, DAMPs induce inflammation to terminate inflammation.

Although the term "DAMPs" is linked to damaged cells, nondamaged cells also produce endogenous ligands of innate immune sensors. For example, fatty acids, phospholipids, and nucleic acids are produced by the metabolism of cells. These metabolites do not induce acute inflammation like PAMPs, but they induce chronic inflammation and may lead to diseases.

To understand the mechanisms of interaction between DAMPs and innate immune sensors, it is important to classify the properties of DAMPs. In this chapter, DAMPs are grouped by their chemical natures and recognized receptors (Table 2.1). The first group includes proteins and fatty acids. They are mainly recognized by cell surface-distributed toll-like receptors (TLRs), such as TLR1, TLR2, TLR6, or TLR4/MD-2. This makes sense because in case of PAMPs recognition, TLR2/TLR1 or TLR2/TLR6 heterodimer recognizes lipoprotein and TLR4/MD-2 recognizes lipopolysaccharide (LPS).[10–17]

The second group consists of nucleic acids, DNA, RNA, and monomers of nucleotides. They are not as diverse as the first group, but they are known as the inducers of various autoimmune diseases.[18,19] The recognition pattern of nucleic acid-sensing sensors is also related to PAMPs, for example, TLR3 recognizes double stranded RNA (dsRNA),[20] TLR7 and TLR8 recognize single stranded RNA (ssRNA),[21,22] TLR9 recognizes DNA,[23–25] and stimulator of interferon genes (STING) recognize cyclic di-guanosine monophosphate (cyclic di-GMP).[26–29]

TABLE 2.1 Type of endogenous ligands and their sensors

DAMP/ metabolite	Chemical nature	Sensor	Reference
Saturated fatty acids	Lipid	TLR4	[42–44]
Oxidized LDL	Lipid	TLR4/TLR6, CD36	[45]
Amyloid-β	Protein (Peptide)	TLR4, TLR6, CD36	[45]
Biglycan	Protein (Proteoglycan)	TLR2, TLR4, NLRP3	[50,51]
Tenascin-C	Protein (Glycoprotein)	TLR4	[47–49]
Fibronectin (Extra domain A)	Protein (Glycoprotein)	TLR4	[52]
Heat shock protein	Protein	TLR4	[55]
SA130	Protein (Ribonucleoprotein)	Micle	[163]
RNA	Nucleic acid	TLR3, TLR7, TLR8	[27,109,219]
DNA	Nucleic acid	TLR9, STING	[26,27,109]
Uric Acid	Nucleic acid	NLRP3	[33]

Although innate immune sensors recognize DAMPs because of their similarity to PAMPs, a nucleotide-binding oligomerization domain containing NOD-like receptor (NLR) in the NLR family, that is, NLR pyrin domain containing 3 (NLRP3), has a broader recognition pattern, activated by proteins, uric acid, and even some crystals (Table 2.1).[30–33]

MODULATION OF METABOLITES RECOGNIZED BY EXTRACELLULAR SENSORS

Lipids (fatty acids, phospholipids, etc.) and proteins can be endogenous ligands of the innate immune system, and exert a great influence on innate immune and inflammatory responses. Since these are mainly recognized by extracellular receptors, such as TLR4/MD-2, their activity for homeostatic inflammation is dependent on the release into the extracellular matrix. It reflects the inflammation in obese adipose tissue, where adipocytes and macrophages interact.[34–38]

The TLR4/MD-2 complex recognizes LPSs as PAMPs. Crystallographic analyses or tests with monoclonal antibody revealed that LPS directly binds to MD-2; furthermore, myristic acid binds to MD-2 as endogenous ligands.[39–41] This is not just binding; myristic acid and other saturated fatty acids, for example, palmitate, stimulate TLR4/MD-2 and induce inflammatory cytokines.[42–44] Saturated fatty acids are taken from foods and synthesized from acetyl coenzyme

A (acetyl-CoA) as part of metabolism. It means that fatty acids continuously stimulate TLR4/MD-2 and induce homeostatic inflammation even in steady state. Of course, overexposure to fatty acids may lead to metabolic syndrome, and it will be described in later sections.

Not only are saturated fatty acids, other lipids, or protein a vast source of endogenous ligands of innate immune sensors. Oxidized low-density lipoprotein (ox-LDL), known as a ligand of scavenger receptor CD36, stimulates a heterodimer of TLR4 and TLR6 in macrophages.[45] CD36–TLR4–TLR6 axis is also shown as amyloid-β-protein recognition system in this report. LDL is a transporter of cholesterol, which is oxidized on vascular endothelial cells, and amyloid-β protein is secreted by the cleavage of amyloid-β precursor protein.[46] These processes are parts of normal metabolism, as far as LDL production and accumulation are limited.

Proteins are recognized by TLR4 much as lipids. Tenascin-C, biglycan, extra domain A of fibronectin, and heat shock proteins (HSPs) are reported as examples.[47–55] HSPs are produced by cellular stress and work as chaperones. Others are glycoproteins, expressed in tendinous tissue (tenascin-C), or as ubiquitous extracellular matrix. Biglycan is also recognized by NLRP3 and causes the release of inflammatory cytokines.[51]

MODIFICATION OF NUCLEIC ACID-SENSING RECEPTORS

Nucleic acids are the most conserved molecules in all organisms, including viruses. The sequences of nucleic acid are totally different between host and microbes, but both sets of genes are constructed from the same nucleotides. As a result, nucleic acid-sensing innate immune receptors may recognize self-derived nucleic acids and induce inflammation.

To avoid excessive inflammation induced by nucleic acids, there are two general modification systems in cells. The former implies modification of nucleic acid-sensing receptors; the latter is involved in the modification of the host's nucleic acids. Nucleic acid-sensing receptors are produced in the endoplasmic reticulum much as other molecules and distributed to the compartments, where they recognize their ligands (Fig. 2.2).[56,57] This is an important tool to control the function of nucleic acid-sensing receptors, and associated molecules ease or suppress recognition.[58]

Nucleic acid-sensing TLRs, TLR3, TLR7, TLR8, TLR9, TLR11, TLR12, and TLR13 require UNC93 homolog B1 (UNC93B1) for response to their ligands.[59–62] UNC93B1 was found as a mammalian homolog of UNC-93, coordinating muscle contraction in *Caenorhabditis elegans*.[63,64] UNC-93 deficient *C. elegans* showed sluggish movement and a characteristic "rubber band," uncoordinated phenotype, thus this molecule was named "UNC." In mammalian cells, the function of UNC93B1 is not related to coordination of muscle contraction. The immunological function of UNC93B1 was found through the analysis of *N*-ethyl-*N*-nitrosourea-induced mutant mice.[59] H412R mutation of

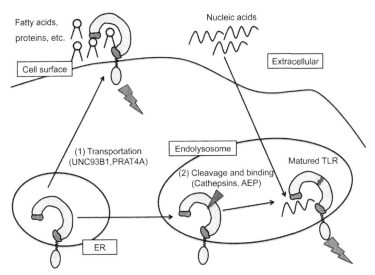

FIGURE 2.2   Modulation of TLRs in cells. TLRs are transported from ER to the cell surface or endolysosomes by accessory molecules.[1] Fatty acids or proteins are recognized on the cell surface, and nucleic acids are recognized in endolysosomes. Nucleic acid-sensing TLRs are cleaved in endolysosomes and cleaved N-terminal region binds to cleaved C-terminal region.[2] This matured form of TLR is able to recognize nucleic acids ligands and induce signal.

UNC93B1 was found in mice susceptible to virus infection, and UNC93B1 was characterized as an essential molecule for TLR3, TLR7, and TLR9. This mutation is called "triple D (3d)," meaning triple defect in these three nucleic acid-sensing TLRs.

UNC93B1 is a multiple transmembrane ER protein, binding to the transmembrane region of these TLRs.[65] UNC93B1 transports TLRs to endolysosomes, where nucleic acid-sensing TLRs recognize their ligands.[56,66] Binding of UNC93B1 to TLRs is upstream of transportation and the H412R mutant is not able to bind to TLRs; as a result, nucleic acid-sensing TLRs in 3d mice are not functional.

UNC93B1 is not only an essential molecule for nucleic acid-sensing TLRs, but also a regulator of them. A D34A mutation in UNC93B1 enhances the response of TLR7 and attenuates the response of TLR9.[67] The response of TLR3 is not affected by this mutation. The D34A mutant UNC93B1 binds more to TLR7 and less to TLR9 compared with wild type UNC93B1, and TLR transportation to endolysosomes reflects the change of binding activity. This data suggest that UNC93B1 reciprocally controls the responses of TLR7 and TLR9, and suppresses the hyperactivity of TLR7. So, it is thought of as a factor of various autoimmune diseases, thus wild type UNC93B1 would prevent excessive exposure of TLR7 to its ligand. The reason why TLR9 has dominance over TLR7 under the control of wild type UNC93B1 has not yet been revealed, but it is predicted to have a protective role of TLR9 for TLR7-dependent autoimmune disease.[68,69]

UNC93B1 transports the nucleic acid-sensing TLR3, TLR7, TLR9, and protein-sensing TLR5 to the cell surface.[70–76] Whereas TLR5 needs transportation to the cell surface for its function, it is still unclear what the functions of nucleic acid-sensing TLRs are on cell surfaces. Interaction of nucleic acid-sensing TLRs with UNC93B1 is an important key to understand the intracellular behavior of these TLRs, thus the details of its mechanisms need to be clarified.

Next, we introduce another molecule for the transportation of nucleic acid-sensing TLRs, that is, protein associated with TLR 4 (PRAT4A). PRAT4A was found to be a transporter of TLR4 from ER to the cell surface for response to LPS, and it is also required for the response of other TLRs.[77–80] Whereas TLR3 function is intact, and responses of TLR2, TLR5, TLR7, and TLR9 are deficient in $Prat4a^{-/-}$ cells.

Requirements of TLR transportation by PRAT4A are different from those of UNC93B1. TLRs requiring UNC93B1 for transportation are TLR3, TLR5, TLR7, TLR8, TLR9, and TLR13, containing acidic amino acid residues in their juxtamembrane region.[70,81] Between the end of the C-terminal-capping module of leucine rich repeat (LRR) and transmembrane regions, a few amino acid residues are inserted into all mammalian TLRs.[82,83] UNC93B1-binding TLRs have one or two acidic amino acids (aspartic acid or glutamic acid) in this conserved region, which is critical for binding to UNC93B1.

The characteristic feature of TLRs using PRAT4A for transportation is not as clear, but they can be grouped according to their adaptor proteins. After recognition of ligands, TLRs activate signaling pathways by recruiting adaptor proteins.[84,85] TLR3 uses TLR adaptor molecule 1 (TICAM-1, TRIF) for signaling,[86–89] whereas all of the other TLRs recruit myeloid differentiation primary response gene 88 (MyD88) for starting their signaling cascade.[23,90–94] TLR4/MD-2 uses both adaptor proteins with toll-interleukin 1 receptor domain-containing adaptor protein (TIRAP, Mal) and TLR adaptor molecule 2 (TICAM-2, TRAM).[95–97]

As described earlier, responses of TLRs through MyD88 is abolished but response of TLR3, independent from MyD88 signaling, is intact in $Prat4a^{-/-}$ mice.[79] Response of TLR4 is partially intact, therefore, MyD88 dependent signaling of TLRs might have deficiency by the lack of PRAT4A. This is a totally different modification system from UNC93B1, and it means multiple mechanisms control the distribution of TLRs and keep correct immune response.

A further modification step of nucleic acid-sensing TLRs is proteolytic cleavage of TLRs, which is performed by proteases in endolysosomes.[57,98] Requirement for cleavage is indicated by finding that response of nucleic acid-sensing TLRs is facilitated by proteases of the cathepsin family.[99,100] These reports showed that members of the cysteine protease family cathepsin K, B, and L are involved in the function of nucleic acid-sensing TLRs. An effect of cathepsins on ligand recognition by TLR9 was revealed, but the substrates of cathepsin were not identified.

In subsequent studies, significant roles of proteolytic cleavage for the function of nucleic acid-sensing TLRs have been recognized. First, two groups reported that proteolytic cleavage and conformational change of TLR9 are essential for their activation.[101,102] According to these reports, the cleavage site of TLR9 is predicted on a flexible loop between LRR14 and LRR15. TLR9 is transported by UNC93B1 from ER to endolysosomes and truncated into a mature form. Truncated TLR9 mainly binds to a ligand, CpG-ODN, and recruits MyD88 for signal transduction. In addition to previously reported cathepsins, cathepsin S, a cysteine protease was implied as a modifier of TLR9 activation, and the enzymatic activity of cathepsins was highlighted.

Thereafter, contribution of protease to TLR9 cleavage was reported in detail.[103,104] In these studies, it is shown that cathepsins and an asparagine-specific cysteine protease, asparagine endopeptidase (AEP), directly cleave TLR9, and this cleavage is a multistep process. Ectodomain of TLR9 is cleaved by AEP or cathepsins first, then cleaved TLR9 is trimmed solely by cathepsins, and changed into its functional form. TLR3 and TLR7 are also cleaved by these processes for their maturation.[103,105]

Finally, the binding of cleaved fragments to their ligands is reported as an indispensable step for functional modification of nucleic acid-sensing TLRs. The modification steps from transportation to binding are common to TLR3, TLR7, and TLR9, but the details of their processes are different. Among these findings, the development of brand new monoclonal antibodies allows to detect nontagged cleaved versus dissociated N-terminal.

About TLR3, human TLR3 and murine TLR3 were analyzed, and the cleaved site of human TLR3 was predicted in LRR12.[106] The cleaved C-terminal of human TLR3 is not dissociated with the N-terminal region, but single expression of the C-terminal region is not functional. In the case of murine TLR3, TLR7, and TLR9, a cleaved site was detected by N-terminal amino acid sequencing.[74,107,108] Their positions were S343, E461, and A462, or T461 and F467, respectively, and coexpression of the C-terminal region and N-terminal region revealed that these murine TLRs require cleavage and following association. Among these TLRs, TLR7 has unique cysteine residues in its ectodomain, whereas C98 and C475 are required for the formation of a disulfide bond.[108] This is accounted for by the fact that TLR7 has only a covalent bond for modification, but this is needed for cleavage and ligand recognition.

DNA AND RNA ARE MODIFIED TO BE RECOGNIZED OR NOT BY INNATE IMMUNE SENSORS

Much as the modification of nucleic acid-sensing sensors, modification of nucleic acid is important for both recognition and ignorance.[109] In this section, modification of nucleic acid is described with both roles of facilitating and suppressing recognition. This two-sided modification reflects the protective and pathogenic roles of interaction with innate immune sensors and metabolites.

To avoid excessive recognition of nucleic acids by innate immune sensors, extracellular self-derived nucleic acids are rapidly digested by enzymes. This is contrary to the recognition of pathogen-derived nucleic acids, to be kept intact for recognition. They are released at intracellular component or cytosol and recognized by nucleic acid sensors.[110]

One well-known clearance system of nucleic acids is DNA digestion by the deoxyribonuclease (DNase) family.[111–113] DNases are expressed in almost all types of cells including macrophages that engulf and digest released DNA. One of the members of the DNase family, DNase I, works in circulation; a neutral environment. This is a protective function of DNase I against systemic lupus erythematosus (SLE).[114,115]

Another member, DNase II, is distributed in cells, and it digests engulfed DNA. DNase II is an essential molecule for the survival of organisms. $Dnase2a^{-/-}$ mice are embryonic lethal with severe anemia, and macrophages are accumulated in lesions of fetal liver.[116,117] In these macrophages, many nucleuses are observed with undigested DNA, released from erythroid precursors.

In the human body, about 100 billion red blood cells are generated every day. At the final stage of differentiation, nucleus is released from red blood cells as a result of enucleation. This is a basic function also for mice, exerted by liver as a blood-forming organ during the embryonic stage. Macrophages in the liver of $Dnase2a^{-/-}$ mice are activated by the DNA and produce excessive interferon (IFN)-β. $Dnase2a^{-/-}$ $Ifnar1^{-/-}$ double mutant mice are rescued from lethal anemia; therefore, digestive modification of DNA by DNase II prevents lethal inflammation in the embryo.

Engulfment of released nucleus by macrophage is dependent on phosphatidylserine expressed on the membrane of the nucleus.[118] Phosphatidylserine is also expressed on apoptotic cells as an "eat-me" signal, and recognized by T cell immunoglobulin and mucin domain-containing molecule 1 (Tim1) and Tim4 on macrophages.[119] From these results, clearance of apoptotic cells by macrophages might be performed much as nucleus is released from erythrocytes.

A factor of the lethal phenotype of $Dnase2a^{-/-}$ mice is thought to activate STING, a sensor of cyclic di-GMP converted from cytosolic DNA.[26,27] Another DNA sensor, TLR9, does not contribute to this phenotype, but DNase II cleaves DNA into the forms recognized by TLR9.[120] DNase II-deficient cells do not respond to several types of TLR9 ligands because of the lack of DNA cleavage activity. One is CpG-A, cleaved by DNase II into 11–12 mer fragments. Treatment of DNase II-deficient cells with precleaved form of CpG-A activates the cells, thus the digestion of DNA ligands is required for TLR9 responses. Not only artificial ligands but also bacterial DNA is cleaved by DNase II for recognition by TLR9. In a strict sense, commensal bacteria are not self but symbiotic organisms, and their components work as metabolites. Based on it, TLR9 signaling induced by gut flora DNA, regulates the balance of T cell populations.[121] In the small intestine of $Trl9^{-/-}$ mice, regulatory T cells are increased and effector T cells are suppressed. DNase II is broadly expressed among the cells, thus gut flora DNA released from commensal bacteria has a potential to be modified by DNase II and to affect the regulation of homeostatic inflammation.

ssRNA is one of the most conserved structures between host and microbes, known as ligand of TLR7 or TLR8.[21,22] These TLRs recognize not only polymer RNA chains, but also small molecules such as imidazoquinolines and nucleoside analogs.[93,122–124] Activity and selectivity for these ligands are different among species; for example, TLR7 works mainly in murine cells but TLR8 does not respond to the ligands strongly. It does not mean that murine TLR8 is not functional, because murine TLR8 is activated by the combination of ligands such as oligodeoxynucleotides and imidazoquinolines.[125,126] In human cells, TLR7 and TLR8 work well; however, ligand binding to each TLR is different from murine TLRs. These are very complicated activation patterns of TLR7 and TLR8, tightly linked to protection against viral or autoimmune diseases. It is therefore important to analyze the functions of TLR7 and TLR8, or the characters of their ligands.

Ribonuclease (RNase) digests RNA into oligonucleotides or mononucleotides for clearance of RNA, and affects the ligand activity of endogenous RNA. TLR7 overexpressing Tg (TLR7-Tg) mice develop SLE-like phenotypes with the production of autoantibody, glomerulonephritis, hepatitis, and splenomegaly.[127,128] These phenotypes are developed spontaneously, but overexpression of RNaseA attenuates inflammation in TLR7-Tg mice.[129]

This means that abundant endogenous RNA ligands exist in circulation, because RNaseA digests RNA in circulation. From these results, TLR7 recognize self-derived RNA polymer chains released into circulation as ligands; meanwhile, endogenous single nucleosides may bind TLR7 or TLR8. Recently, crystal structures of TLR8 in complex with ssRNA and uridine were determined.[130] According to a published report,[130] TLR8 recognizes short oligonucleotides and uridine degraded from uridine- and guanosine-rich ssRNA. These degraded molecules bind to different sites, and both of them are required for activation of TLR8. It implies that TLR8 recognizes both degraded molecules derived from RNA.

PRIMING EFFECT OF NONINFECTIOUS INFLAMMATION ON IMMUNE RESPONSE

Since pathogens may be invading hosts at any time, the immune system should be always ready to protect the hosts. Acquired immunity is a powerful defender but requires several days for activation. The innate immune system is capable of rapid response to pathogens, but their receptor should also be prepared before infection (Fig. 2.3).

For example, expression of TLR7 in B cells is maintained by type I IFNs. IFN-α or IFN-β treatment of B cells enhances mRNA expression of TLR7 and response to TLR7 ligands.[131,132] Type I IFNs signaling deficient *Ifnar1*$^{-/-}$ mice have less TLR7 and treatment of type I IFN does not rescue the expression level

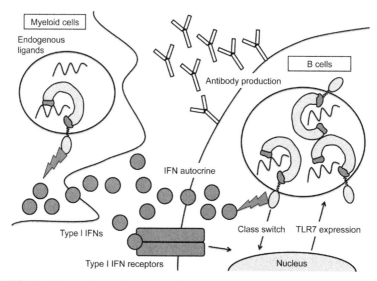

FIGURE 2.3   Priming effect of homeostatic inflammation on the immune system. Endogenous ligands induce type I IFNs in myeloid or B cells. B cells respond to type I IFNs and enhance the transcription of mRNA for TLR7. Expressed TLR7 or other immune sensors induce class switch of immunoglobulin genes and secretion of antibody spontaneously.

of TLR7. These findings suggest that spontaneous production of type I IFN is required for keeping the expression level of TLR7 in B cells. Plasmacytoid DCs (pDCs) are a well-known producer of type I IFN, and B cells also have the potential to produce type I IFNs following stimulation with TLR ligands.[132] Actually, it is not unclear how type I IFNs are produced spontaneously, but the lower expression level of TLR7 in *Ifnar1*$^{-/-}$ B cells implies that homeostatic inflammation induces type I IFNs and primes B cells for maintenance of TLR7 expression.

B cells belong to the acquired immune system by their main role of producing antibodies. Moreover, B cells are primed by metabolites and DAMPs to get ready for the invasion of pathogens. As mentioned earlier, B cells express not only an acquired immune sensor called the B cell receptor (BCR), but also innate immune sensors. These innate immune sensors directly recognize PAMPs and activate B cells without costimulation of BCR.[133–135]

In B cells, the class switch of BCR is induced by activation-induced cytidine deaminase (AID) when B cells are activated by BCR stimulation and cytokines.[136] It is known that TLR ligands facilitate class switch in B cells,[137,138] and even in steady state, spontaneous production of antibodies is dependent on signaling from innate immune sensors. Radioprotective 105 (RP105) is a homolog of TLR4, and expressed on the surface of B cells with MD-1, a homolog of MD-2.[139–142] The heterodimer of RP105/MD-1 is involved in the response of TLR2 and TLR4/MD-2 on B cells, and enhances antibody production from B cells.[143–146]

In the serum of $RP105^{-/-}$ or $MD-1^{-/-}$ mice, concentrations of IgG2b and IgG3 are drastically lower than the level of wild type mice, whereas concentrations of IgM, IgG1, and IgG2c are not changed.[147] Furthermore, IgG3 is only affected by TLR2/TLR4 double deficiency, and IgG2b, IgG2c, and IgG3 are decreased in $Myd88^{-/-}$ mice. These differential patterns of defects in the classes of immunoglobulin imply that spontaneous class switch is controlled by multiple innate immune sensors and each immune sensor induces switching into specific classes. Since antibiotic treatments or germ-free conditions affect spontaneous class switch, cross-talk with commensal bacteria might be an important factor as well.

CORRELATION WITH INFLAMMATORY AND AUTOIMMUNE DISEASES IN ADIPOSE TISSUE

In this chapter, we mainly showed the protective or neutral side of homeostatic inflammation; however, if homeostatic inflammation is out of control, inflammation damages cells and DAMPs are released (Fig. 2.1).[148] A persistent release of DAMPs stimulates innate immune sensors continuously and strongly. Activated innate immune sensors facilitate the production of inflammatory cytokines, and activated cells respond to DAMPs and inflammation. Finally, a vicious circle is constructed among innate immune sensors, inflammation, and DAMPs.

After the vicious circle is constructed, chronic inflammation induced by DAMPs may be associated with disease occurrence. Whereas the response to PAMPs implies an immune response to pathogens, an excessive response to endogenous ligands can lead to autoimmune disease. The correlation between homeostatic inflammation and autoimmune or metabolic diseases is the main topic of these sections. Finally, we present some possible ways to treat diseases based on the control of homeostatic inflammation.

Homeostatic inflammation, driven by lipid/protein-sensing TLRs is related to the metabolic syndrome, and it is tightly linked to obesity and adipose tissue metabolism. Adipose tissue is a connective tissue mainly composed of adipocytes. It stores fatty acids in a steady state, but in adipose tissue of obese subjects production of adipocytokines and chemokines gets increased. According to the interaction between adipocytes and macrophages, obesity is now thought of as a state of inflammation.[149–151] This assumption is corroborated by several findings in obese subjects: (1) metabolites recognized by TLR4 on macrophages (see aforementioned description), (2) expression pattern of innate immune sensors in macrophages, and (3) adipose tissue remodeling as a result of inflammation.

Innate immune sensors are mainly expressed in myeloid cells; for example, dendritic cells and macrophages work as frontlines of the immune system and facilitate the acquired immunity response.[152–156] Among innate immune sensor-expressing cells, macrophage plays a central role in adipose tissue (Fig. 2.4). In obese adipose tissue, production of chemotactic factors, such as monocyte chemoattractant protein-1 (MCP-1), is enhanced, and macrophages infiltrate the

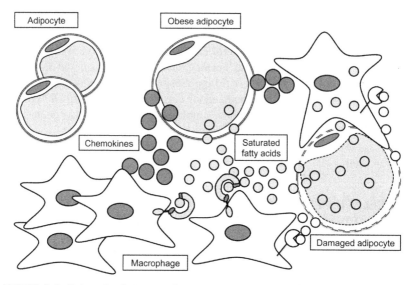

FIGURE 2.4 Interaction between adipocytes and macrophages in adipose tissue. Obese adipocytes release chemokines (dark gray circle) and macrophages infiltrate adipose tissue with their chemokine receptor. Macrophages recognize released saturated fatty acids (light gray circle) by TLR4/MD-2 and get activated. Activated macrophages produce proinflammatory cytokines, which damage adipocytes. These release SA130, a ligand of Mincle (white circle). Attachment of macrophages to damaged adipocytes enhances the recognition of SA130 and macrophages are more activated. Finally, a vicious circle is established between cells and molecules.

tissue after stimulation of chemokine receptor 2 (CCR2), that is, the receptor of MCP-1.[157–159] Infiltrated macrophages are stimulated and activated by saturated fatty acids released from adipocytes, so that large amounts of proinflammatory cytokines are produced and do damage to adipocytes. Damaged adipocytes release more fatty acids as a danger signal and finally a vicious circle is constructed from homeostatic inflammation.

Damaged and dead adipocytes are surrounded by macrophages, and a crown-like structure is formed. Macrophages and adipocytes closely interact in the structure and inflammation is amplified. Macrophage-inducible C-type lectin (Mincle), expressed on macrophages by stimuli, such as LPS or inflammatory cytokines, recognizes mycobacterial glycolipids (trehalose-6,6′-dimycolate, TDM) or a component of fungi.[160–162] In addition to these PAMPs, Mincle recognizes SA130, a nucleoprotein released from dead cells as DAMP.[163] Mincle activates a signal pathway by binding to Fc receptor gamma (FcRγ), an immunoreceptor containing a tyrosine-based activation motif (ITAM motif). SA130 facilitates the binding of Mincle to FcRγ; therefore, Mincle is activated by dead cells. A coculture experiment revealed that direct attachment of macrophages and adipocytes is required for the activation of Mincle, suggesting that tight attachment in the crown-like structure is the core of inflammation in adipose tissue.[164]

EXCESSIVE ACTIVATION OF NUCLEIC ACID-SENSING SENSORS INDUCES AUTOIMMUNE DISEASES

As mentioned in the aforementioned sections, there are multiple controlling systems for nucleic acid-sensing receptors to avoid excessive activation. They vary from the expression of receptors to the feedback after signal transduction, and the collapse of the controlling system results in autoimmune diseases. Here we describe the correlation between homeostatic inflammation and autoimmune diseases, mainly induced by endogenous nucleic acids (Fig. 2.5).

Among nucleic acid-sensing receptors, the contribution of TLR7 to autoimmune disease has been reported frequently. A phenotype of the Yaa mutant mice has been known as a lupus model for about 30 years, and their phenotype is linked to the genetic background and major histocompatibility complex.[165–175] Yaa gene induced autoantibody production and nephritis as observed in SLE patients, but the master gene of Yaa phenotypes had been unclear for a long

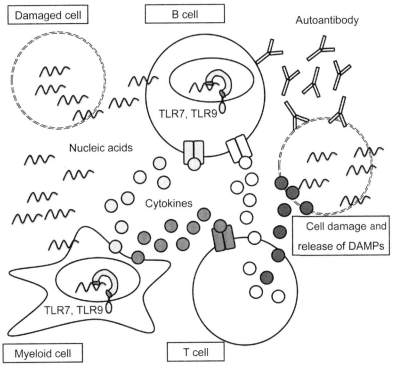

FIGURE 2.5   Homeostatic inflammation and autoimmune diseases. Endogenous nucleic acids (and of course other DAMPs) are released from damaged cells and recognized by nucleic acid-sensing sensors in myeloid and B cells. Activated myeloid cells produce cytokines/IFNs to activate B and T cells, and autoantibodies or T cell-derived cytokines are released, respectively. They damage cells and these damaged cells release DAMPs again. Through these steps, inflammation is amplified and autoimmune diseases are developed.

time. The master gene for the phenotype of Yaa mice was revealed by the expanded investigation into innate immunity. A group found that the TLR7-coding locus is duplicated on Yaa chromosome.[176] TLR7 is an X-linked gene, and the duplicated locus is out of expression control. As a result, response of TLR7 in B cells is enhanced and autoantibody is generated.[177,178] Pathogenic activity of overexpressed TLR7 is reproduced in TLR7 transgenic mice, also giving rise to SLE-like phenotypes like Yaa mice.[127,128]

Even if the expression level of TLR7 is kept normal, TLR7 may underlie autoimmune phenotypes. An imidazoquinolone analog of imiquimod has type I IFN-inducing activity, and is used for antiviral therapy.[179–184] Imiquimod cream is typically used for treatment of papillomavirus, but psoriasis is reported as a side effect. Imiquimod induces type I IFN as an agonist of TLR7, and the side effect of imiquimod is also dependent on TLR7 activation.[185,186] Imiquimod is not a self-derived ligand, but psoriasis is driven by a complex of self-derived RNA and antimicrobial peptide LL37, which is recognized by TLR7 and TLR8 in DCs.[187]

Pathogenicity of TLR9 is more complicated than TLR7, because TLR9 works as an inducer and attenuator of some types of autoimmune diseases. For example, the complex of LL37 and self-derived DNA stimulates TLR9 in pDCs and induces psoriasis.[188,189] Formation of nucleic acid/protein complexes stabilize the ligand activity of nucleic acids and facilitate the recognition by receptors. The immune complex of DNA with antibody or high-mobility group box 1 (HMGB1) stabilizes DNA and induces autoantibody production.[134,190–194]

In addition to these pathogenic sides, TLR9 is involved in the protection and regulation of autoimmune diseases. MRL$^{lpr/lpr}$ mice (lpr mice) are a well-known autoimmune mouse model, harboring a mutation in the locus of *Fas* gene and showing impaired expression of Fas protein.[195] This mutation reduces apoptotic activity and expansion of immature T cells and gives rise to the production of autoantibodies.[196–198]

The phenotype of lpr mice is not directly induced by TLR7 or TLR9, but $Tlr9^{-/-}$ lpr mice produce lower levels of autoantibodies.[199] Interestingly, in spite of impaired autoantibodies, the pathogenic phenotype of $Tlr9^{-/-}$ lpr mice is more severe than that of $Tlr9^{+/+}$ lpr mice, and the phenotype of $Tlr7^{-/-}$ lpr mice is ameliorated.[200,201] These reports suggest that TLR9 has a protective role in lpr mice, by suppressing TLR7-dependent autoantibodies.

The protective role of TLR9 on TLR7-dependent autoinflammation is reported in other autoimmune mice models. In C57BL/6 mice with pathogenic locus of New Zealand Black strain, TLR9 deficiency increases the expression of TLR7 and enhances their diseases.[68]

These are the protective roles of TLR9 in autoimmune models; meanwhile, the response of TLR7 is related to TLR9 even in steady state. As mentioned earlier, UNC93B1 controls the reciprocal response of TLR7 and TLR9 by orchestrating trafficking, so the response of TLR7 is extremely enhanced by the D34A mutation in UNC93B1 whereas the response of TLR9 is impaired.[67]

Dysregulation of TLR7/TLR9 balance in $Unc93b1^{D34A/D34A}$ mice (D34A mice) causes systemic inflammation with splenomegaly, thrombocytopenia, nephritis, and lethal hepatitis.[202] Production of autoantibody is not severe, but B cells play a key role in these phenotypes.

A more direct effect on TLR7 responses is observed in $Tlr8^{-/-}$ or $Tlr9^{-/-}$ mice. A group reported that expression of TLR7 is upregulated in $Tlr8^{-/-}$, $Tlr9^{-/-}$, and $Tlr8/9^{-/-}$ mice.[69,203] Response of TLR7 is enhanced in these mutant mice following an increased expression of TLR7, and autoimmune phenotypes are developed. Single deficiency of TLR8 or TLR9 is able to enhance TLR7 expression and cause autoimmune phenotypes; moreover, double deficiency of TLR8 and TLR9 leads to even more severe phenotypes.

These reports imply that homeostatic inflammation via nucleic acid-sensing TLRs is mutually controlled by each other. The mechanism of interaction among these TLRs has not been fully characterized; however, these aspects are tightly linked to the concept of homeostatic inflammation.

REGULATION OF HOMEOSTATIC INFLAMMATION AND INNATE IMMUNE SENSORS FOR CONTROLLING IMMUNE SYSTEM AND HOMEOSTASIS

Owing to the reasons stated earlier, inflammatory diseases can be treated by modulating the factors of homeostatic inflammation. This is an important concept, which illustrates the need to investigate homeostatic inflammation keeping in mind that adequate induction of homeostatic inflammation is badly needed for environmental adaptation.

One of the strategies to regulate inflammation is to block innate immune sensors.[204,205] Against the pathogenic activity of nucleic acid-sensing TLRs, various antagonistic nucleic acids are tried to treat TLR-associated inflammation.[206–210] In addition to chemical antagonists, a therapeutic effect of anti-TLR7 antibody has been reported.[73] This monoclonal anti-TLR7 blocks the activation of TLR7, and checks the phenotypes developed in D34A mice. Notably, this anti-TLR7 antibody has high specificity and shows efficacy after the symptoms have appeared. These data indicate high validity of therapeutic antibodies against pathogenic homeostatic inflammation.

On the contrary, it was reported that constitutive induction of type I IFN is controlled by TLR7 and protects from hepatitis.[211] TLR7 is thought of as a risk factor of autoimmune diseases, but experimental TLR7-IFN axis is protective against experimentally induced liver fibrosis. Moreover, homeostatic inflammation is critical for controlling endogenous viruses. Retroviral genome is integrated in the host genome and transmitted according to Mendel's principles.[212] Nucleic acid-sensing TLRs contribute to the control of some types of endogenous retrovirus by spontaneous production of antibodies, and TLR7-deficient mice develop tumors following lack of antibodies.[213] For this function, TLR7 plays a central role with the help of TLR3 and TLR9. Taken together, the excessive response of TLR7 is pathogenic but basal homeostatic inflammation by TLR7 and other sensors are important to maintain homeostasis. An ideal therapeutic approach with the suppressor of innate immune sensors should be controlled to keep an appropriate level of activity.

Another approach to regulate homeostatic inflammation is the artificial induction of homeostatic inflammation. If homeostatic inflammation does not progress to a vicious circle stage, it is a part of metabolism. Therefore, the induction of controlled homeostatic inflammation is similar to modification of metabolism.

A promising inducer of homeostatic inflammation is the modulation of commensal bacteria. According to the dramatically accumulating insight into the interaction between commensal bacteria and the immune system, oral administration of commensal bacteria or their component is thought of as a powerful regulator of immunity.[214–217] Among commensal bacteria, lactic acid bacteria (LAB) are broadly used probiotics for oral administration. Abundant LAB is included in fermented foods, and some strains of LAB contain TLR-stimulating nucleic acids.[218] These strains have dsRNA, which stimulates TLR3 and protect mice from dextran sulfate sodium salt-derived colitis. This protection is dependent on the production of IFN-β, induced via TLR3 signaling. Although TLR3 is reported as a factor of lethal radiation-induced gastrointestinal syndrome,[219] TLR3 stimulation by oral treatment is expected as a fine way of controlling the intestinal environment in steady state.

REFERENCES

1. Miyake K, Kaisho T. Homeostatic inflammation in innate immunity. *Curr Opin Immunol* 2014;**30C**:85–90.
2. Kawai T, Akira S. The role of pattern-recognition receptors in innate immunity: update on toll-like receptors. *Nat Immunol* 2010;**11**(5):373–84.
3. Palm NW, Medzhitov R. Pattern recognition receptors and control of adaptive immunity. *Immunol Rev* 2009;**227**(1):221–33.
4. Takeuchi O, Akira S. Pattern recognition receptors and inflammation. *Cell* 2010;**140**(6): 805–20.
5. Mogensen TH. Pathogen recognition and inflammatory signaling in innate immune defenses. *Clin Microbiol Rev* 2009;**22**(2):240–73.
6. Marshak-Rothstein A, Rifkin IR. Immunologically active autoantigens: the role of toll-like receptors in the development of chronic inflammatory disease. *Annu Rev Immunol* 2007;**25**:419–41.
7. Chen GY, Nunez G. Sterile inflammation: sensing and reacting to damage. *Nat Rev Immunol* 2010;**10**(12):826–37.
8. Schaefer L. Complexity of danger: the diverse nature of damage-associated molecular patterns. *J Biol Chem* 2014;**289**(51):35237–45.
9. Piccinini AM, Midwood KS. DAMPening inflammation by modulating TLR signalling. *Mediators Inflamm* 2010;**2010**:672395.
10. Hoshino K, Takeuchi O, Kawai T, Sanjo H, Ogawa T, Takeda Y, et al. Cutting edge: Toll-like receptor 4 (TLR4)-deficient mice are hyporesponsive to lipopolysaccharide: evidence for TLR4 as the Lps gene product. *J Immunol* 1999;**162**(7):3749–52.

11. Takeuchi O, Hoshino K, Kawai T, Sanjo H, Takada H, Ogawa T, et al. Differential roles of TLR2 and TLR4 in recognition of Gram-negative and Gram-positive bacterial cell wall components. *Immunity* 1999;**11**(4):443–51.

12. Takeuchi O, Kawai T, Muhlradt PF, Morr M, Radolf JD, Zychlinsky A, et al. Discrimination of bacterial lipoproteins by Toll-like receptor 6. *Int Immunol* 2001;**13**(7):933–40.

13. Takeuchi O, Kawai T, Sanjo H, Copeland NG, Gilbert DJ, Jenkins NA, et al. TLR6: A novel member of an expanding toll-like receptor family. *Gene* 1999;**231**(1-2):59–65.

14. Takeuchi O, Sato S, Horiuchi T, Hoshino K, Takeda K, Dong Z, et al. Cutting edge: role of Toll-like receptor 1 in mediating immune response to microbial lipoproteins. *J Immunol* 2002;**169**(1):10–4.

15. Nagai Y, Akashi S, Nagafuku M, Ogata M, Iwakura Y, Akira S, et al. Essential role of MD-2 in LPS responsiveness and TLR4 distribution. *Nat Immunol* 2002;**3**(7):667–72.

16. Shimazu R, Akashi S, Ogata H, Nagai Y, Fukudome K, Miyake K, et al. MD-2, a molecule that confers lipopolysaccharide responsiveness on Toll-like receptor 4. *J Exp Med* 1999;**189**(11):1777–82.

17. Poltorak A, He X, Smirnova I, Liu MY, Van Huffel C, Du X, et al. Defective LPS signaling in C3H/HeJ and C57BL/10ScCr mice: mutations in *Tlr4* gene. *Science* 1998;**282**(5396):2085–8.

18. Fukui R, Miyake K. Controlling systems of nucleic acid sensing-TLRs restrict homeostatic inflammation. *Exp Cell Res* 2012;**318**(13):1461–6.

19. Krieg AM, Vollmer J. Toll-like receptors 7, 8 and 9: linking innate immunity to autoimmunity. *Immunol Rev* 2007;**220**:251–69.

20. Alexopoulou L, Holt AC, Medzhitov R, Flavell RA. Recognition of double-stranded RNA and activation of NF-κB by Toll-like receptor 3. *Nature* 2001;**413**(6857):732–8.

21. Diebold SS, Kaisho T, Hemmi H, Akira S, Reis e Sousa C. Innate antiviral responses by means of TLR7-mediated recognition of single-stranded RNA. *Science* 2004;**303**(5663):1529–31.

22. Heil F, Hemmi H, Hochrein H, Ampenberger F, Kirschning C, Akira S, et al. Species-specific recognition of single-stranded RNA via toll-like receptor 7 and 8. *Science* 2004;**303**(5663):1526–9.

23. Hemmi H, Takeuchi O, Kawai T, Kaisho T, Sato S, Sanjo H, et al. A Toll-like receptor recognizes bacterial DNA. *Nature* 2000;**408**(6813):740–5.

24. Bauer S, Kirschning CJ, Hacker H, Redecke V, Hausmann S, Akira S, et al. Human TLR9 confers responsiveness to bacterial DNA via species-specific CpG motif recognition. *Proc Natl Acad Sci USA* 2001;**98**(16):9237–42.

25. Kumagai Y, Takeuchi O, Akira S. TLR9 as a key receptor for the recognition of DNA. *Adv Drug Deliv Rev* 2008;**60**(7):795–804.

26. Burdette DL, Monroe KM, Sotelo-Troha K, Iwig JS, Eckert B, Hyodo M, et al. STING is a direct innate immune sensor of cyclic di-GMP. *Nature* 2011;**478**(7370):515–8.

27. Ahn J, Gutman D, Saijo S, Barber GN. STING manifests self DNA-dependent inflammatory disease. *Proc Natl Acad Sci USA* 2012;**109**(47):19386–91.

28. Ishikawa H, Barber GN. STING is an endoplasmic reticulum adaptor that facilitates innate immune signalling. *Nature* 2008;**455**(7213):674–8.

29. Ishikawa H, Ma Z, Barber GN. STING regulates intracellular DNA-mediated, type I interferon-dependent innate immunity. *Nature* 2009;**461**(7265):788–92.

30. Menu P, Vince JE. The NLRP3 inflammasome in health and disease: the good, the bad and the ugly. *Clin Exp Immunol* 2011;**166**(1):1–15.

31. Naik E, Dixit VM. Modulation of inflammasome activity for the treatment of auto-inflammatory disorders. *J Clin Immunol* 2010;**30**(4):485–90.

32. Ogura Y, Sutterwala FS, Flavell RA. The inflammasome: first line of the immune response to cell stress. *Cell* 2006;**126**(4):659–62.

33. Martinon F, Petrilli V, Mayor A, Tardivel A, Tschopp J. Gout-associated uric acid crystals activate the NALP3 inflammasome. *Nature* 2006;**440**(7081):237–41.

34. Cinti S, Mitchell G, Barbatelli G, Murano I, Ceresi E, Faloia E, et al. Adipocyte death defines macrophage localization and function in adipose tissue of obese mice and humans. *J Lipid Res* 2005;**46**(11):2347–55.

35. Nishimura S, Manabe I, Nagasaki M, Hosoya Y, Yamashita H, Fujita H, et al. Adipogenesis in obesity requires close interplay between differentiating adipocytes, stromal cells, and blood vessels. *Diabetes* 2007;**56**(6):1517–26.

36. Nishimura S, Manabe I, Nagasaki M, Seo K, Yamashita H, Hosoya Y, et al. *In vivo* imaging in mice reveals local cell dynamics and inflammation in obese adipose tissue. *J Clin Invest* 2008;**118**(2):710–21.

37. Weisberg SP, McCann D, Desai M, Rosenbaum M, Leibel RL, Ferrante Jr AW. Obesity is associated with macrophage accumulation in adipose tissue. *J Clin Invest* 2003;**112**(12):1796–808.

38. Xu H, Barnes GT, Yang Q, Tan G, Yang D, Chou CJ, et al. Chronic inflammation in fat plays a crucial role in the development of obesity-related insulin resistance. *J Clin Invest* 2003;**112**(12):1821–30.

39. Ohto U, Fukase K, Miyake K, Satow Y. Crystal structures of human MD-2 and its complex with antiendotoxic lipid IVa. *Science* 2007;**316**(5831):1632–4.

40. Park BS, Song DH, Kim HM, Choi BS, Lee H, Lee JO. The structural basis of lipopolysaccharide recognition by the TLR4-MD-2 complex. *Nature* 2009;**458**(7242):1191–5.

41. Akashi S, Saitoh S, Wakabayashi Y, Kikuchi T, Takamura N, Nagai Y, et al. Lipopolysaccharide interaction with cell surface Toll-like receptor 4-MD-2: higher affinity than that with MD-2 or CD14. *J Exp Med* 2003;**198**(7):1035–42.

42. Suganami T, Mieda T, Itoh M, Shimoda Y, Kamei Y, Ogawa Y. Attenuation of obesity-induced adipose tissue inflammation in C3H/HeJ mice carrying a Toll-like receptor 4 mutation. *Biochem Biophys Res Commun* 2007;**354**(1):45–9.

43. Suganami T, Tanimoto-Koyama K, Nishida J, Itoh M, Yuan X, Mizuarai S, et al. Role of the Toll-like receptor 4/NF-κB pathway in saturated fatty acid-induced inflammatory changes in the interaction between adipocytes and macrophages. *Arterioscler Thromb Vasc Biol* 2007;**27**(1):84–91.

44. Wong SW, Kwon MJ, Choi AM, Kim HP, Nakahira K, Hwang DH. Fatty acids modulate Toll-like receptor 4 activation through regulation of receptor dimerization and recruitment into lipid rafts in a reactive oxygen species-dependent manner. *J Biol Chem* 2009;**284**(40):27384–92.

45. Stewart CR, Stuart LM, Wilkinson K, van Gils JM, Deng J, Halle A, et al. CD36 ligands promote sterile inflammation through assembly of a Toll-like receptor 4 and 6 heterodimer. *Nat Immunol* 2010;**11**(2):155–61.

46. De Strooper B, Vassar R, Golde T. The secretases: enzymes with therapeutic potential in Alzheimer's disease. *Nat Rev Neurol* 2010;**6**(2):99–107.

47. Chiquet-Ehrismann R, Mackie EJ, Pearson CA, Sakakura T. Tenascin: an extracellular matrix protein involved in tissue interactions during fetal development and oncogenesis. *Cell* 1986;**47**(1):131–9.

48. Goh FG, Piccinini AM, Krausgruber T, Udalova IA, Midwood KS. Transcriptional regulation of the endogenous danger signal tenascin-C: a novel autocrine loop in inflammation. *J Immunol* 2010;**184**(5):2655–62.

49. Midwood K, Sacre S, Piccinini AM, Inglis J, Trebaul A, Chan E, et al. Tenascin-C is an endogenous activator of Toll-like receptor 4 that is essential for maintaining inflammation in arthritic joint disease. *Nat Med* 2009;**15**(7):774–80.

50. Schaefer L, Babelova A, Kiss E, Hausser HJ, Baliova M, Krzyzankova M, et al. The matrix component biglycan is proinflammatory and signals through Toll-like receptors 4 and 2 in macrophages. *J Clin Invest* 2005;**115**(8):2223–33.

51. Babelova A, Moreth K, Tsalastra-Greul W, Zeng-Brouwers J, Eickelberg O, Young MF, et al. Biglycan, a danger signal that activates the NLRP3 inflammasome via toll-like and P2X receptors. *J Biol Chem* 2009;**284**(36):24035–48.

52. Gondokaryono SP, Ushio H, Niyonsaba F, Hara M, Takenaka H, Jayawardana ST, et al. The extra domain A of fibronectin stimulates murine mast cells via toll-like receptor 4. *J Leukoc Biol* 2007;**82**(3):657–65.

53. Ohashi K, Burkart V, Flohe S, Kolb H. Cutting edge: heat shock protein 60 is a putative endogenous ligand of the toll-like receptor-4 complex. *J Immunol* 2000;**164**(2):558–61.

54. Roelofs MF, Boelens WC, Joosten LA, Abdollahi-Roodsaz S, Geurts J, Wunderink LU, et al. Identification of small heat shock protein B8 (HSP22) as a novel TLR4 ligand and potential involvement in the pathogenesis of rheumatoid arthritis. *J Immunol* 2006;**176**(11):7021–7.

55. Vabulas RM, Wagner H, Schild H. Heat shock proteins as ligands of toll-like receptors. *Curr Top Microbiol Immunol* 2002;**270**:169–84.

56. Latz E, Schoenemeyer A, Visintin A, Fitzgerald KA, Monks BG, Knetter CF, et al. TLR9 signals after translocating from the ER to CpG DNA in the lysosome. *Nat Immunol* 2004;**5**(2):190–8.

57. Lee BL, Barton GM. Trafficking of endosomal Toll-like receptors. *Trends Cell Biol* 2014;**24**(6):360–9.

58. Lee CC, Avalos AM, Ploegh HL. Accessory molecules for Toll-like receptors and their function. *Nat Rev Immunol* 2012;**12**(3):168–79.

59. Tabeta K, Hoebe K, Janssen EM, Du X, Georgel P, Crozat K, et al. The Unc93b1 mutation 3d disrupts exogenous antigen presentation and signaling via Toll-like receptors 3, 7 and 9. *Nat Immunol* 2006;**7**(2):156–64.

60. Signorino G, Mohammadi N, Patane F, Buscetta M, Venza M, Venza I, et al. Role of Toll-like receptor 13 in innate immune recognition of group B *Streptococci*. *Infect Immun* 2014;**82**(12):5013–22.

61. Pifer R, Benson A, Sturge CR, Yarovinsky F. UNC93B1 is essential for TLR11 activation and IL-12-dependent host resistance to *Toxoplasma gondii*. *J Biol Chem* 2011;**286**(5):3307–14.

62. Itoh H, Tatematsu M, Watanabe A, Iwano K, Funami K, Seya T, et al. UNC93B1 physically associates with human TLR8 and regulates TLR8-mediated signaling. *PLoS One* 2011;**6**(12):e28500.

63. Levin JZ, Horvitz HR. The *Caenorhabditis elegans unc-93* gene encodes a putative transmembrane protein that regulates muscle contraction. *J Cell Biol* 1992;**117**(1):143–55.

64. Chu CC, Paul WE. Expressed genes in interleukin-4 treated B cells identified by cDNA representational difference analysis. *Mol Immunol* 1998;**35**(8):487–502.

65. Brinkmann MM, Spooner E, Hoebe K, Beutler B, Ploegh HL, Kim YM. The interaction between the ER membrane protein UNC93B and TLR3, 7, and 9 is crucial for TLR signaling. *J Cell Biol* 2007;**177**(2):265–75.

66. Kim YM, Brinkmann MM, Paquet ME, Ploegh HL. UNC93B1 delivers nucleotide-sensing toll-like receptors to endolysosomes. *Nature* 2008;**452**(7184):234-L238.

67. Fukui R, Saitoh S, Matsumoto F, Kozuka-Hata H, Oyama M, Tabeta K, et al. Unc93b1 biases Toll-like receptor responses to nucleic acid in dendritic cells toward DNA- but against RNA-sensing. *J Exp Med* 2009;**206**(6):1339–50.

68. Santiago-Raber ML, Dunand-Sauthier I, Wu T, Li QZ, Uematsu S, Akira S, et al. Critical role of TLR7 in the acceleration of systemic lupus erythematosus in TLR9-deficient mice. *J Autoimmun* 2010;**34**(4):339–48.

69. Desnues B, Macedo AB, Roussel-Queval A, Bonnardel J, Henri S, Demaria O, et al. TLR8 on dendritic cells and TLR9 on B cells restrain TLR7-mediated spontaneous autoimmunity in C57BL/6 mice. *Proc Natl Acad Sci USA* 2014;**111**(4):1497–502.

70. Huh JW, Shibata T, Hwang M, Kwon EH, Jang MS, Fukui R, et al. UNC93B1 is essential for the plasma membrane localization and signaling of Toll-like receptor 5. *Proc Natl Acad Sci USA* 2014;**111**(19):7072–7.

71. Pohar J, Pirher N, Bencina M, Mancek-Keber M, Jerala R. The role of UNC93B1 protein in surface localization of TLR3 receptor and in cell priming to nucleic acid agonists. *J Biol Chem* 2013;**288**(1):442–54.

72. Pohar J, Pirher N, Bencina M, Mancek-Keber M, Jerala R. The ectodomain of TLR3 receptor is required for its plasma membrane translocation. *PLoS One* 2014;**9**(3):e92391.

73. Kanno A, Tanimura N, Ishizaki M, Ohko K, Motoi Y, Onji M, et al. Targeting cell surface TLR7 for therapeutic intervention in autoimmune diseases. *Nat Commun* 2015;**6**:6119.

74. Onji M, Kanno A, Saitoh S, Fukui R, Motoi Y, Shibata T, et al. An essential role for the N-terminal fragment of Toll-like receptor 9 in DNA sensing. *Nat Commun* 2013;**4**:1949.

75. Uematsu S, Fujimoto K, Jang MH, Yang BG, Jung YJ, Nishiyama M, et al. Regulation of humoral and cellular gut immunity by lamina propria dendritic cells expressing Toll-like receptor 5. *Nat Immunol* 2008;**9**(7):769–76.

76. Uematsu S, Jang MH, Chevrier N, Guo Z, Kumagai Y, Yamamoto M, et al. Detection of pathogenic intestinal bacteria by Toll-like receptor 5 on intestinal CD11c+ lamina propria cells. *Nat Immunol* 2006;**7**(8):868–74.

77. Kiyokawa T, Akashi-Takamura S, Shibata T, Matsumoto F, Nishitani C, Kuroki Y, et al. A single base mutation in the PRAT4A gene reveals differential interaction of PRAT4A with Toll-like receptors. *Int Immunol* 2008;**20**(11):1407–15.

78. Shibata T, Takemura N, Motoi Y, Goto Y, Karuppuchamy T, Izawa K, et al. PRAT4A-dependent expression of cell surface TLR5 on neutrophils, classical monocytes and dendritic cells. *Int Immunol* 2012;**24**(10):613–23.

79. Takahashi K, Shibata T, Akashi-Takamura S, Kiyokawa T, Wakabayashi Y, Tanimura N, et al. A protein associated with Toll-receptor (TLR) 4 (PRAT4A) is required for TLR-dependent immune responses. *J Exp Med* 2007;**204**(12):2963–76.

80. Wakabayashi Y, Kobayashi M, Akashi-Takamura S, Tanimura N, Konno K, Takahashi K, et al. A protein associated with toll-like receptor 4 (PRAT4A) regulates cell surface expression of TLR4. *J Immunol* 2006;**177**(3):1772–9.

81. Kim J, Huh J, Hwang M, Kwon EH, Jung DJ, Brinkmann MM, et al. Acidic amino acid residues in the juxtamembrane region of the nucleotide-sensing TLRs are important for UNC93B1 binding and signaling. *J Immunol* 2013;**190**(10):5287–95.

82. Matsushima N, Tanaka T, Enkhbayar P, Mikami T, Taga M, Yamada K, et al. Comparative sequence analysis of leucine-rich repeats (LRRs) within vertebrate toll-like receptors. *BMC Genom* 2007;**8**:124.

83. Bell JK, Botos I, Hall PR, Askins J, Shiloach J, Segal DM, et al. The molecular structure of the Toll-like receptor 3 ligand-binding domain. *Proc Natl Acad Sci USA* 2005;**102**(31):10976–80.

84. Kawai T, Akira S. TLR signaling. *Cell Death Differ* 2006;**13**(5):816–25.

85. Takeda K, Akira S. TLR signaling pathways. *Semin Immunol* 2004;**16**(1):3–9.

86. Oshiumi H, Matsumoto M, Funami K, Akazawa T, Seya T. TICAM-1, an adaptor molecule that participates in Toll-like receptor 3-mediated interferon-β induction. *Nat Immunol* 2003;**4**(2):161–7.

87. Sato S, Sugiyama M, Yamamoto M, Watanabe Y, Kawai T, Takeda K, et al. Toll/IL-1 receptor domain-containing adaptor inducing IFN-β (TRIF) associates with TNF receptor-associated factor 6 and TANK-binding kinase 1, and activates two distinct transcription factors, NF-κ B and IFN-regulatory factor-3, in the Toll-like receptor signaling. *J Immunol* 2003;**171**(8):4304–10.

88. Yamamoto M, Sato S, Hemmi H, Hoshino K, Kaisho T, Sanjo H, et al. Role of adaptor TRIF in the MyD88-independent toll-like receptor signaling pathway. *Science* 2003;**301**(5633):640–3.
89. Yamamoto M, Sato S, Mori K, Hoshino K, Takeuchi O, Takeda K, et al. Cutting edge: a novel Toll/IL-1 receptor domain-containing adapter that preferentially activates the IFN-β promoter in the Toll-like receptor signaling. *J Immunol* 2002;**169**(12):6668–72.
90. Adachi O, Kawai T, Takeda K, Matsumoto M, Tsutsui H, Sakagami M, et al. Targeted disruption of the *MyD88* gene results in loss of IL-1- and IL-18-mediated function. *Immunity* 1998;**9**(1):143–50.
91. Kawai T, Adachi O, Ogawa T, Takeda K, Akira S. Unresponsiveness of *MyD88*-deficient mice to endotoxin. *Immunity* 1999;**11**(1):115–22.
92. Takeuchi O, Takeda K, Hoshino K, Adachi O, Ogawa T, Akira S. Cellular responses to bacterial cell wall components are mediated through MyD88-dependent signaling cascades. *Int Immunol* 2000;**12**(1):113–7.
93. Hemmi H, Kaisho T, Takeuchi O, Sato S, Sanjo H, Hoshino K, et al. Small anti-viral compounds activate immune cells via the TLR7 *MyD88*-dependent signaling pathway. *Nat Immunol* 2002;**3**(2):196–200.
94. Sato S, Takeuchi O, Fujita T, Tomizawa H, Takeda K, Akira S. A variety of microbial components induce tolerance to lipopolysaccharide by differentially affecting *MyD88*-dependent and -independent pathways. *Int Immunol* 2002;**14**(7):783–91.
95. Sato N, Takahashi N, Suda K, Nakamura M, Yamaki M, Ninomiya T, et al. MyD88 but not TRIF is essential for osteoclastogenesis induced by lipopolysaccharide, diacyl lipopeptide, and IL-1α. *J Exp Med* 2004;**200**(5):601–11.
96. Yamamoto M, Sato S, Hemmi H, Uematsu S, Hoshino K, Kaisho T, et al. TRAM is specifically involved in the Toll-like receptor 4-mediated *MyD88*-independent signaling pathway. *Nat Immunol* 2003;**4**(11):1144–50.
97. Oshiumi H, Sasai M, Shida K, Fujita T, Matsumoto M, Seya T. TIR-containing adapter molecule (TICAM)-2, a bridging adapter recruiting to toll-like receptor 4 TICAM-1 that induces interferon-β. *J Biol Chem* 2003;**278**(50):49751–62.
98. Lee BL, Moon JE, Shu JH, Yuan L, Newman ZR, Schekman R, et al. UNC93B1 mediates differential trafficking of endosomal TLRs. *Elife* 2013;**2**:e00291.
99. Asagiri M, Hirai T, Kunigami T, Kamano S, Gober HJ, Okamoto K, et al. Cathepsin K-dependent toll-like receptor 9 signaling revealed in experimental arthritis. *Science* 2008;**319**(5863):624–7.
100. Matsumoto F, Saitoh S, Fukui R, Kobayashi T, Tanimura N, Konno K, et al. Cathepsins are required for Toll-like receptor 9 responses. *Biochem Biophys Res Commun* 2008;**367**(3):693–9.
101. Ewald SE, Lee BL, Lau L, Wickliffe KE, Shi GP, Chapman HA, et al. The ectodomain of Toll-like receptor 9 is cleaved to generate a functional receptor. *Nature* 2008;**456**(7222):658–62.
102. Park B, Brinkmann MM, Spooner E, Lee CC, Kim YM, Ploegh HL. Proteolytic cleavage in an endolysosomal compartment is required for activation of Toll-like receptor 9. *Nat Immunol* 2008;**9**(12):1407–14.
103. Ewald SE, Engel A, Lee J, Wang M, Bogyo M, Barton GM. Nucleic acid recognition by Toll-like receptors is coupled to stepwise processing by cathepsins and asparagine endopeptidase. *J Exp Med* 2011;**208**(4):643–51.
104. Sepulveda FE, Maschalidi S, Colisson R, Heslop L, Ghirelli C, Sakka E, et al. Critical role for asparagine endopeptidase in endocytic Toll-like receptor signaling in dendritic cells. *Immunity* 2009;**31**(5):737–48.
105. Garcia-Cattaneo A, Gobert FX, Muller M, Toscano F, Flores M, Lescure A, et al. Cleavage of Toll-like receptor 3 by cathepsins B and H is essential for signaling. *Proc Natl Acad Sci USA* 2012;**109**(23):9053–8.

106. Toscano F, Estornes Y, Virard F, Garcia-Cattaneo A, Pierrot A, Vanbervliet B, et al. Cleaved/associated TLR3 represents the primary form of the signaling receptor. *J Immunol* 2013;**190**(2):764–73.

107. Murakami Y, Fukui R, Motoi Y, Kanno A, Shibata T, Tanimura N, et al. Roles of the cleaved N-terminal TLR3 fragment and cell surface TLR3 in double-stranded RNA sensing. *J Immunol* 2014;**193**(10):5208–17.

108. Kanno A, Yamamoto C, Onji M, Fukui R, Saitoh S, Motoi Y, et al. Essential role for Toll-like receptor 7 (TLR7)-unique cysteines in an intramolecular disulfide bond, proteolytic cleavage and RNA sensing. *Int Immunol* 2013;**25**(7):413–22.

109. Bauer S, Pigisch S, Hangel D, Kaufmann A, Hamm S. Recognition of nucleic acid and nucleic acid analogs by Toll-like receptors 7, 8 and 9. *Immunobiology* 2008;**213**(3-4):315–28.

110. Blasius AL, Beutler B. Intracellular toll-like receptors. *Immunity* 2010;**32**(3):305–15.

111. Nagata S. DNA degradation in development and programmed cell death. *Annu Rev Immunol* 2005;**23**:853–75.

112. Nagata S. Autoimmune diseases caused by defects in clearing dead cells and nuclei expelled from erythroid precursors. *Immunol Rev* 2007;**220**:237–50.

113. Nagata S, Kawane K. Autoinflammation by endogenous DNA. *Adv Immunol* 2011;**110**:139–61.

114. Napirei M, Karsunky H, Zevnik B, Stephan H, Mannherz HG, Moroy T. Features of systemic lupus erythematosus in *Dnase1*-deficient mice. *Nat Genet* 2000;**25**(2):177–81.

115. Yasutomo K, Horiuchi T, Kagami S, Tsukamoto H, Hashimura C, Urushihara M, et al. Mutation of DNASE1 in people with systemic lupus erythematosus. *Nat Genet* 2001;**28**(4):313–4.

116. Okabe Y, Kawane K, Akira S, Taniguchi T, Nagata S. Toll-like receptor-independent gene induction program activated by mammalian DNA escaped from apoptotic DNA degradation. *J Exp Med* 2005;**202**(10):1333–9.

117. Yoshida H, Okabe Y, Kawane K, Fukuyama H, Nagata S. Lethal anemia caused by interferon-beta produced in mouse embryos carrying undigested DNA. *Nat Immunol* 2005;**6**(1):49–56.

118. Yoshida H, Kawane K, Koike M, Mori Y, Uchiyama Y, Nagata S. Phosphatidylserine-dependent engulfment by macrophages of nuclei from erythroid precursor cells. *Nature* 2005;**437**(7059):754–8.

119. Miyanishi M, Tada K, Koike M, Uchiyama Y, Kitamura T, Nagata S. Identification of Tim4 as a phosphatidylserine receptor. *Nature* 2007;**450**(7168):435–9.

120. Chan MP, Onji M, Fukui R, Kawane K, Shibata T, Saitoh S, et al. DNase II-dependent DNA digestion is required for DNA sensing by TLR9. *Nat Commun* 2015;**6**:5853.

121. Hall JA, Bouladoux N, Sun CM, Wohlfert EA, Blank RB, Zhu Q, et al. Commensal DNA limits regulatory T cell conversion and is a natural adjuvant of intestinal immune responses. *Immunity* 2008;**29**(4):637–49.

122. Gibson SJ, Lindh JM, Riter TR, Gleason RM, Rogers LM, Fuller AE, et al. Plasmacytoid dendritic cells produce cytokines and mature in response to the TLR7 agonists, imiquimod and resiquimod. *Cell Immunol* 2002;**218**(1-2):74–86.

123. Jurk M, Heil F, Vollmer J, Schetter C, Krieg AM, Wagner H, et al. Human TLR7 or TLR8 independently confer responsiveness to the antiviral compound R-848. *Nat Immunol* 2002;**3**(6):499.

124. Lee J, Chuang TH, Redecke V, She L, Pitha PM, Carson DA, et al. Molecular basis for the immunostimulatory activity of guanine nucleoside analogs: activation of Toll-like receptor 7. *Proc Natl Acad Sci USA* 2003;**100**(11):6646–51.

125. Gorden KK, Qiu X, Battiste JJ, Wightman PP, Vasilakos JP, Alkan SS. Oligodeoxynucleotides differentially modulate activation of TLR7 and TLR8 by imidazoquinolines. *J Immunol* 2006;**177**(11):8164–70.

126. Gorden KK, Qiu XX, Binsfeld CC, Vasilakos JP, Alkan SS. Cutting edge: activation of murine TLR8 by a combination of imidazoquinoline immune response modifiers and polyT oligode-oxynucleotides. *J Immunol* 2006;**177**(10):6584–7.

127. Deane JA, Pisitkun P, Barrett RS, Feigenbaum L, Town T, Ward JM, et al. Control of toll-like receptor 7 expression is essential to restrict autoimmunity and dendritic cell proliferation. *Immunity* 2007;**27**(5):801–10.

128. Walsh ER, Pisitkun P, Voynova E, Deane JA, Scott BL, Caspi RR, et al. Dual signaling by innate and adaptive immune receptors is required for TLR7-induced B-cell-mediated autoim-munity. *Proc Natl Acad Sci USA* 2012;**109**(40):16276–81.

129. Sun X, Wiedeman A, Agrawal N, Teal TH, Tanaka L, Hudkins KL, et al. Increased ribo-nuclease expression reduces inflammation and prolongs survival in TLR7 transgenic mice. *J Immunol* 2013;**190**(6):2536–43.

130. Tanji H, Ohto U, Shibata T, Taoka M, Yamauchi Y, Isobe T, et al. Toll-like receptor 8 senses degradation products of single-stranded RNA. *Nat Struct Mol Biol* 2015;**22**(2):109–15.

131. Bekeredjian-Ding IB, Wagner M, Hornung V, Giese T, Schnurr M, Endres S, et al. Plasma-cytoid dendritic cells control TLR7 sensitivity of naive B cells via type I IFN. *J Immunol* 2005;**174**(7):4043–50.

132. Green NM, Laws A, Kiefer K, Busconi L, Kim YM, Brinkmann MM, et al. Murine B cell response to TLR7 ligands depends on an IFN-β feedback loop. *J Immunol* 2009;**183**(3):1569–76.

133. Green NM, Marshak-Rothstein A. Toll-like receptor driven B cell activation in the induction of systemic autoimmunity. *Semin Immunol* 2011;**23**(2):106–12.

134. Viglianti GA, Lau CM, Hanley TM, Miko BA, Shlomchik MJ, Marshak-Rothstein A. Activa-tion of autoreactive B cells by CpG dsDNA. *Immunity* 2003;**19**(6):837–47.

135. Miyake K, Nagai Y, Akashi S, Nagafuku M, Ogata M, Kosugi A. Essential role of MD-2 in B-cell responses to lipopolysaccharide and Toll-like receptor 4 distribution. *J Endotoxin Res* 2002;**8**(6):449–52.

136. Muramatsu M, Kinoshita K, Fagarasan S, Yamada S, Shinkai Y, Honjo T. Class switch recom-bination and hypermutation require activation-induced cytidine deaminase (AID), a potential RNA editing enzyme. *Cell* 2000;**102**(5):553–63.

137. Tsukamoto Y, Uehara S, Mizoguchi C, Sato A, Horikawa K, Takatsu K. Requirement of 8-mercaptoguanosine as a costimulus for IL-4-dependent mu to gamma1 class switch recom-bination in CD38-activated B cells. *Biochem Biophys Res Commun* 2005;**336**(2):625–33.

138. Tsukamoto Y, Nagai Y, Kariyone A, Shibata T, Kaisho T, Akira S, et al. Toll-like receptor 7 cooperates with IL-4 in activated B cells through antigen receptor or CD38 and induces class switch recombination and IgG1 production. *Mol Immunol* 2009;**46**(7):1278–88.

139. Miyake K, Shimazu R, Kondo J, Niki T, Akashi S, Ogata H, et al. Mouse MD-1, a molecule that is physically associated with RP105 and positively regulates its expression. *J Immunol* 1998;**161**(3):1348–53.

140. Miyake K, Yamashita Y, Ogata M, Sudo T, Kimoto M. RP105, a novel B cell surface molecule implicated in B cell activation, is a member of the leucine-rich repeat protein family. *J Im-munol* 1995;**154**(7):3333–40.

141. Nagai Y, Shimazu R, Ogata H, Akashi S, Sudo K, Yamasaki H, et al. Requirement for MD-1 in cell surface expression of RP105/CD180 and B-cell responsiveness to lipopolysaccharide. *Blood* 2002;**99**(5):1699–705.

142. Yamashita Y, Miyake K, Miura Y, Kaneko Y, Yagita H, Suda T, et al. Activation mediated by RP105 but not CD40 makes normal B cells susceptible to anti-IgM-induced apoptosis: a role for Fc receptor coligation. *J Exp Med* 1996;**184**(1):113–20.

143. Kimoto M, Nagasawa K, Miyake K. Role of TLR4/MD-2 and RP105/MD-1 in innate recognition of lipopolysaccharide. *Scand J Infect Dis* 2003;**35**(9):568–72.

144. Miura Y, Shimazu R, Miyake K, Akashi S, Ogata H, Yamashita Y, et al. RP105 is associated with MD-1 and transmits an activation signal in human B cells. *Blood* 1998;**92**(8):2815–22.

145. Nagai Y, Kobayashi T, Motoi Y, Ishiguro K, Akashi S, Saitoh S, et al. The radioprotective 105/MD-1 complex links TLR2 and TLR4/MD-2 in antibody response to microbial membranes. *J Immunol* 2005;**174**(11):7043–9.

146. Ogata H, Su I, Miyake K, Nagai Y, Akashi S, Mecklenbrauker I, et al. The toll-like receptor protein RP105 regulates lipopolysaccharide signaling in B cells. *J Exp Med* 2000;**192**(1):23–9.

147. Kobayashi T, Takahashi K, Nagai Y, Shibata T, Otani M, Izui S, et al. Tonic B cell activation by radioprotective105/MD-1 promotes disease progression in MRL/lpr mice. *Int Immunol* 2008;**20**(7):881–91.

148. Medzhitov R. Origin and physiological roles of inflammation. *Nature* 2008;**454**(7203):428–35.

149. Itoh M, Suganami T, Hachiya R, Ogawa Y. Adipose tissue remodeling as homeostatic inflammation. *Int J Inflam* 2011;**2011**:720926.

150. Hotamisligil GS. Inflammation and metabolic disorders. *Nature* 2006;**444**(7121):860–7.

151. Rocha VZ, Libby P. Obesity, inflammation, and atherosclerosis. *Nat Rev Cardiol* 2009;**6**(6):399–409.

152. Gavin AL, Hoebe K, Duong B, Ota T, Martin C, Beutler B, et al. Adjuvant-enhanced antibody responses in the absence of toll-like receptor signaling. *Science* 2006;**314**(5807):1936–8.

153. Barton GM, Medzhitov R. Control of adaptive immune responses by Toll-like receptors. *Curr Opin Immunol* 2002;**14**(3):380–3.

154. Iwasaki A, Medzhitov R. Toll-like receptor control of the adaptive immune responses. *Nat Immunol* 2004;**5**(10):987–95.

155. Edwards AD, Diebold SS, Slack EM, Tomizawa H, Hemmi H, Kaisho T, et al. Toll-like receptor expression in murine DC subsets: lack of TLR7 expression by CD8 alpha+ DC correlates with unresponsiveness to imidazoquinolines. *Eur J Immunol* 2003;**33**(4):827–33.

156. Zarember KA, Godowski PJ. Tissue expression of human Toll-like receptors and differential regulation of Toll-like receptor mRNAs in leukocytes in response to microbes, their products, and cytokines. *J Immunol* 2002;**168**(2):554–61.

157. Ito A, Suganami T, Yamauchi A, Degawa-Yamauchi M, Tanaka M, Kouyama R, et al. Role of CC chemokine receptor 2 in bone marrow cells in the recruitment of macrophages into obese adipose tissue. *J Biol Chem* 2008;**283**(51):35715–23.

158. Kamei N, Tobe K, Suzuki R, Ohsugi M, Watanabe T, Kubota N, et al. Overexpression of monocyte chemoattractant protein-1 in adipose tissues causes macrophage recruitment and insulin resistance. *J Biol Chem* 2006;**281**(36):26602–14.

159. Weisberg SP, Hunter D, Huber R, Lemieux J, Slaymaker S, Vaddi K, et al. CCR2 modulates inflammatory and metabolic effects of high-fat feeding. *J Clin Invest* 2006;**116**(1):115–24.

160. Ishikawa E, Ishikawa T, Morita YS, Toyonaga K, Yamada H, Takeuchi O, et al. Direct recognition of the mycobacterial glycolipid, trehalose dimycolate, by C-type lectin Mincle. *J Exp Med* 2009;**206**(13):2879–88.

161. Yamasaki S, Matsumoto M, Takeuchi O, Matsuzawa T, Ishikawa E, Sakuma M, et al. C-type lectin Mincle is an activating receptor for pathogenic fungus, *Malassezia. Proc Natl Acad Sci USA* 2009;**106**(6):1897–902.

162. Matsumoto M, Tanaka T, Kaisho T, Sanjo H, Copeland NG, Gilbert DJ, et al. A novel LPS-inducible C-type lectin is a transcriptional target of NF-IL6 in macrophages. *J Immunol* 1999;**163**(9):5039–48.

163. Yamasaki S, Ishikawa E, Sakuma M, Hara H, Ogata K, Saito T. Mincle is an ITAM-coupled activating receptor that senses damaged cells. *Nat Immunol* 2008;**9**(10):1179–88.

164. Ichioka M, Suganami T, Tsuda N, Shirakawa I, Hirata Y, Satoh-Asahara N, et al. Increased expression of macrophage-inducible C-type lectin in adipose tissue of obese mice and humans. *Diabetes* 2011;**60**(3):819–26.

165. Izui S, Iwamoto M, Fossati L, Merino R, Takahashi S, Ibnou-Zekri N. The Yaa gene model of systemic lupus erythematosus. *Immunol Rev* 1995;**144**:137–56.

166. Merino R, Iwamoto M, Gershwin ME, Izui S. The Yaa gene abrogates the major histocompatibility complex association of murine lupus in (NZB × BXSB)F1 hybrid mice. *J Clin Invest* 1994;**94**(2):521–5.

167. Izui S, Merino R, Fossati L, Iwamoto M. The role of the Yaa gene in lupus syndrome. *Int Rev Immunol* 1994;**11**(3):211–30.

168. Merino R, Iwamoto M, Fossati L, Muniesa P, Araki K, Takahashi S, et al. Prevention of systemic lupus erythematosus in autoimmune BXSB mice by a transgene encoding I-E alpha chain. *J Exp Med* 1993;**178**(4):1189–97.

169. Merino R, Fossati L, Lacour M, Lemoine R, Higaki M, Izui S. H-2-linked control of the Yaa gene-induced acceleration of lupus-like autoimmune disease in BXSB mice. *Eur J Immunol* 1992;**22**(2):295–9.

170. Merino R, Fossati L, Izui S. The lupus-prone BXSB strain: the Yaa gene model of systemic lupus erythematosus. *Springer Semin Immunopathol* 1992;**14**(2):141–57.

171. Merino R, Fossati L, Lacour M, Izui S. Selective autoantibody production by Yaa + B cells in autoimmune Yaa (+) -Yaa - bone marrow chimeric mice. *J Exp Med* 1991;**174**(5):1023–9.

172. Merino R, Shibata T, De Kossodo S, Izui S. Differential effect of the autoimmune Yaa and *lpr* genes on the acceleration of lupus-like syndrome in MRL/MpJ mice. *Eur J Immunol* 1989;**19**(11):2131–7.

173. Miyawaki S, Nakamura Y, Takeshita T, Yoshida H, Shibata Y, Mitsuoka S. Marked acceleration of the autoimmune disease in MRL-*lpr/lpr* mice by the influence of the Yaa gene from BXSB mice. *Lab Anim Sci* 1988;**38**(3):266–72.

174. Izui S, Higaki M, Morrow D, Merino R. The Y chromosome from autoimmune BXSB/MpJ mice induces a lupus-like syndrome in (NZW × C57BL/6)F1 male mice, but not in C57BL/6 male mice. *Eur J Immunol* 1988;**18**(6):911–5.

175. Gershwin ME, Shultz L. Mechanisms of genetically determined immune dysfunction. *Immunol Today* 1985;**6**(2):36–7.

176. Pisitkun P, Deane JA, Difilippantonio MJ, Tarasenko T, Satterthwaite AB, Bolland S. Autoreactive B cell responses to RNA-related antigens due to TLR7 gene duplication. *Science* 2006;**312**(5780):1669–72.

177. Santiago-Raber ML, Amano H, Amano E, Fossati-Jimack L, Swee LK, Rolink A, et al. Evidence that Yaa-induced loss of marginal zone B cells is a result of dendritic cell-mediated enhanced activation. *J Autoimmun* 2010;**34**(4):349–55.

178. Santiago-Raber ML, Kikuchi S, Borel P, Uematsu S, Akira S, Kotzin BL, et al. Evidence for genes in addition to Tlr7 in the Yaa translocation linked with acceleration of systemic lupus erythematosus. *J Immunol* 2008;**181**(2):1556–62.

179. Weeks CE, Gibson SJ. Induction of interferon and other cytokines by imiquimod and its hydroxylated metabolite R-842 in human blood cells *in vitro*. *J Interferon Res* 1994;**14**(2):81–5.

180. Reiter MJ, Testerman TL, Miller RL, Weeks CE, Tomai MA. Cytokine induction in mice by the immunomodulator imiquimod. *J Leukoc Biol* 1994;**55**(2):234–40.

181. Kono T, Kondo S, Pastore S, Shivji GM, Tomai MA, McKenzie RC, et al. Effects of a novel topical immunomodulator, imiquimod, on keratinocyte cytokine gene expression. *Lymphokine Cytokine Res* 1994;**13**(2):71–6.

182. Bernstein DI, Miller RL, Harrison CJ. Effects of therapy with an immunomodulator (imiquimod, R-837) alone and with acyclovir on genital HSV-2 infection in guinea-pigs when begun after lesion development. *Antiviral Res* 1993;**20**(1):45–55.

183. Bernstein DI, Miller RL, Harrison CJ. Adjuvant effects of imiquimod on a herpes simplex virus type 2 glycoprotein vaccine in guinea pigs. *J Infect Dis* 1993;**167**(3):731–5.

184. Beutner KR, Ferenczy A. Therapeutic approaches to genital warts. *Am J Med* 1997;**102**(5A):28–37.

185. van der Fits L, Mourits S, Voerman JS, Kant M, Boon L, Laman JD, et al. Imiquimod-induced psoriasis-like skin inflammation in mice is mediated via the IL-23/IL-17 axis. *J Immunol* 2009;**182**(9):5836–45.

186. Gilliet M, Conrad C, Geiges M, Cozzio A, Thurlimann W, Burg G, et al. Psoriasis triggered by toll-like receptor 7 agonist imiquimod in the presence of dermal plasmacytoid dendritic cell precursors. *Arch Dermatol* 2004;**140**(12):1490–5.

187. Ganguly D, Chamilos G, Lande R, Gregorio J, Meller S, Facchinetti V, et al. Self-RNA-antimicrobial peptide complexes activate human dendritic cells through TLR7 and TLR8. *J Exp Med* 2009;**206**(9):1983–94.

188. Gilliet M, Lande R. Antimicrobial peptides and self-DNA in autoimmune skin inflammation. *Curr Opin Immunol* 2008;**20**(4):401–7.

189. Lande R, Gregorio J, Facchinetti V, Chatterjee B, Wang YH, Homey B, et al. Plasmacytoid dendritic cells sense self-DNA coupled with antimicrobial peptide. *Nature* 2007;**449**(7162):564–9.

190. Yanai H, Ban T, Wang Z, Choi MK, Kawamura T, Negishi H, et al. HMGB proteins function as universal sentinels for nucleic-acid-mediated innate immune responses. *Nature* 2009;**462**(7269):99–103.

191. Tian J, Avalos AM, Mao SY, Chen B, Senthil K, Wu H, et al. Toll-like receptor 9-dependent activation by DNA-containing immune complexes is mediated by HMGB1 and RAGE. *Nat Immunol* 2007;**8**(5):487–96.

192. Marshak-Rothstein A, Busconi L, Lau CM, Tabor AS, Leadbetter EA, Akira S, et al. Comparison of CpG s-ODNs, chromatin immune complexes, and dsDNA fragment immune complexes in the TLR9-dependent activation of rheumatoid factor B cells. *J Endotoxin Res* 2004;**10**(4):247–51.

193. Avalos AM, Busconi L, Marshak-Rothstein A. Regulation of autoreactive B cell responses to endogenous TLR ligands. *Autoimmunity* 2010;**43**(1):76–83.

194. Kruse K, Janko C, Urbonaviciute V, Mierke CT, Winkler TH, Voll RE, et al. Inefficient clearance of dying cells in patients with SLE: anti-dsDNA autoantibodies, MFG-E8, HMGB-1 and other players. *Apoptosis* 2010;**15**(9):1098–113.

195. Adachi M, Watanabe-Fukunaga R, Nagata S. Aberrant transcription caused by the insertion of an early transposable element in an intron of the *Fas* antigen gene of *lpr* mice. *Proc Natl Acad Sci USA* 1993;**90**(5):1756–60.

196. Sobel ES, Katagiri T, Katagiri K, Morris SC, Cohen PL, Eisenberg RA. An intrinsic B cell defect is required for the production of autoantibodies in the *lpr* model of murine systemic autoimmunity. *J Exp Med* 1991;**173**(6):1441–9.

197. Davignon JL, Arnold LW, Cohen PL, Eisenberg RA. CD3 expression, modulation and signalling in T-cell subpopulations from MRL/Mp-*lpr/lpr* mice. *J Autoimmun* 1991;**4**(6):831–44.

198. Cohen PL, Eisenberg RA. *Lpr* and *gld*: single gene models of systemic autoimmunity and lymphoproliferative disease. *Annu Rev Immunol* 1991;**9**:243–69.

199. Christensen SR, Kashgarian M, Alexopoulou L, Flavell RA, Akira S, Shlomchik MJ. Toll-like receptor 9 controls anti-DNA autoantibody production in murine lupus. *J Exp Med* 2005;**202**(2):321–31.

200. Christensen SR, Shupe J, Nickerson K, Kashgarian M, Flavell RA, Shlomchik MJ. Toll-like receptor 7 and TLR9 dictate autoantibody specificity and have opposing inflammatory and regulatory roles in a murine model of lupus. *Immunity* 2006;**25**(3):417–28.

201. Nickerson KM, Christensen SR, Shupe J, Kashgarian M, Kim D, Elkon K, et al. TLR9 regulates TLR7- and MyD88-dependent autoantibody production and disease in a murine model of lupus. *J Immunol* 2010;**184**(4):1840–8.

202. Fukui R, Saitoh S, Kanno A, Onji M, Shibata T, Ito A, et al. Unc93B1 restricts systemic lethal inflammation by orchestrating Toll-like receptor 7 and 9 trafficking. *Immunity* 2011;**35**(1):69–81.

203. Demaria O, Pagni PP, Traub S, de Gassart A, Branzk N, Murphy AJ, et al. TLR8 deficiency leads to autoimmunity in mice. *J Clin Invest* 2010;**120**(10):3651–62.

204. Kanzler H, Barrat FJ, Hessel EM, Coffman RL. Therapeutic targeting of innate immunity with Toll-like receptor agonists and antagonists. *Nat Med* 2007;**13**(5):552–9.

205. Li J, Wang X, Zhang F, Yin H. Toll-like receptors as therapeutic targets for autoimmune connective tissue diseases. *Pharmacol Ther* 2013;**138**(3):441–51.

206. Shukla NM, Malladi SS, Day V, David SA. Preliminary evaluation of a 3H imidazoquinoline library as dual TLR7/TLR8 antagonists. *Bioorg Med Chem* 2011;**19**(12):3801–11.

207. Shukla NM, Mutz CA, Malladi SS, Warshakoon HJ, Balakrishna R, David SA. Toll-like receptor (TLR)-7 and -8 modulatory activities of dimeric imidazoquinolines. *J Med Chem* 2012;**55**(3):1106–16.

208. Barrat FJ, Meeker T, Chan JH, Guiducci C, Coffman RL. Treatment of lupus-prone mice with a dual inhibitor of TLR7 and TLR9 leads to reduction of autoantibody production and amelioration of disease symptoms. *Eur J Immunol* 2007;**37**(12):3582–6.

209. Pawar RD, Ramanjaneyulu A, Kulkarni OP, Lech M, Segerer S, Anders HJ. Inhibition of Toll-like receptor-7 (TLR-7) or TLR-7 plus TLR-9 attenuates glomerulonephritis and lung injury in experimental lupus. *J Am Soc Nephrol* 2007;**18**(6):1721–31.

210. Martin HJ, Lee JM, Walls D, Hayward SD. Manipulation of the toll-like receptor 7 signaling pathway by Epstein–Barr virus. *J Virol* 2007;**81**(18):9748–58.

211. Roh YS, Park S, Kim JW, Lim CW, Seki E, Kim B. Toll-like receptor 7-mediated type I interferon signaling prevents cholestasis- and hepatotoxin-induced liver fibrosis. *Hepatology* 2014;**60**(1):237–49.

212. Feschotte C, Gilbert C. Endogenous viruses: insights into viral evolution and impact on host biology. *Nat Rev Genet* 2012;**13**(4):283–96.

213. Yu P, Lubben W, Slomka H, Gebler J, Konert M, Cai C, et al. Nucleic acid-sensing Toll-like receptors are essential for the control of endogenous retrovirus viremia and ERV-induced tumors. *Immunity* 2012;**37**(5):867–79.

214. Furusawa Y, Obata Y, Fukuda S, Endo TA, Nakato G, Takahashi D, et al. Commensal microbe-derived butyrate induces the differentiation of colonic regulatory T cells. *Nature* 2013;**504**(7480):446–50.

215. Jeon SG, Kayama H, Ueda Y, Takahashi T, Asahara T, Tsuji H, et al. Probiotic *Bifidobacterium breve* induces IL-10-producing Tr1 cells in the colon. *PLoS Pathog* 2012;**8**(5):e1002714.

216. Mazmanian SK, Round JL, Kasper DL. A microbial symbiosis factor prevents intestinal inflammatory disease. *Nature* 2008;**453**(7195):620–5.

217. Shida K, Nanno M. Probiotics and immunology: separating the wheat from the chaff. *Trends Immunol* 2008;**29**(11):565–73.

218. Kawashima T, Kosaka A, Yan H, Guo Z, Uchiyama R, Fukui R, et al. Double-stranded RNA of intestinal commensal but not pathogenic bacteria triggers production of protective interferon-β. *Immunity* 2013;**38**(6):1187–97.

219. Takemura N, Kawasaki T, Kunisawa J, Sato S, Lamichhane A, Kobiyama K, et al. Blockade of TLR3 protects mice from lethal radiation-induced gastrointestinal syndrome. *Nat Commun* 2014;**5**:3492.

Chapter 3

The Molecular Basis of the Immune Response to Stressed Cells and Tissues

Segundo González,* Carlos López-Larrea,** Alejandro López-Soto*,**
*Departamento de Inmunología, Hospital Universitario Central de Asturias, Oviedo, Asturias, Spain; **Departamento de Biología Funcional, Inmunología, Universidad de Oviedo, Instituto Universitario de Oncología del Principado de Asturias, Asturias, Spain

Cells and tissues are constantly exposed to harmful conditions, which are potential sources of malignancies and illnesses, when the damage is not detected and repaired in time. Given the relevance of the action of such environmental and endogenous stressors for the viability of any biological system, a plethora of mechanisms devoted to reverting the damage are needed to maintain the physiological parameters within a controlled range, which is commonly defined as homeostasis. Thus, different forms of stresses specifically activate a number of proteins, which are highly conserved in all organisms in an attempt to revert their potential effects in the stressed cell. Under danger conditions, these sensors regulate key cellular functions, including cell cycle, DNA and protein stability, or trigger cell clearance processes by activating apoptosis when the damage cannot be repaired.[1] Significantly, in addition to these intrinsic mechanisms, cell stress also results in the activation of the a host's immune response, leading to the recognition and elimination of stressed cells to prevent any further cellular or systemic complication. This means, a potential consequence of disturbing cellular or tissue homeostasis can be the increment of the immunogenicity of the cell, at least in part, through the expression of stress-regulated molecules, which are ligands for activating immune receptors. The fact that immune response of the host is a cell-extrinsic mechanism that collaborates with those activated inside the damaged cell to cope with harmful conditions, is crucial to preserve the homeostasis, mainly when such intrinsic responses are somehow impaired. Given this relevance, in this chapter we will summarize the key molecular mechanisms underpinning the innate immune surveillance associated with cellular response to stress, with a focus on how the expression and biogenesis of immune-relevant molecules are regulated by stress and disease. The immune responses to different types of stresses will be detailed, as well.

INNATE IMMUNE RESPONSES: RECEPTORS AND LIGANDS

The first line of the host's defense is constituted by innate immunity, which basically includes natural killer (NK) cells, macrophages, and dendritic cells (DCs). Innate immune cells are responsible for early immune responses to pathogens and environmental stressors, which typically lead to inflammatory conditions in order to control and eradicate infection or cellular damage.[2] In this sense, a growing body of evidence demonstrates a key role for NK cell-mediated surveillance in the immune response to diverse stressors. Unlike T lymphocytes of adaptive immunity, cells of the innate immune system have been typically considered to be nonspecific. For instance, NK cells, which are lymphocytes of the innate immunity, do not express antigen-specific receptors. Instead, they respond rapidly to damaged or infected cells by monitoring the surface of the target cell for the expression of molecules, which are ligands for NK cell-activating and inhibitory receptors.[3] Thus, inhibitory receptors, such as the killer cell immunoglobulin (Ig)-like receptors (KIRs) and the leukocyte Ig-like receptors (LIRs), bind MHC class I molecules, which are abundantly present on the membrane of healthy cells. So, the absence of such self-proteins, which are commonly observed during infectious or tumorigenic processes, lift NK-cell inhibition imposed by these receptors, that is a recognition strategy known as "missing-self."[4] Additionally, NK cells are strongly activated when germline encoded activating receptors are engaged by molecules whose expression gets dramatically increased in stressed or damaged cells, which is known as the "induced-self" recognition. Examples of NK cell-activating receptors are DNAX accessory molecule-1 (DNAM-1), also known as CD226, natural cytotoxicity receptors (NCRs, including NKp30, NKp44, and NKp46), and NK group 2, member D (NKG2D),[5] which has been described further. Overall, the activity against a target cell strictly depends on the final balance between inhibitory and stimulatory signals, that such NK cells receive and integrate through these receptors (Fig. 3.1). Hence, an activated NK cell responds by releasing preformed lytic granules containing granzymes and perforin, thus inducing the apoptotic death of the target cell.[6,7] Likewise, NK cells are known to interact with DCs and macrophages, which influence subsequent immune responses. Thus, NK cell activation also leads to the production of immunomodulatory molecules, such as interferon-γ (IFN-γ), tumor necrosis factor-α (TNF-α), and other proinflammatory molecules, which are able to regulate innate and adaptive immunity.

STRESS-MEDIATED REGULATION OF IMMUNE RECEPTORS AND LIGANDS: AN OVERVIEW

As stated earlier, a link between cellular or tissue stress and regulation of immune responses to deal with the damage can be established, given that a vast majority of ligands for NK-cell activating receptors are stress-regulated molecules. Consequently, knowledge of the precise molecular and cellular mechanisms

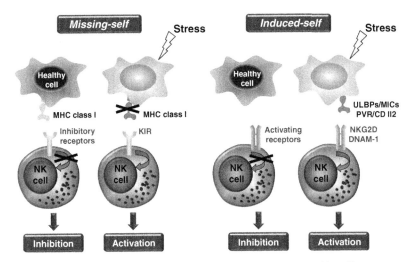

FIGURE 3.1 Recognition strategies that regulate NK-Cell activity. Healthy cells are protected from getting eliminated by autologous NK cells by expressing high surface levels of MHC class I molecules, which bind KIR inhibitory receptors on NK cells, resulting in inhibition of cytotoxic responses of the latter. Cells undergoing stress, such as transformed and infected cells, express much lower levels of MHC class I molecules ("missing-self recognition"), thereby impairing KIR-dependent inhibition and, eventually triggering the NK-mediated elimination of damaged cells. Additionally, NK cell activity is regulated by activating receptors (e.g., NKG2D and DNAM-1), whose ligands (MICs/ULBPs and PVR/CD112, respectively) are self-molecules upregulated under a plethora of cellular stresses, such as those typically associated with tumorigenesis and infection, thus allowing the recognition and elimination of diseased cells by CD8$^+$ T lymphocytes and, chiefly NK cells ("induced-self recognition").

by which an injurious condition modulates the expression of such receptors and ligands, is crucial to understand the immune surveillance of stressed and damaged cells.

NKG2D is a C-type lectin-like activating receptor with a prominent role in the immune response to stress and disease. It is expressed on the surface of all human NK and NKT cells and in cells of adaptive immunity, including CD8$^+$ T cells, γδ T cells, and in certain subsets of CD4$^+$ T cells.[8] In order to be expressed on the cell surface, NKG2D needs to interact with adaptor proteins (DNAX-activating protein of 10 kDa, DAP10, in humans, and DAP10 or DAP12 in mice), which are also required for a proper signaling through the NKG2D receptor[9,10] (Fig. 3.2). An immunoreceptor tyrosine-based activation motif (ITAM) is present on DAP12, which upon NKG2D engagement is phosphorylated by Src family kinases, leading to the recruitment and the activation of tyrosine kinase ζ-chain associated protein of 70 kDa (Zap70) in NK cells, or of spleen tyrosine kinase (Syk) in myeloid cells.[9,11] Conversely, no ITAM domain is found on DAP10 adaptor protein, so that its signaling pathway differs from that of DAP12. Thus, after tyrosine phosphorylation, DAP10 recruits

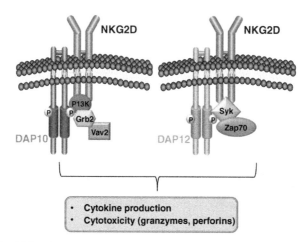

FIGURE 3.2 **Molecular signaling through NKG2D receptor.** NKG2D-activating receptor binds to adaptor molecules for its correct assembly on the cell surface and for a proper signaling transduction upon receptor engagement, the latter leading to cytokine secretion and release of cytotoxic granules with granzymes and perforin. In humans, NKG2D binds to DAP10 adaptor protein resulting in activation of the p85 subunit of PI3K and also the Grb2–Vav1 complex. In mouse, a short isoform of NKG2D is expressed in activated NK cells, which also interacts with DAP12, an adaptor protein that signals through Zap70 and Syk.

phosphatidylinositol-3 kinase (PI3K) and a Grb2-Vav1 complex, which are required for full cell activation.[12,13]

In humans, two families of NKG2D ligands have been described: (1) the MHC class I-related molecules A and B (MICA and MICB) and (2) the family of UL16-binding proteins (ULBP1-6).[14,15] Although these molecules are mainly absent or scarcely expressed in healthy tissues and cells, their expression is substantially induced on the surface of infected and transformed cells.[16] It is noteworthy that NKG2D ligands are highly polymorphic, while they are exclusively recognized by a single receptor. Such variability has been hypothesized to reflect a strategy to circumvent potential mechanisms of immune evasion, thus warranting that infected or diseased cells are detected and eliminated by the immune system.[17,18]

DNAM-1 (CD226) is a member of the Ig superfamily of receptors constitutively expressed on the majority of NK cells, T cells, platelets, and monocytes.[19] The DNAM-1 receptor is involved in leukocyte adhesion and also stimulates NK cell activity by interacting with its ligands, poliovirus receptor (PVR, also known as CD155), and Nectin-2 (CD112), which are both modulated by stress and pathological conditions.[20] Significantly, DNAM-1 ligands are also bound by T cell immunoreceptor with Ig, ITIM domains (TIGIT), and CD96 inhibitory receptors, limiting NK cell functions and counteracting DNAM-1-mediated activation.[21-23] Likewise, the NKp30 receptor triggers immune responses by recognizing the expression of natural cytotoxicity triggering receptor 3

(NCR3 or B7-H6) and HLA-B-associated transcript 3 (BAT3) on the target, mainly transformed cells.[24]

The exacerbated presence of these ligands of activating receptors as danger molecules allows specific immune recognition and elimination of damaged and cancerous cells, which are thus discriminated from healthy cells.[25] In this sense, experimental findings and clinical observations strongly support a key role for NK-cell activating receptors in the immune response during different pathologies, including cancer. As an example, NK cell infiltration was associated with a favorable outcome in colorectal cancer patients.[26] A relevant piece of information demonstrating the surveillance of primary tumors by an NK cell receptor, was obtained upon the generation of mice deficient in *Klrk1* gene, which encodes for murine NKG2D. These mice were found to be more susceptible to cancer development in two models of spontaneous tumorigenesis, albeit signaling through other NK cell activating receptors was not affected.[27] Furthermore, DNAM-1-deficient mice showed increased tumor growth and mortality in chemical models of carcinogenesis, and upon inoculation of a methylcholanthrene-induced fibrosarcoma cell line.[28,29] Moreover, the absence of NKp46 in mice resulted in an impaired cell line-specific rejection of lymphomas, and led to an enhanced formation of tumor metastases established by two different cancer cell models.[30,31]

A myriad of forms of stress and harmful conditions affecting cells and tissues have been reported to regulate immunity by upregulating the expression of ligands for activating immune receptors. Such interplay between stress and immunity is perhaps highlighted by the fact that this regulation occurs at multiple levels of biogenesis of NKG2D and DNAM-1 ligands.

Transcriptional Regulation of NK-Cell Activating Ligands Modulated by Stress Responses

MICA and *MICB* were initially identified as genes induced by heat shock conditions upon binding of heat shock factor 1 (HSF1) transcription factor to consensus DNA binding elements present on the promoters of these ligands.[32,33] Accordingly, pharmacological and small interfering RNA (siRNA)-mediated inhibition of HSF1 completely blocked MICA and MICB surface expression, and NK-dependent cytotoxicity.

Additionally, the transcription of several human NKG2D ligands (*MICA, MICB,* and *ULBP1*) were found to be regulated by Sp1/Sp3 factors in cancer, which are stress-inducible transcription factors that recognize GC boxes in the regulatory regions of their target genes.[33–36] The importance of Sp1-transcription factors is also evidenced by the dependence of NKG2D ligand regulation during transdifferentiation processes such as epithelial-to-mesenchymal transition (EMT). In this regard, it has been reported that tumor cells undergoing an EMT, which are typically associated with malignant progression and metastasis, display higher levels of NKG2D ligands, thereby enhancing the recognition and elimination of these cells by NK cells. Of note, such upregulation was found to be strictly dependent on the transcriptional activity of Sp1, as evidenced by the use of specific inhibitors and siRNA-mediated depletion of the endogenous level of this transcription factor.[37,38]

AP-1 is another example of a transcriptional regulator that is induced by environmental stresses, such as short wavelength UV radiation, with a role in modulating immunity.[39] In this regard, it was shown that AP-1 stimulates the promoter activity and protein expression of DAP10, an adaptor molecule that, as we stated earlier, is required for NKG2D membrane expression and signaling.[40] Moreover, the AP-1 subunit JunB regulates the expression of a mouse ligand of NKG2D (RAE-1ε) and NK-cell cytotoxic functions.[41]

Epigenetic modifications provide a possible link between environmental extrinsic stimuli and alterations in gene expression.[42] These alterations – mainly chromatin modifications (histone acetylation and methylation) and DNA methylation are key regulators of the expression of a vast number of genes.[43] NKG2D ligands are dramatically induced in cell lines derived from different types of cancer, upon exposure to histone deacetylase (HDAC) inhibitors. For instance, valproic acid increases NKG2D ligand expression in acute myeloid leukemia (AML) patient samples, hepatoma, osteosarcoma, and bladder cancer cell lines.[44–46] Accordingly, HDAC3 represses ULBP expression in epithelial cancer cell lines by getting recruited into their promoter regions by Sp3 transcription factor, resulting in histone deacetylation in the vicinity of ULBP promoters, and leading to the inhibition of NK cell-mediated cytotoxic functions.[47] Conversely, a study shows that B7-H6 expression correlates with HDAC3 in samples of follicular lymphoma and hepatocellular cancer, and that HDAC inhibition reduced NKp30-dependent degranulation of NK cells.[48] DNA promoter hypermethylation also reduces the expression of several NKG2D ligands in cancer. Thus, MICB expression was increased upon treatment with DNA methyltransferase inhibitors in hepatoma cells.[49] Analysis of bisulfite genomic sequencing revealed that, *ULBP2* promoter was aberrantly methylated in a colorectal tumor cell line.[50] However, a recent study did not find hypermethylation of NKG2D ligand promoter regions in a cohort of 44 colorectal cancer patients, although *MICA*, *ULBP1*, and *ULBP2* gene methylation was reported in AML patients.[51] Altogether, these studies support that epigenetic mechanisms are a crucial trait of tumors to impair and evade anticancer immune responses mediated by NKG2D receptors.

Posttranscriptional Regulation of Stress-Controlled NK-Cell Activating Ligands

A striking feature of NKG2D ligand biogenesis is that, many cells and tissues display a marked mRNA expression of these molecules, whereas little or absent protein expression can be frequently detected, which suggests the existence of posttranscriptional mechanisms of regulation.[32] Significantly, this observation has been linked to the existence of a preformed cellular pool of NKG2D ligand transcripts, which under stress ensures a rapid protein translation and immune activation.[52] MicroRNAs (miRNAs) are small noncoding RNAs that mediate specific regulation of gene expression.[53] Notably, miRNAs play a pivotal role in mediating stress responses, being the biogenesis of miRNAs itself modulated by such stress stimuli.[54] Consequently, NKG2D ligand expression has been shown to be controlled by a number of miRNAs. In healthy cells, *MICA* and *MICB* mRNA levels were found to be maintained under a certain threshold by a group of endogenous cellular miRNAs (miR-20a, miR-93, miR-106b; and miR-10b in the case of *MICB*). Upon short-term stresses such as heat shock, the upregulation of MICA/B transcription was suggested to overcome the repressive effects of these miRNAs, leading to increased protein expression and immune responses.[55,56] These observations are supported by recent findings revealing that several NKG2D ligands are downregulated in glioma cells by the activity of miR-20a, miR-93, and miR-106b, which contribute to the impaired immunogenicity of this tumor.[57] Furthermore, a report shows that tumor suppressive miRNAs regulated by p53 (miR-34a and miR-34c) target the 3'-untraslated region of the *ULBP2* gene, reducing its expression.[58] NKG2D signaling may be also affected by miR-145, which attenuates NKG2D receptor expression in NK cells, representing an additional mechanism of subversion of antitumor immune surveillance in cancer.[59]

Translational and Posttranslational Regulation of Stress-Modulated NK-Cell Activating Ligands

It has been shown that overexpression of oncogene H-RASV12 modestly increased the transcription of the *Rae1* family of mouse NKG2D ligands, although a strong induction of RAE-1 protein levels was detected. Further experiments unveiled that such increments in protein expression were mediated, at least in part, by enhanced translation initiation involving the factor eIF4E.[60] This factor is crucial in the regulation of immune responses via translational control.[61] For instance, Toll-like receptor (TLR) engagement stimulates eIF4E-mediated protein translation of interferon regulatory factor 7 (IRF7), a master regulator of IFN immune responses, which has been linked to innate immunity to cellular stress.[62,63] Contrarily, diverse physiological stresses inhibit translational initiation by reducing the cellular availability and function of eIF4E, suggesting that this mode of regulation of immune-related molecules is not likely to be a universal mechanism under stress conditions.[64]

Several mechanisms that regulate protein stability and turnover of relevant components of innate immune responses to stress have been reported. In healthy cells, transcripts of the mouse NKG2D ligand MULT1 are frequently detected, which is not accompanied by the expected protein levels on the cell surface. Such a discrepancy is due to the fact that, under normal conditions, MULT1 is polyubiquitinated by a MARCH family of transmembrane E3 ubiquitin ligases and, consequently, it is degraded. However, under stress conditions, such as UV-irradiation and heat shock, the association between MULT1 and the MARCH ligase is reverted, leading to a lower level of ubiquitination. This prevents MULT1 degradation and results in enhanced NK-cell activity against the stressed cell.[65,66] Additionally, human cancer cell lines were reported to be more susceptible to NK-mediated cytotoxicity due to the upregulation of NKG2D and DNAM-1 ligand expression by treatment with proteasome inhibitors bortezomib and MG132.[67,68]

The proteolytic shedding of stress-regulated ligands of NK-cell activating receptors is a major immunomodulatory mechanism frequently observed in different pathologies. Indeed, soluble forms of multiple NKG2D ligands have been reported in a variety of tumor types as well as in diseases such as renal insufficiency.[69,70] Also, a recent report shows that increased levels of soluble NKp30 ligand B7-H6 are detected in sera of malignant melanoma patients compared with healthy individuals.[71] Such soluble cell-free NKG2D ligands strongly impair immune activity, as their binding leads to the endocytosis and subsequent degradation of NKG2D receptor, and they also compete with cell-bound ligands for the engagement of NKG2D.[72] In fact, the presence of soluble NKG2D ligands in the sera of patients, is a prognostic indicator in a number of cancer types, including melanoma, lung and pancreatic cancers, and chronic lymphocytic leukemia.[73–76] In sharp contrast, it has recently been shown that soluble MULT1 accumulated in the blood sera of patients with tumors and inflammatory diseases, can promote NK-cell activation, rather than inhibition of immune activity against stressed cells.[77] Compelling pieces of evidence demonstrate that members of the matrix metalloproteinase (MMP) and, chiefly, of the "A disintegrin and metalloproteinase domain" families of proteases are crucially involved in the molecular mechanisms underpinning the shedding of NKG2D and NKp30 ligands. Thus, MMP-9 and MMP-14 mediate MICA and MICB ectodomain cleavage in osteosarcoma cells, and ADAM10 and ADAM17 were reported to shed MICA/B and B7-H6 in tumors ranging from pancreatic cancer to malignant melanoma.[71,78] Notably, MICA was shown to interact with the disulfide isomerase endoplasmic reticulum (ER) protein 5 (ERp5) on the cell surface, which leads to the reduction of a disulfide bond located in the $\alpha 3$ domain of MICA, a process that seems to be required for the proteolytic cleavage of the ligand.[79] ERp5 (also known as protein disulfide isomerase A6, PDIA6) as well as many proteases are under the regulation of stress-dependent molecular pathways, suggesting that harmful conditions are likely to stimulate the proteolytic shedding of these immune-relevant molecules.

Exosomes are endosomal-derived vesicles secreted by many immune cell types, including macrophages, DCs, platelets, and B and T cells. Likewise, stressed cells also release exosomes bearing intercellular mediators in the form of proteins, miRNAs, or mRNAs. Many studies support a key role for endosomes in modulating immune activity under both physiological and disease conditions.[80] Thus, it was found that DCs released exosomes expressing

MHC class I and class II proteins and T cell costimulatory molecules with immunomodulatory activity, which supported the use of exosomes as vaccines to transfer antigens during infections and cancer.[81] Moreover, exosome vesicles from antigen-presenting cells (APCs) bearing B7 and intercellular adhesion molecule-1 (ICAM-1) were able to stimulate naïve T cells even in the absence of APCs, challenging the idea that the immune synapse between the T cell and the APC is mandatory for immune activation.[82] NKG2D and NKp30 ligands can also be incorporated into exosomes and transferred to CD8⁺ T and NK cells, where they downregulate NKG2D receptor expression and immune activity.[83,84] Remarkably, it was suggested that alterations in the composition and secretion of exosomes mediate the cellular response to environmental stress. Hence, exposure of B cells to heat stress conditions increased the presence of heat shock proteins (HSPs) and the release of exosomes, without affecting MHC expression.[85] Furthermore, thermal and oxidative stress were found to increase tumor-derived exosomes bearing NKG2D ligands, as a mechanism evolved by cancer cells to impair immune responses.[86]

DIFFERENT FORMS OF STRESS REGULATE INNATE IMMUNITY

A thorough knowledge of the immune responses triggered by different kinds of stresses is imperative for the complete understanding of the relationship between stress and immunity. Therefore, we will now detail how specific forms of environmental and internal stress modulate the expression and activity of pivotal mediators of innate immune responses to threatening conditions.

Osmotic Stress

Eukaryotic cells and tissues are exposed to physiologic fluids containing variable concentrations of a set of electrolytes. Changes in the composition of such fluids strongly influence the structure of cytoplasmic membrane and cellular viability. Therefore, cells under osmotic pressure need to trigger rapid responses to adapt to the harmful environment in order to protect themselves from unrepairable damage. For instance, cells of the renal medulla are endowed with a higher osmotic tolerance, because they are exposed to concentrations of NaCl and urea higher than those found in other interstitial fluids, a consequence of the physiological function of that area. Such hypertonic conditions can be lethal for the cell, as they are able to activate apoptotic programs. However, kidney medullar cells are adapted to hypertonic environments by accumulating organic osmolytes, such as sorbitol, taurine, free aminoacids, or glycerophosphocholine (GPC), which restores intracellular homeostatic conditions.[87] In addition to the mechanisms that involve transport of solutes across the cell membrane, a regulation of the immune system occurs under abnormal osmotic pressure to cope with this stress. Secretion of proinflammatory cytokines (including IL-1α, IL-1β, IL-6, and IL-8) and immune functions are stimulated in peripheral blood mononuclear cells and human leukocytes exposed to hypertonic conditions.[88–90] Of relevance, hypertonic solutions have been used as fluids to help critically injured patients to recover, which causes excessive inflammatory conditions. This results in organ injury and requires later treatment with immunosuppressants.[91,92] Also, an increased level of proinflammatory mediators and T cell response is detected in patients with chronic renal failure after dialysis with hypertonic solutions.[93] Moreover, a linkage between modulation of immune responses and several diseases involving local osmotic pressure can be established, the latter including diabetes mellitus, inflammatory bowel disease, and hypernatremia.[94] A relevant study shows that a decrease in extracellular osmotic pressure activates caspase 1 (CASP1) expression in macrophages. This CASP, also known as the IL-1β converting enzyme, is involved in the cleavage of pro-IL-1β and the production of the mature form of the cytokine, which is required for its secretion and extracellular activities.[95] Accordingly, such a response was found to be dependent on NLRP3 inflammasome activation, which thus functions as a sensor of changes in the cellular volume, as a molecular strategy to recover normality under altered osmotic pressure conditions. The authors also found that macrophages from mice deficient in NLRP3 did not activate CASP1 expression or IL-1β processing, which led to the hypothesis that this mechanism was evolutionarily conserved from fish to mammals.[96] Furthermore, several studies illustrate a key role for nuclear factor of activated T cells 5 (NFAT5) transcription factor in the modulation of immune responses upon hypertonic stimuli.[94] Hence, osmotic stress leads to the dimerization of NFAT5 in lymphocytes, a process required for its transcriptional activity, resulting in cytokine (including TNF-α) production, which was suggested to be important as a protective response to pathological conditions where osmotic stress is observed.[97] Activation of NFAT5 by extracellular hyperosmolarity involves a pathway that translates the extracellular stress signal leading to B cell differentiation and production of Igs. This signaling cascade is regulated by the guanine nucleotide exchange factor (GEF) Brx and requires p38α mitogen-activated protein kinase (MAPK) activation.[98] Immune cells in the lymphoid microenvironment are subject to osmotic stress, a phenomenon that is decisive for viability during T cell development. Mouse models of partial NFAT5 loss of function demonstrated that this osmosensitive transcription factor is indispensable to counteract the deleterious effects of osmotic stress on T cells in lymphoid tissues.[99,100]

Thermal Stress

Body temperature must be under a tight control to preserve the homeostatic molecular functions of macromolecules and tissue integrity. Mammals and birds are homeothermic animals endowed with an internal source of temperature to keep their temperature constant. The main organ involved in thermogenesis in mammals is the brown adipose tissue. Facing a demand of heat production, the sympathetic nervous system releases catecholamines, mainly the neurotransmitter norepinephrine, which binds to β3-adrenergic receptors in the adipocyte thereby activating protein kinase A (PKA) and triggering the breakage and combustion of triglycerides accumulated in the brown adipose tissue.[101] Interestingly, phagocytes can be a source of catecholamines as well.[102] Following this line of evidence, recent research revealed that the innate immune system is also involved in an alternative node of regulation of the thermogenic process. Thus, in response to cold temperature stress, macrophages of the adipose tissue respond secreting catecholamines that enhance the lipolysis and the expression of thermogenic proteins in the fat tissue. Such macrophage activation resembles an alternative anti-inflammatory profile of activation and, accordingly, impairment of IL-4 signaling in the phagocytes led to a dramatic reduction in the thermogenic response initiated to adapt to the cold environment.[103] At the molecular level, a complex of HSPs, which will be deeply reviewed in Chapter 5, by Lacetera et al., is activated in a cell, among other stimuli, upon improper increase of the temperature. These conditions can lead to the accumulation of proteins with a wrong folding pattern, sometimes resulting in cell death. To avoid this, cells respond to stress conditions by stimulating the expression of HSPs, which bind and prevent the aggregation of such misfolded proteins.[104] Additionally, several HSPs, including HSP60, HSP70, and HSP90, have been linked to antigen presentation through binding to antigenic peptides and delivery to the surface MHC class I molecules.[105] Furthermore, HSPs can bind to TLR receptors inducing the maturation of DCs and the production of proinflammatory cytokines by monocytes/macrophages.[106,107] The transcription of HSPs is induced by binding of HSF1 to heat shock elements (HSE) located in the DNA promoter regions of HSP genes. HSF1 is the main transcription factor underlying cellular responses to physiological and environmental stressors. Under normal conditions, HSF1 is present in the cytosol as a monomer repressed by interaction with HSP40, HSP70, and HSP90. Upon stress conditions, HSPs are activated and released from HSF1 binding, which is then phosphorylated by a RAS-dependent mechanism, resulting in the formation of HSF1 homotrimers that translocate into the nucleus to bind the promoters of target genes and activate their transcription.[108–110] As pointed out earlier, one of the genes stimulated by HSF1 under heat shock conditions is *MICA*, whose 5′-regulatory region displays HSE similar to those found in *HSP70* genes.[32,33] Accordingly, pharmacological inhibition of HSP90 increases MICA surface expression, rendering stressed cells more susceptible to NK-mediated cytotoxicity.[111]

Genotoxic Stress

Our cells, tissues, and entire body face the threat of many exogenous and endogenous DNA-damaging agents, leading to mutations, DNA breaks, and chromosomal rearrangements that put genome stability and homeostasis at risk. Sources of genetic damage are physical (UV light and ionizing radiations) and chemical agents, such as mutagens and those frequently used in anticancer chemotherapies. Likewise, routine errors in DNA replication and recombination can account for lesions in the DNA with deleterious consequences for the cell. For instance, DNA double strand breaks (DSBs) are severe lesions caused when a replication fork encounters a damaged template or following exposure to genotoxic agents such as ionizing radiations or anticancer drugs.[112] To counteract the harmful effects of these agents, cells have evolved a complex molecular system to quickly sense the genetic damage, which modulates fundamental cellular processes to prevent any irreversible damage to the cell. For instance, the presence of DNA lesions is recognized in cells undergoing a genotoxic stress by factors of the DNA damage response (DDR), which induce cell cycle arrest to allow the reparation of such lesions or, when these are incorrigible, the apoptotic death of the cell. These factors are mainly members of the PI3K-like protein kinases (PIKKs) family, which includes the ataxia-telangiectasia mutated (ATM)- and Rad3-related (ATR) kinases and DNA-dependent protein kinase (DNA-PK), and members of the poly(ADP-ribose) polymerase (PARP) family.[113] DSBs are detected by "sensor" proteins, such as the Mre11-Rad50-Nbs1 (MRN) complex, resulting in the recruitment of inactive homodimers of ATM to the broken DNA molecules and the monomerization of ATM.[114] In this scenario, intermolecular autophosphorylations of ATM at different residues, chiefly Ser1981, are triggered, which are essential for the retention of ATM at DSBs sites and the activation of the kinase.[115,116] The global impact of the ATM-driven modulation of the cellular transcriptome and proteome makes this kinase a master regulator of the cellular response to stress. Indeed, upon DSBs-dependent activation, hundreds of ATM substrates with key roles in crucial aspects of cellular functions are phosphorylated, being a number of them also kinases, which markedly amplifies the regulatory landscape of ATM during the DDR. This complex form of regulation is, for instance, illustrated by the stabilization and the induction of p53 activity in response to genotoxic stress.[117] Significantly, genome integrity is also ensured by immune surveillance mechanisms that detect and eliminate cells suffering a DNA damage stress.[118] Thus, genotoxic agents were found to induce the expression of human and mouse NKG2D ligands in healthy and tumor cells, thus allowing the NK cell-mediated recognition and the elimination of stressed cells. Pharmacological and siRNA-mediated inhibition experiments demonstrated that ATM and ATR kinases were essential for the enhanced NKG2D ligand expression.[119] Recent research revealed that DNAM-1 ligands are also upregulated by therapeutic agents that activate DDR, supporting the idea that ATM/ATR kinases are master regulators of NK-cell activating ligand expression to cope with genetic stress leading to DNA damage.[68] Given that the DDR is already activated in the early stages of cancerous premalignant lesions,[120,121] these pieces of evidence might explain the wide pattern of expression of NKG2D and DNAM-1 ligands observed in tumor cells. Looking at the molecular mediators downstream of ATM involved in the regulation of NKG2D ligands after DDR signaling, activation of checkpoint kinase 1 (Chk1), which regulates DNA damage-induced G2/M arrest,[122] was found to be required for the upregulation of these molecules.[119,123] Interestingly, p53 was not necessary for the induction of NKG2D ligand expression in mouse cell lines,[119] albeit further research revealed that transcription of the human ligands *ULBP1* and *ULBP2* is stimulated by forced expression of wild-type p53, and not by a DNA-binding deficient p53 mutant (R175H), in a p53-null, non-small-cell lung cancer cell line.[124] Accordingly, pharmacological reactivation of p53 was reported to stimulate NK-cell cytotoxic activity by increasing *ULBP2* transcription upon binding of p53 to a response element present in its promoter region.[125] Similarly, DNA damage may also modulate inflammatory responses through the p53-dependent regulation of TLR expression in primary human T-cells, alveolar macrophages, and cancer cell lines. Thus, several p53-binding sites were found in the promoter regions of all human *TLR* genes, except *TLR7*, which were bound by p53 upon DNA damage conditions, resulting in enhanced cytokine production, with different effects exerted by several p53 mutants on the expression of *TLR* gene family.[126,127] Besides, genotoxic stress by chemical agents induces the expression of DR5, a death cell receptor that induces apoptosis through its binding to TRAIL expressed on the surface of NK and T cells, by p53-dependent and -independent mechanisms.[128,129]

DNA-damaging agents have been shown to lead to the accumulation of single- and double-stranded DNA in the cytosol of the cell, in a mechanism dependent on ATM and ATR function. Cytosolic DNA can be detected by the stimulator of interferon genes (STING) sensor pathway, which activates TANK-binding kinase 1 (TBK1) and interferon regulatory factor 3 (IRF3), leading to the upregulation of TLR and the retinoic acid early inducible-1 (RAE-1) family of mouse NKG2D ligands expression.[130,131] In addition, STING signaling in DCs has been shown to mediate the recognition of DNA released by dying cells, leading to IFN-dependent priming of immune responses.[132] Further clues evidencing that ATM signaling is an essential regulator of innate immune responses come from the discovery that IFN signaling can be stimulated by DNA-damaging agents in a mechanism dependent on ATM activity and that the cellular IFN-response signaling can be impaired by siRNA-mediated knockdown of ATM.[133–135]

Collectively, all these observations support the idea that the DDR constitutes a switch that triggers immune responses to collaborate with intrinsic mechanisms activated by genotoxic stress.

Oxidative Stress

A main consequence of the activity of the cellular metabolism is the generation of by-products, the reactive oxygen species (ROS), which can cause DNA oxidative damage, resulting in mutagenesis and leading to genetic alterations and, even more, to cell death. When the endogenous levels of ROS exceed the capacity of intrinsic mechanisms that neutralize these species, the cell undergoes an oxidative stress, with dramatic consequences for the cellular and tissue homeostasis. Sources of ROS are multiple, ranging from exogenous UV radiation and γ-irradiation, to the activity of endogenous organelles (principally the ER and mitochondria), and of several enzymes associated with them, such as cyclooxygenases, cytochrome p450 enzymes, and NADPH oxidases.[136] Given the strong relationship between oxidative stress and hypoxia, which is the subject of a different chapter of this book, we will just briefly introduce the molecular mechanisms regulating innate immunity upon oxidative stress. The interaction between this form of stress and immune response may occur even at a structural level, given that TLR and MyD88 activation in macrophages influences the assemble and function of the NADPH complex.[137,138] It is also known that activity of nuclear factor-kappa B (NF-κB), a family of transcription factors with a central role in inflammation and immunity, is regulated by ROS at multiple levels.[139] Due to the fact that ROS can lead to DNA damage and other forms of cellular stress, the NKG2D receptor/ligand system is also regulated by oxidative stress.[140] Strikingly, many immunosuppressive mechanisms have been shown to affect this signaling. Thus, patients with end-stage renal disease undergoing chronic dialysis, display reduced levels of NKG2D-expressing NK and T cells, the downregulation of NKG2D expression being dependent on the presence of ROS.[141] Additionally, oxidative stress enhances the release of exosomes bearing NKG2D ligands, which abrogates NK-cell-mediated cytotoxic responses in hematopoietic-malignancy models.[86] Conversely, H_2O_2-induced oxidative stress stimulates NKG2D ligand expression and innate immune activities in human airway epithelial cells and colorectal cancer cells.[142,143]

Endoplasmic Reticulum Stress

The ER is a specialized organelle with a central role in many cellular aspects, including the achievement of the initial checkpoints of protein folding and assembly of most proteins of the secretory pathway. To ensure the correct maturation of proteins, the ER stress is enriched in a set of chaperones involved in the posttranslational and molecular modifications that are required to this end. Perturbation of proper ER functions leads to the deleterious accumulation of unfolded and misfolded proteins, which is referred to as ER stress. To cope with this, cells activate the unfolded-protein response (UPR) leading to the upregulation of ER molecular chaperone expression, such as GRP78/BiP and GRP94, and the reduction of protein translation. In mammals, the UPR involves three molecular branches initiated by ER-resident sensor proteins: (1) the activating transcription factor 6 (ATF6), (2) inositol-requiring enzyme 1α (IRE1α), and (3) double-stranded RNA-dependent protein kinase (PKR)-like ER kinase (PERK).[144] However, if cells cannot recover from such a harmful situation, the apoptotic cell death program is activated to eliminate the damaged cell.[145] Now we know that, in addition, a variety of molecules that alert and elicit immune responses are modulated in cells undergoing an ER stress. In fact, ER stress is typically observed in a number of inflammatory and autoimmune diseases, which is thought to determine the extent of the immune activation, and proteins involved in ER stress responses have even been postulated as autoantigens.[146-148] Moreover, it has been shown that such ER stress mediator proteins may also act downstream of immune receptors such as TLR2 and TLR4, which activate the IRE1α axis. Thus, macrophages undergoing an ER stress were found to be hyper-responsive to TLR stimulation through activation of X box-binding protein 1 (XBP1), a transcription factor that regulates the expression of IRE1α target genes, resulting in a sustained production of proinflammatory cytokines.[149] Furthermore, mice lacking XBP1 displayed markedly reduced numbers of both conventional and plasmacytoid DCs, most likely due to an increased sensitivity to apoptotic cell death during differentiation.[150]

As mentioned earlier, the MMP-mediated shedding of MICA requires the binding and the activity on the cell surface of the ER chaperone and disulfide isomerase ERp5/PDIA6, which makes it likely that a triggering ER stress may enhance the formation of soluble forms of MICA. Furthermore, mass spectrophotometric analysis revealed that GRP78 was another MICA-interacting protein on the cell membrane. Supporting this, high surface expression of ERp5 and GRP78 ER chaperones correlated with enhanced levels of serum MICA in chronic lymphocytic leukemia patients.[151]

A computational analysis revealed the presence of putative binding sites for ATF6 in the promoter regions of several human NKG2D ligands, including *MICA*, *ULBP1*, and *ULBP2*, suggesting that activation of the ATF6 axe of the UPR might regulate NKG2D ligand expression in cancer cells.[152] In this regard, exposure to tunicamycin (a pharmacological inducer of the UPR by inhibiting protein N-glycosylation, leading to the accumulation of unfolded proteins in the ER) was shown to regulate the expression of several immune molecules. For instance, this inhibitor reduces MHC class I surface expression in thyroid cells[153] and NKG2D receptor levels in NK cells, but not in CD3$^+$ T cells.[154]

Significantly, a new mechanism of immune surveillance of tumors involving the detection and elimination of hyperploid cancer cells has been reported. Such polyploid tumor cells exhibited higher levels of ER stress than counterparts with a normal DNA content, resulting in an increased surface expression of an ER-resident protein named calreticulin (CRT), which enhances the engulfment of hyperploid cancer cells by antigen-presenting cells and, eventually, stimulates specific antitumor immune responses.[155]

Stress-Induced Senescence

Cells under stress can also respond by entering an irreversible growth arrest, a process known as cellular senescence. The stimuli that induce the transition to a senescent phenotype are multiple, including oncogenic stress, or oncogene-induced senescence, DNA damage, and oxidative stress. The induction of cellular senescence is observed in certain stem cell pools, and it is a typical hallmark of aging; nevertheless, one of the main biological consequences of this process is the blockade of the proliferation of malignant cells as a cellular strategy to block tumorigenesis.[156,157] A key feature of senescent cells is the acquisition of a secretory phenotype, which profoundly alters the surrounding stroma by the activity of a myriad of factors, mostly inflammatory mediators. Thus, TNF-α, interleukin 6 (IL-6), monocyte chemoattractant protein-1 (MCP-1), and IL-1α are highly expressed in senescent tissues.[158,159] In this sense, restoration of p53 function in a model of hepatocellular carcinoma resulted in cellular senescence and tumor regression through a mechanism not involving apoptosis; it involves instead a strong production of proinflammatory cytokines that recruit innate immune cells (neutrophils, macrophages, and NK cells), which reject the developing tumor.[160] Subsequent research revealed that p53 reactivation resulted in the expression of several chemokines that are known to recruit NK cells, including the chemokine (C-C motif) ligand-2 (CCL2), and chemokines (C-X-C motif) ligand 1 (CXCL1) and CXCL2; as well as cytokines that activate the cytotoxic activity of NK cells (IL-12, IL-15, and IL-18). No significant differences in the expression of mouse NKG2D ligands were, however, detected in senescent versus actively proliferating cells.[161] Additional work from the Lowe group showed that senescent, activated hepatic stellate cells express enhanced levels of NKG2D (MICA and ULBP2) and DNAM-1 (PVR) ligands, which leads to NK-mediated rejection of these cells in a model of liver fibrosis.[162] Conversely, cellular senescence also impairs immune surveillance and activities.[163] Hence, phagocytic function is strongly reduced in neutrophils from elderly donors due, at least in part, to the downregulation of Fc receptor CD16 expression.[164] In addition, senescence induced by a novel oncogene, *SENEX*, that activates *p16* expression, is characterized by a strong anti-inflammatory phenotype in endothelial cells, making them highly resistant to TNF-α-induced apoptosis.[165]

IMMUNOGENIC CELL DEATH: PUTTING ALL THE THINGS TOGETHER

Most of the forms of stress that we have depicted in this chapter are integrated in certain pathologies, mainly in cancer. Thus, cells undergoing a tumorigenic transformation frequently display a strong baseline level of ER stress, oxidative stress, and genotoxic stress and, in some cases, they are pushed to a senescent phenotype. Likewise, a complex interplay between stress and activation of specific immune responses occurs during the immunogenic cell death (ICD) process. For a long time, apoptosis was considered a tolerogenic (nonimmunogenic) form of cell death, which does not induce an inflammatory response. However, accumulating evidence has shown that certain chemical and physical agents that are commonly used in anticancer therapies elicit innate and adaptive immune responses upon triggering cell death.[166] In this regard, treatments with anthracyclines and oxaliplatin, as well as exposure to ionizing-irradiation not only cause cell death by activating intrinsic mechanisms, but also promote the expression of mediators that induce the host's immune response. Thus, antineoplastic agents cause DNA damage that can directly kill the cell through activation of apoptosis, or by enhancing the expression of stress-regulated NK-cell activating ligands (e.g., those for NKG2D and DNAM-1 receptors), rendering malignant cells more susceptible to an immune-mediated rejection (Fig. 3.3). Likewise, preapoptotic cells expose the ER protein CRT on the membrane, which acts as an "eat-me" signal for phagocytic cells by binding to the internalization receptor LRP1/CD91, leading to the engulfment of dying cells.[167] To recruit such phagocytes, tumor cells undergoing ICD secrete high levels of ATP, thereby functioning as a "find-me" signal and also to enhance the clearance process by activating the purinergic receptors P2RX7 in DCs and macrophages.[168,169] Moreover, cells under late stages (secondary) of apoptosis passively release high-mobility group box 1 (HMGB1), a damage-associated molecular patterns (DAMPs) immunomodulatory molecule that binds TLR4 and the receptor for

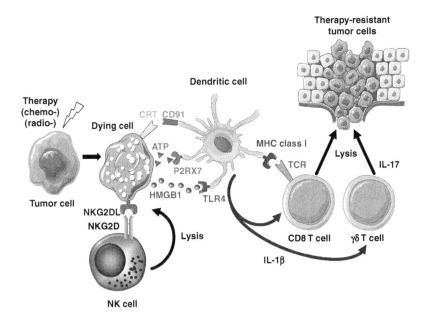

FIGURE 3.3 Cellular and molecular mechanisms involved in the immunogenic cancer cell death. Cancer cells exposed to physical and chemical antineoplastic agents can be killed by the inducement of intrinsic mechanisms of apoptotic cell death. Likewise, treated tumor cells trigger a number of stress responses that upregulate the expression of NKG2D ligands (NKG2DL), resulting in immune elimination by NK cells. Significantly, preapoptotic cells expose the ER protein CRT on their surface, an "eat me" signal for DCs that upon binding to CD91 receptor, stimulates the phagocytosis of dying cancer cells. This engulfment is also enhanced by the ATP-mediated recruitment of phagocytes, which eventually leads to optimal antigen presentation to CD8+ T cells, a process heightened by HMGB1 released by late apoptotic cancer cells. Moreover, DCs secrete IL-1β, further contributing to the activation of cytotoxic T lymphocytes and of IL-17-producing-γδ T cells, which collectively elicit strong antitumor responses targeting the malignant cancer population resistant to the therapeutic agents used.

advanced glycosylation end products (RAGE) on phagocytes, which strongly potentiates their antigen-presenting function.[170] Of relevance, CRT surface exposure was mediated by ER stress responses, and ATP secretion was strictly dependent on autophagy, therefore, these two forms of cellular stress are essential for ICD.[171,172] Additionally, recent research shows that ionizing radiation, a form of therapy that induces ICD, stimulates type I interferon antitumor responses that require the activity of STING receptor as a pathway that senses cytosolic DNA.[173,174]

Consequent to the engulfment of dying cells by phagocytes, antigens associated with apoptotic cells are presented to cytotoxic CD8$^+$ T cells in a mechanism dependent on MHC class I molecules, resulting in strong specific adaptive immune responses.[175] Besides, activated mature DCs produce and release proinflammatory cytokines, such as IL-1β, which recruits γδ T cells that produce IL-17, a cytokine that plays a decisive role in triggering ICD upon chemotherapy.[176] It is worth mentioning that studies performed using spontaneous mammary tumor models found that the adaptive immune system was dispensable for the efficacy of certain chemotherapeutics, supporting a pivotal role for the innate immunity in rejecting tumors after treatment with antineoplastic drugs.[177]

During the last years, great efforts have been made to implement the chemotherapeutic approaches to treat cancer patients. Thus, different forms of chemotherapy that preferentially induce the death of cancer cells have been successfully used in patients with different types of cancer. Nonetheless, no treatment is able to eliminate all the malignant population, which eventually leads to the progression of the disease. Of relevance, the stimulation of specific immune responses upon the ICD-mediated killing of sensitive cancer cells could reflect a crucial strategy to reach and reject such resistant tumors, impairing the malignant development. Therefore, the study of molecular and cellular mechanisms underlying the immunogenic cancer cell death may be of great relevance for the establishment of new therapeutic approaches designed to overcome tumor cell resistance to therapy.

REFERENCES

1. Kultz D. Molecular and evolutionary basis of the cellular stress response. *Ann Rev Physiol* 2005;**67**:225–57.
2. Mogensen TH. Pathogen recognition and inflammatory signaling in innate immune defenses. *Clin Microbiol Rev* 2009;**22**:240–73.
3. Long EO, Kim HS, Liu D, Peterson ME, Rajagopalan S. Controlling natural killer cell responses: integration of signals for activation and inhibition. *Ann Rev Immunol* 2013;**31**:227–58.
4. Karre K. Natural killer cell recognition of missing self. *Nat Immunol* 2008;**9**:477–80.
5. Huergo-Zapico L, Acebes-Huerta A, Lopez-Soto A, Villa-Alvarez M, Gonzalez-Rodriguez AP, Gonzalez S. Molecular bases for the regulation of NKG2D ligands in cancer. *Front Immunol* 2014;**5**:106.
6. Raulet DH, Vance RE. Self-tolerance of natural killer cells. *Nat Rev Immunol* 2006;**6**:520–31.

7. Lanier LL. Up on the tightrope: natural killer cell activation and inhibition. *Nat Immunol* 2008;**9**:495–502.

8. Lopez-Soto A, Huergo-Zapico L, Acebes-Huerta A, Villa-Alvarez M, Gonzalez S. NKG2D signaling in cancer immunosurveillance. *Int J Cancer* 2015;**136**:1741–50.

9. Rosen DB, Araki M, Hamerman JA, Chen T, Yamamura T, Lanier LL. A structural basis for the association of DAP12 with mouse, but not human, NKG2D. *J Immunol* 2004;**173**:2470–8.

10. Lanier LL. DAP10- and DAP12-associated receptors in innate immunity. *Immunol Rev* 2009;**227**:150–60.

11. Gilfillan S, Ho EL, Cella M, Yokoyama WM, Colonna M. NKG2D recruits two distinct adapters to trigger NK cell activation and costimulation. *Nat Immunol* 2002;**3**:1150–5.

12. Wu J, Song Y, Bakker AB, et al. An activating immunoreceptor complex formed by NKG2D and DAP10. *Science* 1999;**285**:730–2.

13. Billadeau DD, Upshaw JL, Schoon RA, Dick CJ, Leibson PJ. NKG2D-DAP10 triggers human NK cell-mediated killing via a Syk-independent regulatory pathway. *Nat Immunol* 2003;**4**:557–64.

14. Groh V, Steinle A, Bauer S, Spies T. Recognition of stress-induced MHC molecules by intestinal epithelial γδ T cells. *Science* 1998;**279**:1737–40.

15. Cosman D, Mullberg J, Sutherland CL, et al. ULBPs, novel MHC class I-related molecules, bind to CMV glycoprotein UL16 and stimulate NK cytotoxicity through the NKG2D receptor. *Immunity* 2001;**14**:123–33.

16. Gonzalez S, Lopez-Soto A, Suarez-Alvarez B, Lopez-Vazquez A, Lopez-Larrea C. NKG2D ligands: key targets of the immune response. *Trends Immunol* 2008;**29**:397–403.

17. Eagle RA, Trowsdale J. Promiscuity and the single receptor: NKG2D. *Nat Rev Immunol* 2007;**7**:737–44.

18. Stephens HA. *MICA* and *MICB* genes: can the enigma of their polymorphism be resolved? *Trends Immunol* 2001;**22**:378–85.

19. Shibuya A, Campbell D, Hannum C, et al. DNAM-1, a novel adhesion molecule involved in the cytolytic function of T lymphocytes. *Immunity* 1996;**4**:573–81.

20. Bottino C, Castriconi R, Pende D, et al. Identification of PVR (CD155) and Nectin-2 (CD112) as cell surface ligands for the human DNAM-1 (CD226) activating molecule. *J Exp Med* 2003;**198**:557–67.

21. Chan CJ, Martinet L, Gilfillan S, et al. The receptors CD96 and CD226 oppose each other in the regulation of natural killer cell functions. *Nat Immunol* 2014;**15**:431–8.

22. Stanietsky N, Simic H, Arapovic J, et al. The interaction of TIGIT with PVR and PVRL2 inhibits human NK cell cytotoxicity. *Proc Natl Acad Sci USA* 2009;**106**:17858–63.

23. Martinet L, Smyth MJ. Balancing natural killer cell activation through paired receptors. *Nat Rev Immunol* 2015;**15**:243–54.

24. Koch J, Steinle A, Watzl C, Mandelboim O. Activating natural cytotoxicity receptors of natural killer cells in cancer and infection. *Trends Immunol* 2013;**34**:182–91.

25. Lopez-Larrea C, Suarez-Alvarez B, Lopez-Soto A, Lopez-Vazquez A, Gonzalez S. The NKG2D receptor: sensing stressed cells. *Trends Mol Med* 2008;**14**:179–89.

26. Coca S, Perez-Piqueras J, Martinez D, et al. The prognostic significance of intratumoral natural killer cells in patients with colorectal carcinoma. *Cancer* 1997;**79**:2320–8.

27. Guerra N, Tan YX, Joncker NT, et al. NKG2D-deficient mice are defective in tumor surveillance in models of spontaneous malignancy. *Immunity* 2008;**28**:571–80.

28. Gilfillan S, Chan CJ, Cella M, et al. DNAM-1 promotes activation of cytotoxic lymphocytes by nonprofessional antigen-presenting cells and tumors. *J Exp Med* 2008;**205**:2965–73.

29. Iguchi-Manaka A, Kai H, Yamashita Y, et al. Accelerated tumor growth in mice deficient in DNAM-1 receptor. *J Exp Med* 2008;**205**:2959–64.

30. Halfteck GG, Elboim M, Gur C, Achdout H, Ghadially H, Mandelboim O. Enhanced *in vivo* growth of lymphoma tumors in the absence of the NK-activating receptor NKp46/NCR1. *J Immunol* 2009;**182**:2221–30.

31. Glasner A, Ghadially H, Gur C, et al. Recognition and prevention of tumor metastasis by the NK receptor NKp46/NCR1. *J Immunol* 2012;**188**:2509–15.

32. Groh V, Bahram S, Bauer S, Herman A, Beauchamp M, Spies T. Cell stress-regulated human major histocompatibility complex class I gene expressed in gastrointestinal epithelium. *Proc Natl Acad Sci USA* 1996;**93**:12445–50.

33. Venkataraman GM, Suciu D, Groh V, Boss JM, Spies T. Promoter region architecture and transcriptional regulation of the genes for the MHC class I-related chain A and B ligands of NKG2D. *J Immunol* 2007;**178**:961–9.

34. Rodriguez-Rodero S, Gonzalez S, Rodrigo L, et al. Transcriptional regulation of MICA and MICB: a novel polymorphism in MICB promoter alters transcriptional regulation by Sp1. *Eur J Immunol* 2007;**37**:1938–53.

35. Lopez-Soto A, Quinones-Lombrana A, Lopez-Arbesu R, Lopez-Larrea C, Gonzalez S. Transcriptional regulation of ULBP1, a human ligand of the NKG2D receptor. *J Biol Chem* 2006;**281**:30419–30.

36. Ryu H, Lee J, Zaman K, et al. Sp1 and Sp3 are oxidative stress-inducible, antideath transcription factors in cortical neurons. *J Neurosci* 2003;**23**:3597–606.

37. Lopez-Soto A, Huergo-Zapico L, Galvan JA, et al. Epithelial-mesenchymal transition induces an antitumor immune response mediated by NKG2D receptor. *J Immunol* 2013;**190**:4408–19.

38. Lopez-Soto A, Zapico LH, Acebes-Huerta A, Rodrigo L, Gonzalez S. Regulation of NKG2D signaling during the epithelial-to-mesenchymal transition. *Oncoimmunology* 2013;**2**:e25820.

39. Shaulian E, Karin M. AP-1 in cell proliferation and survival. *Oncogene* 2001;**20**:2390–400.

40. Marusina AI, Burgess SJ, Pathmanathan I, Borrego F, Coligan JE. Regulation of human DAP10 gene expression in NK and T cells by Ap-1 transcription factors. *J Immunol* 2008;**180**:409–17.

41. Nausch N, Florin L, Hartenstein B, Angel P, Schorpp-Kistner M, Cerwenka A. Cutting edge: the AP-1 subunit JunB determines NK cell-mediated target cell killing by regulation of the NKG2D-ligand RAE-1ε. *J Immunol* 2006;**176**:7–11.

42. Jirtle RL, Skinner MK. Environmental epigenomics and disease susceptibility. *Nat Rev Genet* 2007;**8**:253–62.

43. Esteller M. Cancer epigenomics: DNA methylomes and histone-modification maps. *Nat Rev Genet* 2007;**8**:286–98.

44. Diermayr S, Himmelreich H, Durovic B, et al. NKG2D ligand expression in AML increases in response to HDAC inhibitor valproic acid and contributes to allorecognition by NK-cell lines with single KIR-HLA class I specificities. *Blood.* 2008;**111**:1428–36.

45. Yamanegi K, Yamane J, Kobayashi K, et al. Sodium valproate, a histone deacetylase inhibitor, augments the expression of cell-surface NKG2D ligands, MICA/B, without increasing their soluble forms to enhance susceptibility of human osteosarcoma cells to NK cell-mediated cytotoxicity. *Oncol Rep* 2010;**24**:1621–7.

46. Suzuki T, Terao S, Acharya B, et al. The antitumour effect of γδ T-cells is enhanced by valproic acid-induced up-regulation of NKG2D ligands. *Anticancer Res* 2010;**30**:4509–13.

47. Lopez-Soto A, Folgueras AR, Seto E, Gonzalez S. HDAC3 represses the expression of NKG2D ligands ULBPs in epithelial tumour cells: potential implications for the immunosurveillance of cancer. *Oncogene* 2009;**28**:2370–82.

48. Fiegler N, Textor S, Arnold A, et al. Downregulation of the activating NKp30 ligand B7-H6 by HDAC inhibitors impairs tumor cell recognition by NK cells. *Blood* 2013;**122**:684–93.

49. Tang KF, He CX, Zeng GL, et al. Induction of MHC class I-related chain B (MICB) by 5-aza-2′-deoxycytidine. *Biochem Biophys Res Commun* 2008;**370**:578–83.

50. Sers C, Kuner R, Falk CS, et al. Down-regulation of HLA Class I and NKG2D ligands through a concerted action of MAPK and DNA methyltransferases in colorectal cancer cells. *Int J Cancer* 2009;**125**:1626–39.

51. Baragano Raneros A, Martin-Palanco V, Fernandez AF, et al. Methylation of NKG2D ligands contributes to immune system evasion in acute myeloid leukemia. *Genes Immun* 2015;**16**:71–82.

52. Stern-Ginossar N, Mandelboim O. An integrated view of the regulation of NKG2D ligands. *Immunology* 2009;**128**:1–6.

53. Ha M, Kim VN. Regulation of microRNA biogenesis. *Nat Rev Mol Cell Biol* 2014;**15**:509–24.

54. Leung AK, Sharp PA. MicroRNA functions in stress responses. *Mol Cell* 2010;**40**:205–15.

55. Stern-Ginossar N, Gur C, Biton M, et al. Human microRNAs regulate stress-induced immune responses mediated by the receptor NKG2D. *Nat Immunol* 2008;**9**:1065–73.

56. Tsukerman P, Stern-Ginossar N, Gur C, et al. MiR-10b downregulates the stress-induced cell surface molecule MICB, a critical ligand for cancer cell recognition by natural killer cells. *Cancer Res* 2012;**72**:5463–72.

57. Codo P, Weller M, Meister G, et al. MicroRNA-mediated down-regulation of NKG2D ligands contributes to glioma immune escape. *Oncotarget* 2014;**5**:7651–62.

58. Heinemann A, Zhao F, Pechlivanis S, et al. Tumor suppressive microRNAs miR-34a/c control cancer cell expression of ULBP2, a stress-induced ligand of the natural killer cell receptor NKG2D. *Cancer Res* 2012;**72**:460–71.

59. Espinoza JL, Takami A, Yoshioka K, et al. Human microRNA-1245 down-regulates the NK-G2D receptor in natural killer cells and impairs NKG2D-mediated functions. *Haematologica* 2012;**97**:1295–303.

60. Liu XV, Ho SS, Tan JJ, Kamran N, Gasser S. Ras activation induces expression of Raet1 family NK receptor ligands. *J Immunol* 2012;**189**:1826–34.

61. Piccirillo CA, Bjur E, Topisirovic I, Sonenberg N, Larsson O. Translational control of immune responses: from transcripts to translatomes. *Nat Immunol* 2014;**15**:503–11.

62. Colina R, Costa-Mattioli M, Dowling RJ, et al. Translational control of the innate immune response through IRF-7. *Nature* 2008;**452**:323–8.

63. Liang Q, Deng H, Sun CW, Townes TM, Zhu F. Negative regulation of IRF7 activation by activating transcription factor 4 suggests a cross-regulation between the IFN responses and the cellular integrated stress responses. *J Immunol* 2011;**186**:1001–10.

64. Clemens MJ. Translational regulation in cell stress and apoptosis. Roles of the eIF4E binding proteins. *J Cell Mol Med* 2001;**5**:221–39.

65. Nice TJ, Coscoy L, Raulet DH. Posttranslational regulation of the NKG2D ligand Mult1 in response to cell stress. *J Exp Med* 2009;**206**:287–98.

66. Nice TJ, Deng W, Coscoy L, Raulet DH. Stress-regulated targeting of the NKG2D ligand Mult1 by a membrane-associated RING-CH family E3 ligase. *J Immunol* 2010;**185**:5369–76.

67. Vales-Gomez M, Chisholm SE, Cassady-Cain RL, Roda-Navarro P, Reyburn HT. Selective induction of expression of a ligand for the NKG2D receptor by proteasome inhibitors. *Cancer Res* 2008;**68**:1546–54.

68. Soriani A, Zingoni A, Cerboni C, et al. ATM-ATR-dependent up-regulation of DNAM-1 and NKG2D ligands on multiple myeloma cells by therapeutic agents results in enhanced NK-cell susceptibility and is associated with a senescent phenotype. *Blood* 2009;**113**:3503–11.

69. Chitadze G, Bhat J, Lettau M, Janssen O, Kabelitz D. Generation of soluble NKG2D ligands: proteolytic cleavage, exosome secretion and functional implications. *Scand J Immunol* 2013;**78**:120–9.

70. Holdenrieder S, Eichhorn P, Beuers U, et al. Soluble NKG2D ligands in hepatic autoimmune diseases and in benign diseases involved in marker metabolism. *Anticancer Res* 2007;**27**:2041–5.

71. Schlecker E, Fiegler N, Arnold A, et al. Metalloprotease-mediated tumor cell shedding of B7-H6, the ligand of the natural killer cell-activating receptor NKp30. *Cancer Res* 2014;**74**:3429–40.

72. Groh V, Wu J, Yee C, Spies T. Tumour-derived soluble MIC ligands impair expression of NKG2D and T-cell activation. *Nature* 2002;**419**:734–8.

73. Paschen A, Sucker A, Hill B, et al. Differential clinical significance of individual NKG2D ligands in melanoma: soluble ULBP2 as an indicator of poor prognosis superior to S100B. *Clin Cancer Res* 2009;**15**:5208–15.

74. Yamaguchi K, Chikumi H, Shimizu A, et al. Diagnostic and prognostic impact of serum-soluble UL16-binding protein 2 in lung cancer patients. *Cancer Sci* 2012;**103**:1405–13.

75. Chang YT, Wu CC, Shyr YM, et al. Secretome-based identification of ULBP2 as a novel serum marker for pancreatic cancer detection. *PLoS One* 2011;**6**:e20029.

76. Nuckel H, Switala M, Sellmann L, et al. The prognostic significance of soluble NKG2D ligands in B-cell chronic lymphocytic leukemia. *Leukemia* 2010;**24**:1152–9.

77. Deng W, Gowen BG, Zhang L, et al. A shed NKG2D ligand that promotes natural killer cell activation and tumor rejection. *Science* 2015;**348**(6230):136–9.

78. Chitadze G, Lettau M, Bhat J, et al. Shedding of endogenous MHC class I-related chain molecules A and B from different human tumor entities: heterogeneous involvement of the "a disintegrin and metalloproteases" 10 and 17. *Int J Cancer* 2013;**133**:1557–66.

79. Kaiser BK, Yim D, Chow IT, et al. Disulphide-isomerase-enabled shedding of tumour-associated NKG2D ligands. *Nature* 2007;**447**:482–6.

80. Thery C, Zitvogel L, Amigorena S. Exosomes: composition, biogenesis and function. *Nat Rev Immunol* 2002;**2**:569–79.

81. Zitvogel L, Regnault A, Lozier A, et al. Eradication of established murine tumors using a novel cell-free vaccine: dendritic cell-derived exosomes. *Nat Med* 1998;**4**:594–600.

82. Hwang I, Shen X, Sprent J. Direct stimulation of naive T cells by membrane vesicles from antigen-presenting cells: distinct roles for CD54 and B7 molecules. *Proc Natl Acad Sci USA* 2003;**100**:6670–5.

83. Clayton A, Mitchell JP, Court J, Linnane S, Mason MD, Tabi Z. Human tumor-derived exosomes down-modulate NKG2D expression. *J Immunol* 2008;**180**:7249–58.

84. Reiners KS, Topolar D, Henke A, et al. Soluble ligands for NK cell receptors promote evasion of chronic lymphocytic leukemia cells from NK cell anti-tumor activity. *Blood* 2013;**121**:3658–65.

85. Clayton A, Turkes A, Navabi H, Mason MD, Tabi Z. Induction of heat shock proteins in B-cell exosomes. *J Cell Sci* 2005;**118**:3631–8.

86. Hedlund M, Nagaeva O, Kargl D, Baranov V, Mincheva-Nilsson L. Thermal- and oxidative stress causes enhanced release of NKG2D ligand-bearing immunosuppressive exosomes in leukemia/lymphoma T and B cells. *PLoS One* 2011;**6**:e16899.

87. Burg MB, Ferraris JD, Dmitrieva NI. Cellular response to hyperosmotic stresses. *Physiol Rev* 2007;**87**:1441–74.

88. Shapiro L, Dinarello CA. Osmotic regulation of cytokine synthesis *in vitro*. *Proc Natl Acad Sci USA* 1995;**92**:12230–4.

89. Shapiro L, Dinarello CA. Hyperosmotic stress as a stimulant for proinflammatory cytokine production. *Exp Cell Res* 1997;**231**:354–62.

90. Junger WG, Liu FC, Loomis WH, Hoyt DB. Hypertonic saline enhances cellular immune function. *Circ Shock* 1994;**42**:190–6.

91. Gushchin V, Stegalkina S, Alam HB, Kirkpatrick JR, Rhee PM, Koustova E. Cytokine expression profiling in human leukocytes after exposure to hypertonic and isotonic fluids. *J Trauma* 2002;**52**:867–71.

92. Bulger EM, Jurkovich GJ, Nathens AB, et al. Hypertonic resuscitation of hypovolemic shock after blunt trauma: a randomized controlled trial. *Arch Surg* 2008;**143**:139–48.

93. Descamps-Latscha B, Herbelin A, Nguyen AT, et al. Balance between IL-1 β, TNF-α, and their specific inhibitors in chronic renal failure and maintenance dialysis. Relationships with activation markers of T cells, B cells, and monocytes. *J Immunol* 1995;**154**:882–92.

94. Neuhofer W. Role of NFAT5 in inflammatory disorders associated with osmotic stress. *Curr Genom* 2010;**11**:584–90.

95. Dinarello CA. Immunological and inflammatory functions of the interleukin-1 family. *Ann Rev Immunol* 2009;**27**:519–50.

96. Compan V, Baroja-Mazo A, Lopez-Castejon G, et al. Cell volume regulation modulates NLRP3 inflammasome activation. *Immunity* 2012;**37**:487–500.

97. Lopez-Rodriguez C, Aramburu J, Jin L, Rakeman AS, Michino M, Rao A. Bridging the NFAT and NF-κB families: NFAT5 dimerization regulates cytokine gene transcription in response to osmotic stress. *Immunity* 2001;**15**:47–58.

98. Kino T, Takatori H, Manoli I, et al. Brx mediates the response of lymphocytes to osmotic stress through the activation of NFAT5. *Sci Signal* 2009;**2**:ra5.

99. Trama J, Go WY, Ho SN. The osmoprotective function of the NFAT5 transcription factor in T cell development and activation. *J Immunol* 2002;**169**:5477–88.

100. Go WY, Liu X, Roti MA, Liu F, Ho SN. NFAT5/TonEBP mutant mice define osmotic stress as a critical feature of the lymphoid microenvironment. *Proc Natl Acad Sci USA* 2004;**101**:10673–8.

101. Cannon B, Nedergaard J. Brown adipose tissue: function and physiological significance. *Physiol Rev* 2004;**84**:277–359.

102. Flierl MA, Rittirsch D, Nadeau BA, et al. Phagocyte-derived catecholamines enhance acute inflammatory injury. *Nature* 2007;**449**:721–5.

103. Nguyen KD, Qiu Y, Cui X, et al. Alternatively activated macrophages produce catecholamines to sustain adaptive thermogenesis. *Nature* 2011;**480**:104–8.

104. Tsan MF, Gao B. Heat shock protein and innate immunity. *Cell Mol Immunol* 2004;**1**:274–9.

105. Murshid A, Gong J, Calderwood SK. The role of heat shock proteins in antigen cross presentation. *Front Immunol* 2012;**3**:63.

106. Asea A, Kraeft SK, Kurt-Jones EA, et al. HSP70 stimulates cytokine production through a CD14-dependant pathway, demonstrating its dual role as a chaperone and cytokine. *Nat Med* 2000;**6**:435–42.

107. Friedland JS, Shattock R, Remick DG, Griffin GE. Mycobacterial 65-kD heat shock protein induces release of proinflammatory cytokines from human monocytic cells. *Clin Exp Immunol* 1993;**91**:58–62.

108. Guo Y, Guettouche T, Fenna M, et al. Evidence for a mechanism of repression of heat shock factor 1 transcriptional activity by a multichaperone complex. *J Biol Chem* 2001;**276**:45791–9.

109. Neef DW, Jaeger AM, Thiele DJ. Heat shock transcription factor 1 as a therapeutic target in neurodegenerative diseases. *Nat Rev Drug Discov* 2011;**10**:930–44.

110. Zou J, Guo Y, Guettouche T, Smith DF, Voellmy R. Repression of heat shock transcription factor HSF1 activation by HSP90 (HSP90 complex) that forms a stress-sensitive complex with HSF1. *Cell* 1998;**94**:471–80.

111. Fionda C, Soriani A, Malgarini G, Iannitto ML, Santoni A, Cippitelli M. Heat shock protein-90 inhibitors increase MHC class I-related chain A and B ligand expression on multiple myeloma cells and their ability to trigger NK cell degranulation. *J Immunol* 2009;**183**:4385–94.

112. Harper JW, Elledge SJ. The DNA damage response: ten years after. *Mol Cell* 2007;**28**:739–45.

113. Ciccia A, Elledge SJ. The DNA damage response: making it safe to play with knives. *Mol Cell* 2010;**40**:179–204.

114. Lee JH, Paull TT. ATM activation by DNA double-strand breaks through the Mre11-Rad50-Nbs1 complex. *Science* 2005;**308**:551–4.

115. Bakkenist CJ, Kastan MB. DNA damage activates ATM through intermolecular autophosphorylation and dimer dissociation. *Nature* 2003;**421**:499–506.

116. So S, Davis AJ, Chen DJ. Autophosphorylation at serine 1981 stabilizes ATM at DNA damage sites. *J Cell Biol* 2009;**187**:977–90.

117. Shiloh Y, Ziv Y. The ATM protein kinase: regulating the cellular response to genotoxic stress, and more. *Nat Rev Mol Cell Biol* 2013;**14**:197–210.

118. Chatzinikolaou G, Karakasilioti I, Garinis GA. DNA damage and innate immunity: links and trade-offs. *Trends Immunol* 2014;**35**:429–35.

119. Gasser S, Orsulic S, Brown EJ, Raulet DH. The DNA damage pathway regulates innate immune system ligands of the NKG2D receptor. *Nature* 2005;**436**:1186–90.

120. Gorgoulis VG, Vassiliou LV, Karakaidos P, et al. Activation of the DNA damage checkpoint and genomic instability in human precancerous lesions. *Nature* 2005;**434**:907–13.

121. Bartkova J, Horejsi Z, Koed K, et al. DNA damage response as a candidate anti-cancer barrier in early human tumorigenesis. *Nature* 2005;**434**:864–70.

122. Smith J, Tho LM, Xu N, Gillespie DA. The ATM-Chk2 and ATR-Chk1 pathways in DNA damage signaling and cancer. *Adv Cancer Res* 2010;**108**:73–112.

123. Leung WH, Vong QP, Lin W, Janke L, Chen T, Leung W. Modulation of NKG2D ligand expression and metastasis in tumors by spironolactone via RXRgamma activation. *J Exp Med* 2013;**210**:2675–92.

124. Textor S, Fiegler N, Arnold A, Porgador A, Hofmann TG, Cerwenka A. Human NK cells are alerted to induction of p53 in cancer cells by upregulation of the NKG2D ligands ULBP1 and ULBP2. *Cancer Res* 2011;**71**:5998–6009.

125. Li H, Lakshmikanth T, Garofalo C, et al. Pharmacological activation of p53 triggers anticancer innate immune response through induction of ULBP2. *Cell Cycle* 2011;**10**:3346–58.

126. Menendez D, Shatz M, Azzam K, Garantziotis S, Fessler MB, Resnick MA. The Toll-like receptor gene family is integrated into human DNA damage and p53 networks. *PLoS Genet* 2011;**7**:e1001360.

127. Shatz M, Menendez D, Resnick MA. The human TLR innate immune gene family is differentially influenced by DNA stress and p53 status in cancer cells. *Cancer Res* 2012;**72**:3948–57.

128. Wu GS, Burns TF, McDonald 3rd ER, et al. KILLER/DR5 is a DNA damage-inducible p53-regulated death receptor gene. *Nat Genet* 1997;**17**:141–3.

129. Sheikh MS, Burns TF, Huang Y, et al. p53-dependent and -independent regulation of the death receptor KILLER/DR5 gene expression in response to genotoxic stress and tumor necrosis factor alpha. *Cancer Res* 1998;**58**:1593–8.

130. Hartlova A, Erttmann SF, Raffi FA, et al. DNA damage primes the type I interferon system via the cytosolic DNA sensor STING to promote anti-microbial innate immunity. *Immunity* 2015;**42**:332–43.

131. Lam AR, Le Bert N, Ho SS, et al. RAE1 ligands for the NKG2D receptor are regulated by STING-dependent DNA sensor pathways in lymphoma. *Cancer Res* 2014;**74**:2193–203.

132. Klarquist J, Hennies CM, Lehn MA, Reboulet RA, Feau S, Janssen EM. STING-mediated DNA sensing promotes antitumor and autoimmune responses to dying cells. *J Immunol* 2014;**193**:6124–34.

133. Brzostek-Racine S, Gordon C, Van Scoy S, Reich NC. The DNA damage response induces IFN. *J Immunol* 2011;**187**:5336–45.

134. Pamment J, Ramsay E, Kelleher M, Dornan D, Ball KL. Regulation of the IRF-1 tumour modifier during the response to genotoxic stress involves an ATM-dependent signalling pathway. *Oncogene* 2002;**21**:7776–85.

135. Watling D, Carmo CR, Kerr IM, Costa-Pereira AP. Multiple kinases in the interferon-γ response. *Proc Natl Acad Sci USA* 2008;**105**:6051–6.

136. Fang J, Seki T, Maeda H. Therapeutic strategies by modulating oxygen stress in cancer and inflammation. *Adv Drug Deliv Rev* 2009;**61**:290–302.

137. Park HS, Jung HY, Park EY, Kim J, Lee WJ, Bae YS. Cutting edge: direct interaction of TLR4 with NAD(P)H oxidase 4 isozyme is essential for lipopolysaccharide-induced production of reactive oxygen species and activation of NF-κ B. *J Immunol* 2004;**173**:3589–93.

138. Laroux FS, Romero X, Wetzler L, Engel P, Terhorst C. Cutting edge: MyD88 controls phagocyte NADPH oxidase function and killing of Gram-negative bacteria. *J Immunol* 2005;**175**:5596–600.

139. Morgan MJ, Liu ZG. Crosstalk of reactive oxygen species and NF-κB signaling. *Cell Res* 2011;**21**:103–15.

140. Chan CJ, Smyth MJ, Martinet L. Molecular mechanisms of natural killer cell activation in response to cellular stress. *Cell Death Diff* 2014;**21**:5–14.

141. Peraldi MN, Berrou J, Dulphy N, et al. Oxidative stress mediates a reduced expression of the activating receptor NKG2D in NK cells from end-stage renal disease patients. *J Immunol* 2009;**182**:1696–705.

142. Borchers MT, Harris NL, Wesselkamper SC, Vitucci M, Cosman D. NKG2D ligands are expressed on stressed human airway epithelial cells. *Am J Physiol* 2006;**291**:L222–31.

143. Yamamoto K, Fujiyama Y, Andoh A, Bamba T, Okabe H. Oxidative stress increases *MICA* and *MICB* gene expression in the human colon carcinoma cell line (CaCo-2). *Biochim Biophys Acta* 2001;**1526**:10–2.

144. Ron D, Walter P. Signal integration in the endoplasmic reticulum unfolded protein response. *Nat Rev Mol Cell Biol* 2007;**8**:519–29.

145. Hetz C. The unfolded protein response: controlling cell fate decisions under ER stress and beyond. *Nat Rev Mol Cell Biol* 2012;**13**:89–102.

146. Zhang K, Kaufman RJ. From endoplasmic-reticulum stress to the inflammatory response. *Nature* 2008;**454**:455–62.

147. Todd DJ, Lee AH, Glimcher LH. The endoplasmic reticulum stress response in immunity and autoimmunity. *Nat Rev Immunol* 2008;**8**:663–74.

148. Kaser A, Lee AH, Franke A, et al. XBP1 links ER stress to intestinal inflammation and confers genetic risk for human inflammatory bowel disease. *Cell* 2008;**134**:743–56.

149. Martinon F, Chen X, Lee AH, Glimcher LH. TLR activation of the transcription factor XBP1 regulates innate immune responses in macrophages. *Nat Immunol* 2010;**11**:411–8.

150. Iwakoshi NN, Pypaert M, Glimcher LH. The transcription factor XBP-1 is essential for the development and survival of dendritic cells. *J Exp Med* 2007;**204**:2267–75.

151. Huergo-Zapico L, Gonzalez-Rodriguez AP, Contesti J, et al. Expression of ERp5 and GRP78 on the membrane of chronic lymphocytic leukemia cells: association with soluble MICA shedding. *Cancer Immunol* 2012;**61**:1201–10.

152. Eagle RA, Traherne JA, Ashiru O, Wills MR, Trowsdale J. Regulation of NKG2D ligand gene expression. *Human Immunol* 2006;**67**:159–69.

153. Ulianich L, Terrazzano G, Annunziatella M, Ruggiero G, Beguinot F, Di Jeso B. ER stress impairs MHC Class I surface expression and increases susceptibility of thyroid cells to NK-mediated cytotoxicity. *Biochim Biophys Acta* 2011;**1812**:431–8.

154. Berrou J, Fougeray S, Venot M, et al. Natural killer cell function, an important target for infection and tumor protection, is impaired in type 2 diabetes. *PLoS One* 2013;**8**:e62418.

155. Senovilla L, Vitale I, Martins I, et al. An immunosurveillance mechanism controls cancer cell ploidy. *Science* 2012;**337**:1678–84.

156. Lopez-Otin C, Blasco MA, Partridge L, Serrano M, Kroemer G. The hallmarks of aging. *Cell* 2013;**153**:1194–217.

157. Campisi J, d'Adda di Fagagna F. Cellular senescence: when bad things happen to good cells. *Nat Rev Mol Cell Biol* 2007;**8**:729–40.

158. Kuilman T, Michaloglou C, Vredeveld LC, et al. Oncogene-induced senescence relayed by an interleukin-dependent inflammatory network. *Cell* 2008;**133**:1019–31.

159. Tchkonia T, Zhu Y, van Deursen J, Campisi J, Kirkland JL. Cellular senescence and the senescent secretory phenotype: therapeutic opportunities. *J Clin Invest* 2013;**123**:966–72.

160. Xue W, Zender L, Miething C, et al. Senescence and tumour clearance is triggered by p53 restoration in murine liver carcinomas. *Nature* 2007;**445**:656–60.

161. Iannello A, Thompson TW, Ardolino M, Lowe SW, Raulet DH. p53-Dependent chemokine production by senescent tumor cells supports NKG2D-dependent tumor elimination by natural killer cells. *J Exp Med* 2013;**210**:2057–69.

162. Krizhanovsky V, Yon M, Dickins RA, et al. Senescence of activated stellate cells limits liver fibrosis. *Cell* 2008;**134**:657–67.

163. Hoenicke L, Zender L. Immune surveillance of senescent cells – biological significance in cancer- and non-cancer pathologies. *Carcinogenesis* 2012;**33**:1123–6.

164. Butcher SK, Chahal H, Nayak L, et al. Senescence in innate immune responses: reduced neutrophil phagocytic capacity and CD16 expression in elderly humans. *J Leukoc Biol* 2001;**70**:881–6.

165. Coleman PR, Hahn CN, Grimshaw M, et al. Stress-induced premature senescence mediated by a novel gene, SENEX, results in an anti-inflammatory phenotype in endothelial cells. *Blood* 2010;**116**:4016–24.

166. Kroemer G, Galluzzi L, Kepp O, Zitvogel L. Immunogenic cell death in cancer therapy. *Ann Rev Immunol* 2013;**31**:51–72.

167. Gardai SJ, McPhillips KA, Frasch SC, et al. Cell-surface calreticulin initiates clearance of viable or apoptotic cells through trans-activation of LRP on the phagocyte. *Cell* 2005;**123**:321–34.

168. Ma Y, Adjemian S, Mattarollo SR, et al. Anticancer chemotherapy-induced intratumoral recruitment and differentiation of antigen-presenting cells. *Immunity* 2013;**38**:729–41.

169. Martins I, Tesniere A, Kepp O, et al. Chemotherapy induces ATP release from tumor cells. *Cell Cycle* 2009;**8**:3723–8.

170. Apetoh L, Ghiringhelli F, Tesniere A, et al. Toll-like receptor 4-dependent contribution of the immune system to anticancer chemotherapy and radiotherapy. *Nat Med* 2007;**13**:1050–9.

171. Obeid M, Tesniere A, Ghiringhelli F, et al. Calreticulin exposure dictates the immunogenicity of cancer cell death. *Nat Med* 2007;**13**:54–61.

172. Michaud M, Martins I, Sukkurwala AQ, et al. Autophagy-dependent anticancer immune responses induced by chemotherapeutic agents in mice. *Science* 2011;**334**:1573–7.

173. Woo SR, Fuertes MB, Corrales L, et al. STING-dependent cytosolic DNA sensing mediates innate immune recognition of immunogenic tumors. *Immunity* 2014;**41**:830–42.

174. Deng L, Liang H, Xu M, et al. STING-dependent cytosolic DNA sensing promotes radiation-induced type I interferon-dependent antitumor immunity in immunogenic tumors. *Immunity* 2014;**41**:843–52.

175. Green DR, Ferguson T, Zitvogel L, Kroemer G. Immunogenic and tolerogenic cell death. *Nat Rev Immunol* 2009;**9**:353–63.

176. Ma Y, Aymeric L, Locher C, et al. Contribution of IL-17-producing gamma delta T cells to the efficacy of anticancer chemotherapy. *J Exp Med* 2011;**208**:491–503.

177. Ciampricotti M, Hau CS, Doornebal CW, Jonkers J, de Visser KE. Chemotherapy response of spontaneous mammary tumors is independent of the adaptive immune system. *Nat Med* 2012;**18**:344–6.

Chapter 4

Modulation of Innate Immunity by Hypoxia

Elena Riboldi,* Antonio Sica*,**

*Department of Pharmaceutical Sciences, Università del Piemonte Orientale "Amedeo Avogadro," Novara, Italy; **Department of Inflammation and Immunology, Humanitas Clinical and Research Center, Rozzano, Italy

HYPOXIA

Oxygen (O_2) is a key component of all major biomolecules of living organisms and a fundamental element for many cellular reactions. In fact, oxygen is indispensable for oxidative phosphorylation, which is the most efficient process to generate ATP that is needed to power physiochemical cellular reactions. Homeostasis of oxygen level is finely regulated and, if the concentration of oxygen decreases, a stress condition called hypoxia is generated. Hypoxia is the result of a combination of events, including high cell proliferation rates and blood vessel leakiness.[1]

Air contains 21% oxygen, 78% nitrogen, and low amounts of carbon dioxide, argon, and helium. Since air has a total pressure of 760 mmHg (1 atm = 760 mmHg = 760 Torr = 101 kPa), the partial pressure of oxygen (pO_2) at sea level is 159 mmHg ($21/100 \times 760 = 159$). The pO_2 in the trachea reaches 150 mmHg, at the pulmonary alveolus it falls to 100 mmHg (16% O_2), thereafter, it decreases and in most organs of the body is $\sim$40 mmHg (6% O_2).[2]

Tissue oxygen levels can be measured in several ways.[3] The oxygen electrode developed in the 1950s by Leland Clark allowed demonstrating that wounded, infected, and inflamed tissues are characterized by reduced oxygen tension.[4–7] Hypoxia can be identified *in vivo* using 2-nitroimidazol derivatives. When these chemicals are injected into animals, if O_2 levels are lower than $\sim$10 mmHg ($\sim$1.3% O_2), they form adducts with proteins that can be detected by immunohistochemistry in tissue specimens. This method was used to reveal hypoxia in inflamed gut mucosa.[8,9] The newest techniques to quantify tissue oxygenation levels are based on the luminescence quenching of dyes. Luminescence-based optical oxygen imaging techniques have the advantage of allowing repetitive noninvasive measurement both in animals and in humans.[10]

Hypoxia and inflammation are closely linked. Individuals suffering mountain sickness have increased blood levels of inflammatory cytokines. Also, healthy volunteers exposed to hypoxia at high altitudes (>3400 m) upregulate the levels of the cytokine IL-6.[11] The continuous activation of the hypoxic signaling in individuals, who live at a high altitude, can lead to reduced activity of inflammatory pathways. This seems to be the explanation of the increased prevalence of *Helicobacter pylori* infection in Tibetan monks.[12]

Immune cells drive inflammation by secreting various proinflammatory cytokines and inflammatory mediators in order to eliminate the pathogen or the causative threat. However, inflammation can cause collateral injury to tissues. Damages to endothelial cells and microcirculation, as well as clogging, can cause an interruption of normal blood and oxygen supply that results in local tissue hypoxia. Hypoxia is associated with inflammation in a variety of pathological conditions including rheumatoid arthritis (RA) (8–78 mmHg/~1.1–10.5% O_2),[13–16] inflammatory bowel disease (IBD) (~10 mmHg/~1.3% O_2),[8,9] atherosclerosis (<10 mmHg/1.3% O_2),[17,18] and ischemia induced by reduced blood perfusion.[19]

It has been estimated that 50–60% of solid tumors contain areas of hypoxic and/or anoxic (no oxygen) tissues that develop as a result of an imbalance between oxygen supply and consumption in proliferating tumors.[20] Several studies provide evidence that the presence of hypoxia within the tumor mass is an independent marker of poor prognosis for patients with various types of cancer, including carcinoma of the cervix, carcinoma of the breast, carcinoma of the head and neck, soft-tissue sarcoma, cutaneous melanoma, and prostatic adenocarcinoma.[21] Intratumor hypoxia is associated with a malignant phenotype characterized by uncontrolled tumor growth, angiogenesis, and increased risk of metastasis.[22]

Hypoxia can cause oxidative stress. Oxidative stress occurs when free radicals and other reactive species overwhelm the availability of antioxidants. Imbalance between oxidants and antioxidants may provoke pathological reactions causing a range of nonrespiratory and respiratory diseases, particularly chronic obstructive pulmonary disease.[23] In animals, oxidative stress can also be the result of genetic selection. As an example, pig husbandry selected highly inbred lines with extremely fast growth rates (up to 120 kg body weight in the first 6 months of age) and reduced fat content.[24] These animals have an impaired balance between muscular mass and cardiocirculatory system, as well as high levels of constitutive-oxidative stress.

HYPOXIA SENSING

Hypoxia is perceived, at a cellular level, through oxygen sensor relays that operate inside the cell and can lead to the activation of transcriptional activators. The hypoxia-inducible factor (HIF) and nuclear factor κB (NF-κB) families of transcriptional factors have been identified as crucial regulators of this metabolic adaptation.[25,26] In addition, other factors (e.g., AP-1 and Egr-1) have been implicated in shaping the hypoxic phenotype of the cells.[27]

Hypoxia-Inducible Factors

HIF is a heterodimer composed of the constitutively expressed β subunit and an α subunit, whose stability depends on the oxygen level.[25] Each subunit contains basic helix–loop–helix-PAS (bHLH-PAS) domains required for dimerization and DNA binding.[28] In mammals, three closely related transcription factor complexes exist: HIF-1, HIF-2, and HIF-3. HIF-1α is the first α subunit identified and the most studied. HIF-2α can functionally overlap HIF-1α, but its expression is more restricted and in some cases it can mediate distinct biological functions. HIF-3α seems to have regulatory functions as it can act as competitive inhibitor of the HIF-1α–HIF-1β interaction.[29] Under normoxic conditions, the α subunit is hydroxylated by prolyl hydroxylases (PHDs), recognized by the protein product of the Von Hippel–Lindau (VHL) tumor-suppressor gene, ubiquitinated and degraded by the proteasome. Under hypoxic conditions, PHDs are not active and consequently HIF-α is not degraded but it can translocate to the nucleus, and can dimerize with the β subunit. Factor inhibiting HIF (FIH) provides another level of regulation by hydroxylating asparaginyl residues in the α subunit and blocking the formation of the active transcriptional complex.[30] PHDs and FIH require α-ketoglutarate as a limiting electron donor cosubstrate. Ferrous iron and ascorbate are also required for hydroxylation reactions.[30] Reactive oxygen species (ROS) can activate HIF-1α promoter and regulate FIH hydroxylase function.[30] ROS generation stabilizes HIF-1α.[31] HIFs can be stabilized and exert their activity under normoxic conditions, in response to bacterial products, cytokines, inflammatory mediators, and stress. Pathogen-associated molecules that can stabilize HIF-1α include lipopolysaccharide (LPS), lipoteichoic acid, cytosine-phosphatidyl-guanine oligodeoxynucleotides, and trehalose dimycolate.[3,32] Hypoxia-independent stabilization of HIF-2α by inflammatory stimuli has also been demonstrated.[3] Exogenous HIF-inducers include dimethyloxalylglycine (DMOG), a competitive antagonist of α-ketoglutarate, iron chelators (e.g., desferrioxamine), and cobalt chloride, which displaces iron from the catalytic center.[28]

HIFs induce the transcription of genes mediating cellular adaptation to a low oxygen environment.[25] HIF target genes contain hypoxia-response elements (HREs) with a conserved G/ACGTG core sequence in their promoter or enhancer.[33] Target genes are involved in a broad range of functions including angiogenesis, erythropoiesis, metabolism, autophagy, and apoptosis. Hundreds of genes are directly controlled by HIF binding to HRE, as demonstrated by RNA interference and chromatin immunoprecipitation assay. Interestingly, HIF reduces the expression of hundreds of genes without directly binding the transcriptional factor to the genes. In this case, HIF transcriptional regulation seems to depend on indirect mechanisms such as the expression of transcriptional repressor and micro-RNA.[28]

One of the most important activities of HIF is the promotion of glycolysis to produce ATP, as low tissue oxygenation impairs oxidative phosphorylation. HIF-1 mediates the transition from oxidative to glycolytic metabolism through the regulation of four factors, namely, pyruvate dehydrogenase (PDK1), lactate dehydrogenase A (LDHA), BCL2/adenovirus E1B 19 kDa interacting protein 3 (BNIP3), and BNIP3-like (BNIP3L).[28] Glycolysis is less efficient than oxidative phosphorylation in producing ATP. The switch from oxidative phosphorylation to glycolysis is considered a mechanism to prevent ROS-mediated damages to the cell. In fact, under hypoxic conditions, mitochondria would generate an excess of ROS because of a reduction in the efficiency of electronic transfer.[28]

Normal cells can adapt their metabolism to environmental pO_2, whereas tumor cells always favor glycolysis regardless of oxygen availability (the "Warburg effect").[34] The gene responsible for this "aerobic glycolysis" is the pyruvate kinase isoenzyme type M2 (M2-PK), an HIF-dependent gene, and the upregulation of M2-PK is attributable to oncogene-mediated, hypoxia-independent HIF-1 stabilization.[35]

HIFs directly activate the expression of several proangiogenic factors, including vascular endothelial growth factors (VEGFs), VEGF receptors (VEG-FRs), plasminogen activator inhibitor 1 (PAI-1), angiopoietins, platelet-derived growth factor B (PDGFB), surface receptor tunica internal endothelial kinase 2 (Tie-2), and matrix metalloproteinase-2 and -9 (MMP-2 and MMP-9).[20] Mononuclear phagocytes exposed to hypoxia express high levels of several proinflammatory cytokines (e.g., IL-1, TNF-α) and adhesion molecules.[36,37] HIF-responsive elements are present in the genes encoding toll-like receptors (TLRs), including TLR2 and TLR6, which are pattern-recognition receptors that are upregulated in response to hypoxia.[38]

HIF-1α and HIF-2α gene deletion is lethal. Mice that are homozygous for a null allele at the locus encoding HIF-1α die by embryonic day 10.5 with cardiac malformations, vascular defects, and impaired erytropoiesis.[39,40] Depending on the genetic background, mice lacking HIF-2α die by embryonic day 12.5 with vascular defects or bradycardia, due to deficient catecholamine production;[41,42] die as neonates due to impaired lung maturation;[43] or die as adults due to ROS-mediated multiorgan failure.[44] Hence, it is necessary to use conditional cell-specific knockout mice for *in vivo* studies. Many studies took advantage of the Cre/LoxP recombination system. In these transgenic mice, LoxP sites are introduced in the desired gene. Simultaneous cell-type-specific expression of the Cre recombinase *in vivo* allows for selective deletion of the LoxP-floxed target gene. Conditional knockout of HIF-1α demonstrated the importance of this molecule in chondrogenesis, osteogenesis, adipogenesis, B lymphocyte development, T lymphocyte differentiation, and innate immunity.[28]

Hypoxia signaling pathway is overexpressed in many human cancers. Significant associations between HIF-1α overexpression and patient mortality have been shown in cancers of the brain, breast, cervix, oropharynx, ovary, and uterus.[45] As a prognostic marker, high HIF-2α relates to advanced stage and/or poor patient outcome in nonsmall-cell lung cancer, breast cancer, bladder cancer, colorectal cancer, and neuroblastoma.[46] A number of HIF-inducible genes mediate key steps in tumorigenesis.[20] Therefore, HIF represents a suitable molecular target for cancer therapy.[47]

The PHD isoform PHD3 has been shown to control neutrophils and macrophage survival.[48,49] Interestingly, these effects are independent of HIF stabilization, suggesting that other hypoxia pathways are active in myeloid cells.[48–52] Some mechanisms by which the stabilized isoforms can influence the activity of other signaling pathways independent of the HIF heterodimer or an HRE include the regulation of Notch, c-Myc, and p53 signaling.[29]

Nuclear Factor κB

In mammals, the NF-κB family is composed of five members: (1) RelA (p65), (2) RelB, (3) cRel, (4) NF-κB1 (p50 and its precursor p105), and (5) NF-κB2 (p52 and its precursor p100).[53] These proteins form homodimeric and heterodimeric complexes. Under nonstimulated conditions, NF-κB is sequestered in the cytoplasm through interaction with inhibitory proteins of the IκB family. Following stimulation with a broad range of stimuli, such as inflammatory cytokines, microbial components, genotoxic agents, and ionizing radiation, the IκB molecules are phosphorylated at specific serine residues by the IκB kinase (IKK) complex (containing three catalytic subunits termed IKK-α, -β, and -γ), which leads to their ubiquitylation and degradation by the proteasome. NF-κB dimers are subsequently released and translocate to the nucleus, where they activate the transcription of various target genes. This pathway has a major role in the control of innate immunity and inflammation.

Hypoxia has long been shown to stimulate NF-κB-mediated signaling and several pieces of evidence indicate that both HIF and NF-κB proteins are redox-sensitive proteins regulated by the same oxygen sensors.[54] HIF and NF-κB have several common target genes, common regulators, and common stimuli. It was shown that ROS activates the HIF-1α promoter via a functional NF-κB site.[55] In macrophages, the increased production of ROS due to hypoxia promotes NF-κB activation and the synergy between hypoxia and LPS.[56] In contrast, inhibition of PHDs suppresses the LPS-induced expression of TNF-α in macrophages, through NF-κB inhibition.[57] It has been shown that hypoxia leads to NF-κB activation through decreased PHD-dependent hydroxylation of IKK-β, whereas ablation of IKK-β impairs HIF-1α accumulation in hypoxia, suggesting that NF-κB transcriptionally regulates HIF-1α.[26,58] A physical interaction between IKK-γ (i.e., NEMO) and HIF-2α enhances HIF-2α transcriptional activity.[59] NF-κB can stabilize HIF-1α in hypoxia and in inflammation.[60] In addition, HIF-1α can inhibit NF-κB under inflammatory conditions.[9,29] A basal NF-κB activity is required for HIF-1α mRNA transcription.[26,60] NF-κB-dependent induction of the micro-RNA miR155, in response to LPS can target HIF-1α for silencing.[61] A synergistic relationship between HIF and NF-κB contributes to myeloid-cell responses against pathogens. Macrophages infected with Gram-positive or -negative bacteria reveal a marked defect in HIF-1α expression following the deletion of the NF-κB activity regulator IKK-β.[26] Interestingly, the continuous activation of HIF in individuals who live at a high altitude, can lead to reduced NF-κB activity. Evidence supporting a negative effect on the immune response is the increased prevalence of *H. pylori* infection in Tibetan monks.[12]

HYPOXIA EFFECTS ON LEUKOCYTES

Myeloid Cells

Hypoxia is an important noninfectious stressor for cells, stimulating innate immunity (Fig. 4.1). A seminal study by Cramer et al. showed that monocyte and granulocyte development as well as differentiation are not affected by HIF-1α deletion.[62] By using myeloid-specific HIF-1α conditional knockout mice, Cramer et al. demonstrated that this transcription factor is essential for myeloid cell activities such as cell aggregation, motility, invasiveness, and bacterial killing.[62] On the contrary, mice lacking HIF-1α in myeloid cells are more resistant to sterile endotoxemia induced with LPS or lipoteichoic acid/peptidoglycan, displaying lower levels of proinflammatory cytokines and prolonged survival.[63] Similar effects were observed in myeloid-specific HIF-2α conditional knockout mice. Also in this case, HIF-deficient macrophages showed reduced migration, invasion, proinflammatory cytokines production, and mice were resistant to LPS-induced endotoxemia.[64]

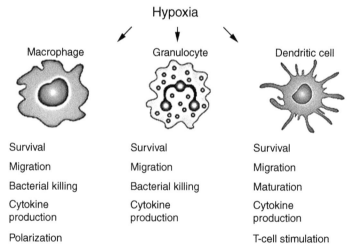

FIGURE 4.1   Effects of hypoxia on monocytes/macrophages, granulocytes, and dendritic cells. See text for description.

Hypoxia has detrimental effects on myeloid cell-driven antimicrobial defense.[3] In fact, many enzymes with antimicrobial and immune-modulatory effects can function only in the presence of oxygen such as phagocyte NADPH oxydase (PHOX),[65] type 2 nitric oxide synthase (NOS2), and indoleamine 2,3 dioxygenase (IDO).[66–68] However, hypoxia can induce antimicrobial peptides such as cathelicidins and beta defensin 2.[69,70] Hypoxia-induced release of beta defensin 2 by macrophages inhibits intracellular growth of *Mycobacterium tuberculosis*.[70] Therefore, divergent effects on the antimicrobial mechanism of myeloid cells can be observed in different infections.

Hypoxia can have different effects in tissue injuries depending on their acute or chronic nature.[3] Myeloid HIF-1α is needed in the early stages of wound repair. In this context, HIF-1α induces soluble growth factors or adhesion proteins to restore oxygen homeostasis. On the contrary, the absence of HIF-1α in myeloid cells has been shown to favor a faster wound closure in secondary dermal wound healing, possibly through reduced nitric oxide activity on keratinocytes.[71] Similarly, myeloid cell-derived HIF-1α responses can be different depending on the injured organ. HIF-1α activation in myeloid cells contributes to the development of fibrosis in a model of chronic liver injury.[72] In contrast, myeloid cell-derived HIF-1α attenuated kidney inflammation by facilitating tissue repair in a model of kidney injury.[73] Therefore, the context of HIF activation in myeloid cells is determining the final effect on homeostatic immune functions.[3]

Myeloid-derived suppressor cells (MDSCs) represent a heterogeneous population of cells, whose common characteristics are an immature state and the ability to suppress T-cell responses *in vitro* and *in vivo*.[74] In healthy individuals, immature myeloid cells differentiate in mature granulocytes, macrophages or dendritic cells (DCs); whereas in pathological conditions they expand into MDSCs. MDSCs have been observed in cancer, chronic infectious diseases, and autoimmunity. Exposure of spleen MDSC to hypoxia resulted in an HIF-1α-dependent conversion of these cells into macrophages.[75] Moreover, HIF-1α has been shown to induce a glycolytic metabolic reprogramming in MDSCs and to regulate the high expression of PD-L1 on MDSC.[76,77]

Monocytes/Macrophages

Immature monocytes are generated in the bone marrow, where stem cells survive in "hypoxic niches" of hematopoietic tissue.[78] After leaving the relatively high oxygen concentration of the blood circulation, they reach peripheral tissues where they adapt to the hypoxic microenvironment of pathological tissues. Hypoxia prolongs cell survival of human monocytes because it enhances glucose uptake and induces the expression of glycolytic-gene expression.[79] Transcriptome analysis of human monocytes exposed to hypoxia showed the induction of genes related to glucose transport (e.g., solute carrier family member 1, *SLC2A1*), glycolytic metabolism (e.g., *enolase 2*), angiogenesis (*VEGF*), apoptosis (e.g., *Bcl2*), and matrix remodeling (e.g., *MMP9*).[80,81] In monocytes hypoxia also regulates chemotactic factors. The production of the chemokine CCL20 by hypoxic monocytes recruits in the hypoxic region of the inflamed tissues other leukocytes expressing the CCR6 receptor, namely, immature DCs, effector/memory T lymphocytes, and naïve B cells.[80] In this context CCL20 expression is regulated by p50 NF-κB.[82] Hypoxic monocytes upregulate the receptor CXCR4 and increase chemotactic responsiveness to its specific ligand CXCL12.[83] The gene for CXCL12 (otherwise known as SDF-1), is regulated by HIF-1 in endothelial cells, resulting in the expression of the chemokines in ischemic tissue in direct proportion to reduced oxygen tension.[84] CXCR4 induction by hypoxia is also HIF-1α-dependent. Hypoxia-driven expression of CXCR4 is seen in different cell types (monocytes, monocyte-derived macrophages, tumor-associated macrophages (TAMs), endothelial cells, and cancer cells) and may regulate trafficking in and out of hypoxic-tissue microenvironments. In addition, the CCL2–CCR5 axis is inhibited in mouse macrophages in response to hypoxia.[85] The regulation of chemokines and their receptors, is a way to retain/concentrate recruited macrophages at hypoxic sites. Monocytes/macrophages migrate until they reach a hypoxic area and they are inhibited from progressing further.

Macrophages are characterized by considerable diversity and plasticity.[86,87] In tissues, mononuclear phagocytes respond to environmental cues (e.g., microbial products, damaged cells, and activated lymphocytes) with the acquisition of distinct functional phenotypes, differentially affecting disease onset and progression.[74] In response to various signals, macrophages may undergo classical M1 activation (stimulated by TLR ligands and IFN-γ) or alternative M2 activation (stimulated by IL-4/IL-13). These states mirror the Th1 versus Th2 polarization of T cells. M1 macrophages have antimicrobial activity and stimulate adaptive immunity, while M2 macrophages promote wound healing, angiogenesis, and tumor growth. Macrophage polarization results in differential expression of HIF-1α and HIF-2α, with HIF-1α associated with M1 activation, and HIF-2α associated with M2 activation of macrophages.[88,89] NOS2 is regulated by HIF-1α, whereas arginase 1 expression is controlled by HIF-2α. Therefore, NO homeostasis is controlled in macrophages by the antagonism of HIF-1α and HIF-2α.[33] Proinflammatory monocytes acquire an altered, immunosuppressive phenotype, during human sepsis.[90] Hypoxic regions of solid tumors are often characterized by high accumulation of macrophages, which contribute to tumor angiogenesis and development.[91] This trophic action of tumor hypoxia on TAMs is clinically relevant, as a high TAM number is considered a negative prognostic marker in several human malignancies, including Hodgkin's disease, glioma, colangiocarcinoma, and breast carcinoma.[87,92] HIF-1α induces VEGF and CXCL12 that synergistically recruit bone-marrow-derived myeloid cells including macrophages and Tie2-expressing monocytes.[93] These cells secrete MMP-9 that mobilizes VEGF from the extracellular matrix. This event promotes vascular remodeling and neovascularization. Hypoxia can induce the expression of endothelin-2, a vasoactive peptide, which can recruit macrophages at tumor sites.[33,94] Another axis that contributes to the accumulation of TAMs into hypoxic areas of tumors is semaphorin3A (Sema3A)-neuropilin-1 (Nrp-1). Nrp-1 expression on macrophages is downregulated by hypoxia. Deletion of Nrp-1 prevents TAM infiltration, resulting in delayed tumor growth because of impaired vascularization and improved antitumor immunity.[95] It was reported that lactic acid produced by tumor cells, as a by-product of aerobic or anaerobic glycolysis, has a critical function in inducing the expression of VEGF and the M2-like polarization of TAMs.[96]

HIF-1α drives macrophage production of VEGF, whereas HIF-2α drives macrophage production of soluble VEGFR-1 (sVEGFR-1). Therefore, specific and independent roles for HIF-1 and HIF-2 regulate the production of antiangiogenic molecules from mononuclear phagocytes in a GM-CSF-rich environment.[97] Angiogenic monocytes expressing *Tie-2*, the so called Tie-2+ monocytes, are mainly clustered in hypoxic areas of solid tumors, in close proximity to nascent tumor vessels, where they are recruited by hypoxia-inducible hemotactic factors such as the CXCR4 ligand CXCL12 and angiopoietin 2 (Ang-2).[98,99]

Low oxygen tension activates macrophages to release proinflammatory cytokines and to upregulate pattern-recognition receptors and costimulatory molecules.[100–102] A recent report showed that LPS increases the levels of the tricarboxylic-acid cycle intermediate succinate, which stabilizes HIF-1α and enhances IL-1β production by macrophages.[103]

Immunological memory is a cardinal feature of the adaptive-immune system, but there is growing evidence that innate immune cells can also show memory-like behavior.[104] Epigenetic and metabolic changes are necessary for trained immunity in monocytes. Switch to glycolysis has been shown to be necessary for monocyte training by β-glucan and it seems to depend on the activation of mammalian target of rapamycin (mTOR) through a dectin 1-AKT–HIF1α-dependent pathway.[105]

An important role of PHD3 in the control of macrophage survival was described recently.[48] PHD3-deficient bone-marrow-derived macrophages (BMDMs) showed no altered HIF-1α or HIF-2α stabilization or increased HIF target gene expression in normoxia or hypoxia. Macrophage M1 and M2 polarization was unchanged likewise. However, PHD3-deficient BMDMs showed reduced apoptosis, indicating that this enzyme is crucial for macrophage survival under stress conditions.

Granulocytes

Notably, blood neutrophils can contribute to the development of local tissue hypoxia by enhancing plasmatic coagulation. When they are attracted by perivascular macrophages to inflamed tissues, neutrophils release serine proteases and extracellular nucleosomes activating clotting. In infections, this event impairs tissue perfusion and prevents systemic spreading of the bacteria.[106,107]

Moreover, the oxygen demand of transmigrating polymorphonuclear cells (PMNs) can reduce local oxygen availability and induce tissue hypoxia, as seen in the gut mucosa.[8]

Hypoxia promotes granulocyte survival.[108] In humans, neutrophils isolated from individuals harboring a heterozygous germline mutation of the *VHL* gene displayed reduced apoptosis and enhanced bacterial phagocytosis.[109] Both HIF-1α (that induces NF-κB prosurvival activity) and HIF-2α are implicated in neutrophil increased lifespan.[110,111] HIF-1α and HIF-2α seem to intervene in different phases of inflammation, with HIF-2α predominating in the resolution phases.[110] It has emerged that PHD3 also plays a pivotal role in the prolongation of PMN survival.[49] PHD3 expression is increased in neutrophils subjected to hypoxia or isolated from RA patients.

As macrophage chemotaxis in hypoxia involves the neuronal guidance protein Sema3A, another member of the family was seen to contribute to the migration of neutrophils, that is, semaphorin7A (Sema7A).[112]

HIF-1α is crucial for bactericidal activity of neutrophils. HIF-1α-deficient neutrophils have reduced levels of granule proteases and cathelicidin antimicrobial peptide.[69] In response to inflammatory stimuli and pathogens, neutrophils form neutrophil extracellular traps (NETs), which capture and kill extracellular microbes. mTOR has been shown to regulate NET formation by post-transcriptional control of expression of HIF-1α.[113] Inhibition of mTOR and HIF-1α inhibits NET-mediated extracellular bacterial killing.

Finally, hypoxia and HIF can modulate the activities of basophils and eosinophils, as investigated in studies that highlight the functional roles of HIF in asthma and allergy.[114–116]

Dendritic Cells

Dendritic cells are professional antigen-presenting cells. They act as the sentinels of innate immunity and activate the adaptive-immune response. The effects of hypoxia and HIF activation on DCs are not completely clear. HIF-1α signaling affects maturation, activation, migration, and antigen presentation of DCs.[117–120] Our group reported that low oxygen pressure modulates the activation of DCs.[121] Hypoxia strongly enhances the innate immune functions of DCs by inhibiting their maturation, while increasing the production of inflammatory cytokines and their chemotactic response toward chemokines that are selectively expressed at peripheral sites of inflammation.[121] Partially contrasting studies from other groups report that DC stimulation with LPS in hypoxia can upregulate costimulatory molecules, induce proinflammatory cytokines production, and also activate allogeneic lymphocyte proliferation.[117,122] Hypoxia can promote the upregulation of pattern-recognition receptors, components of complement receptors, and immunoregulatory receptors on DCs.[33,123,124]

Interestingly, different sets of target genes are induced by HIF-1α in response to hypoxia or TLR ligands.[125] Hypoxia, in the absence of inflammatory stimuli, promotes HIF-1α-dependent apoptosis of DCs.[126] Recently, it was reported that HIF-1α is a negative regulator of the development of a particular subset of DCs, plasmacytoid DCs.[127] HIF-1α activation in DCs is also controlled by Sirtuin 1 (SIRT1), a type III histone deacetylase. The SIRT1-HIF-1α axis promotes the activation of proinflammatory Th1 cells while restraining anti-inflammatory regulatory T cells (Tregs).[76]

The role of HIF-2α in DCs has not been characterized so far. Experiments performed in our laboratory suggest that HIF-2α has a marginal role in DC biology. Mouse bone-marrow-derived DCs lacking HIF-2α normally upregulated maturation markers in response to LPS and did not differ from wild-type DCs in terms of proinflammatory cytokines production, antigen uptake, and T cell activation.[128]

Lymphoid Cells

An extensive analysis of the impact of hypoxia on B and T lymphocytes is beyond the scope of this book, which focuses on innate immunity. However, as the two arms of the immune system act together, we will briefly present some of the effects of the hypoxic environment on cells involved in adaptive immunity. First of all, it must be said that innate immune cells are better equipped to maintain their viability and functions in hypoxia, as compared to adaptive-immune cells.[129] In fact, it has been described that non-antigen-specific proliferation is defective if T cells are cultured in hypoxic conditions.[130] HIF-1α constitutive activation represses T cell receptor signal transduction, while HIF-1α deletion enhances T cell responses.[131–133] HIF-1α affects CD4+ cell differentiation, by promoting Th17 differentiation and downregulating Tregs development.[134] One proposed mechanism for Treg downregulation is that HIF directly binds FOXP3, targeting it for degradation.[134] On the contrary, HIF-1α-dependent production of CCL28 and TGF-β promotes Treg recruitment to the tumor site.[135,136] In tumors, hypoxia is associated with the accumulation of extracellular adenosine.[137] Adenosine binding to A2A receptors promotes the generation of cAMP that inhibits T cell receptor-triggered proliferation and the production of cytokines such as IFN-γ and TNFα,[138] which establishes a powerful correlation between hypoxia and suppression of adaptive-immune responses. TCR cross-linking and cytokines (namely, IL-2 and IL4) stabilize HIF-1α and HIF-2α in activated CD8+ cells.[89,139] VHL-deficient CD8+ T cells are resistant to exhaustion due to chronic antigen exposure and have increased effector functions.[140] Moreover, HIF-1α drives CTLA-4 expression on CD8+ T cells.[140]

Chimeric mice, obtained by injecting embryonic stem cells with a homozygous disruption of the gene encoding HIF-1α into blastocysts of $Rag2^{-/-}$ or $Rag2^{+/+}$ wild-type mice, show dramatic defects in the development of B lymphocytes and autoimmunity.[141] Using B cell-specific conditional knockout, it was demonstrated that HIF-1α is a major regulator of cell cycle arrest in B cells during hypoxia.[142]

HYPOXIA, MYELOID CELLS, AND DISEASES

Low tissue oxygenation and/or HIF signaling pathway activation have been observed in several pathological conditions. Some of the pathologies in which myeloid cells are important players have been reviewed here.

Pulmonary Hypertension (PH)

PH is the result of pulmonary artery remodeling. The correlation among chronic hypoxia, PH, medial hypertrophy of the small pulmonary arteries, and right ventricular hypertrophy was first recognized due to studies in the early 1900s on brisket disease (bovine high mountain disease).[143] In fact, among mammalian species, cattle exhibit the most severe chronic hypoxic PH. A seminal study by Glover and Newsom reported that altitude was the chief causative factor of brisket disease, which was associated with "exhaustion of the heart."[144] Atmospheric hypoxia causes pulmonary changes leading to increased resistance to circulation through the lungs, consequent dilation, and failure of the right ventricle. The susceptibility to PH due to the intensity of pulmonary vascular response to hypoxia allows classifying "hyperresponders" and "hyporesponders." Among animal species, cattle and pigs are hyperresponders; sheep, dog, rabbit, and guinea pig are hyporesponders; rats are moderate responders. An intraspecies variability exists also in the human population, with some individuals displaying a minimal response to hypoxia, and others exhibiting a vigorous response.[143]

Macrophage accumulation is a critical component of PH etiopathogenesis. Using *in vivo* (bovine and rat models of hypoxia-induced PH) and *in vitro* (animal, human macrophages, and fibroblasts) approaches, El Kasmi et al. observed that adventitial fibroblasts derived from hypertensive pulmonary arteries (bovine and human) regulate macrophage activation.[145] HIF-1α is responsible for skewing macrophages toward a proinflammatory and profibrotic phenotype that can be involved in PH progression. The finding that presence of M2 macrophage is associated with the proliferation of smooth-muscle cells in the *in vitro* pulmonary artery and the development of PH *in vivo* suggests that these macrophages may play a significant role in the etiopathogenesis of PH.[146] In agreement with this hypothesis, Th2 cytokines, which are involved in M2 polarization, and Fizz-1, an M2 marker, have been also implicated in the development of PH.[146–148]

Rheumatoid Arthritis

Macrophages are more abundant in RA synovium, compared to other arthropathies such as psoriatic arthritis.[149] Number of activated synovial macrophages is predictive of the gravity of erosive damage seen in radiographs, suggesting a direct role of macrophages in the erosive process.[150] Depletion of macrophages from synovial cell cultures reduces the production of cytokines and MMPs.[151] Moreover, CD68$^+$ macrophage number in the synovium has been validated as the most relevant tissue biomarker of response to therapy in RA.[152] In RA, HIF-1α is abundantly expressed by macrophages. In fact, myeloid-specific HIF-1α knockout mice show reduced swelling of the joints and a better clinical score in a mouse model of arthritis.[62] HIF-1α is also involved in osteoclast activity. The hypoxic environment of bones promotes HIF stabilization and osteoclast-mediated progression of osteoarthritic diseases.[153,154]

NF-κB is highly activated in the synovium of RA. Proinflammatory signals, which sustain chronic inflammation, are enhanced by a positive feedback loop controlled by NF-κB.[29] Myeloid activation of NF-κB leads to the release of many cytokines, chemokines, and metalloproteases that sustain chronic and persistent inflammation.

Inflammatory Bowel Disease

In IBD, Crohn's disease, and ulcerative colitis, HIF has a protective role. Local inflammation in the gut menaces mucosal integrity. Hypoxia-induced HIF-1α stabilization helps to preserve barrier functions through the expression of barrier-protective genes.[155] Transmigrating neutrophils (that consume large amounts of oxygen during the production of hydrogen peroxide by PHOX) contribute in the generation of hypoxia in IBD and help to resolve inflammatory foci.[8]

NF-κB is crucial in the inflammation associated with IBD. Activation of NF-κB has been demonstrated in intestinal macrophages and epithelial cells.[156] NF-κB activation in macrophages potentiates inflammation, thereby leading to IBD. Conversely, NF-κB signaling in epithelial cells is protective against the development of colitis.[157,158] Local administration of p65 NF-κB-antisense phosphorothioate oligonucleotides abrogated clinical and histological signs of colitis in mouse models of Crohn's disease.[156] Several treatments have been proposed to target NF-κB in IBD. However, all these approaches faced significant systemic toxicity due to the broad role of NF-κB.[29]

Atherosclerosis

Atherosclerosis arises in the context of chronic inflammation of arterial vessels. The thickening of arteriosclerotic plaques and local inflammation determine HIF stabilization. Moreover, oxidized low-density lipoproteins can lead to HIF-1α accumulation in macrophages through a mechanism that involves ROS.[159] HIF-1α has a crucial role in promoting atherosclerosis progression.[17] HIF-1α expression is upregulated in activated macrophages within the plaque and is associated with an atheromatous inflammatory phenotype.[160] In plaque macrophages, HIF can drive the release of angiogenic factor and lipid accumulation.[3] Evidence from a mouse model of atherosclerosis indicates that local HIF activation can promote neointima formation.[161]

Ischemia

Hypoxia and/or anoxia are the natural consequences of ischemic processes. In postischemic reperfusion injury, ROS production is at first due to vascular cells, whereas a second burst of ROS production is thought to originate from phagocytic myeloid cells.[162] Transplanted organs are inflamed organs due to ROS-induced injury occurring in the donor under brain death condition and in the recipient during postischemic reperfusion.[162] Ischemia in organ grafts increases the risk of graft failure or organ rejection.[163]

Macrophages contribute to tissue repair and remodeling during acute and chronic ischemic vascular diseases. Macrophages accumulate in cardiac tissue in myocardial infarction.[164] HIF-1 and HIF2 are upregulated in macrophages in damaged tissues where they orchestrate postinfarction remodeling.[165] In the central nervous system, resident macrophages (microglia) and infiltrating macrophages participate in responses to hypoxia.[166] The region surrounding the infarct core, known as the ischemic penumbra, is characterized by moderate ischemic conditions. In this setting, HIF is activated and microglia can function in a neuroprotective manner and promote regeneration by releasing growth factors and modulating the immune response.[167] The idea of a neuroprotective function for myeloid cells in the acute phase of ischemic stroke was supported by a study using a transgenic mouse model that allows selective ablation of proliferating microglia/macrophages.[168]

Preeclampsia

Preeclampsia is a pathological condition secondary to decreased oxygenated blood supply. Fetoplacental macrophages influence placental development and function through the synthesis and secretion of cytokines and growth factors.[169] Overproduction of inflammatory cytokines in response to hypoxia is thought to lead to increased plasma levels, higher endothelial activation, and dysfunction in preeclampsia.

Allergy

In allergy, myeloid-cell-derived HIF-1α exerts immunoregulatory functions. A recent report showed that, in a mouse model of airway allergy, HIF-1α prevented hypersensitivity through macrophage-mediated immunoregulation.[170]

Cancer

Tumors are an important milieu, where hypoxia shapes the myeloid cell phenotype and functions. Hypoxia-driven HIF activation in myeloid cells promotes tumor progression as seen in murine models of breast carcinoma.[64,139] HIF-1α activation in TAMs promotes angiogenesis and impairs T cell responses.[88,139] Immunosuppression in cancer microenvironment is also mediated by MDSCs.[171]

In these cells hypoxia-induced HIF-1α signaling is responsible for the upregulation of PD-L1, a B7-family coinhibitory molecule contrasting T cell activation.[77]

THERAPEUTIC TARGETING OF HYPOXIC SIGNALING

Therapeutic approaches aimed at the modulation of tissue oxygenation or hypoxic signaling can be applied to several diseases. Significantly, responses to hypoxia are strictly dependent on the context of local inflammation. Therefore, benefits of lowering or increasing tissue oxygenation and HIF activity will depend on the local conditions. For example, hydroxylase inhibitors have a protective effect in a model of endotoxic shock, while a detrimental effect in a model of polymicrobial sepsis.[172] Moreover, HIF-α subunits can exert divergent effects. HIF-1α and HIF-2α mediate proinflammatory signaling cascades in myeloid cells. However, when HIF signaling is skewed toward HIF-1α, the response against *M. tuberculosis* is favored, thanks to NOS2 activation and antimicrobial nitrosative stress.[173] Therefore, specific targeting of HIF isoforms could be exploited to obtain the desired effect.

Due to their natural ability to accumulate in hypoxic areas, macrophages can be exploited to deliver HIF-regulated therapeutic genes to otherwise inaccessible areas in tumors. A new approach has been designed that selectively targets oncolytic adenovirus to hypoxic areas of prostate tumors, resulting in intratumoral spread and a lasting therapeutic effect.[174] Alongside this, interfering with specific chemotactic pathways (e.g., VEGF and CXCL12) and macrophage recruitment in the hypoxic areas of tumors would provide therapeutic benefits.[83,91,175] By analogy, inhibition of the hypoxia-inducible gene *Ang-2* may restrain the recruitment of Tie-2$^+$ proangiogenic monocytes.[176] Elucidation of the molecular pathways underlying macrophage adaptation to hypoxia is expected to provide novel therapeutic strategies. From this perspective, the therapeutic use of selected HIF inhibitors may potentially modulate macrophage polarization to elicit more beneficial macrophage phenotypes, associated with anti-infective, regulatory, and anticancer activities.

HIF Activators

Pharmacological inactivation of PHDs stabilizes HIF-1α.[177] However, drugs such as the 2-oxoglutarate analog DMOG are nonspecific with respect to PHD isoforms, so efforts are needed to generate specific inhibitors. Several PHD classes have been described, including iron chelators and PHD active site blockers.[177]

In ischemia, activation of HIF signaling would be expected to be of benefit to patients. Similarly, in anemia HIF-driven erythropoietin expression is desirable. Activation of the transcriptional activity of HIFs in angiogenic monocytes would benefit vasculature reconstitution. Recent evidence indicates that PHD2 inhibitors may favor tissue healing and arteriogenesis.[178]

Treatment with hydroxylase inhibitors showed a positive impact in disease progression in models of renal pathologies including ischemia reperfusion, subtotal nephrectomy, and kidney transplant.[179] PHD inhibitors FG-4592, AKB-6548, and GSK1278863 are in ongoing clinical trials in anemia-associated chronic kidney disease.[177]

A positive role for hypoxia signaling has been identified in IBD. The stabilization of HIF in the mucosa obtained by oral treatment with PHD inhibitors, can protect mice in murine models of colitis.[180–182]

Because of the positive effect on the antimicrobial activity of macrophages, HIF agonists could potentially be used alongside conventional antibiotics in localized infections.

HIF Inhibitors

HIFs represent a suitable molecular target for cancer therapy and several HIF inhibitors have been identified so far.[28,45,183] These include inhibitors of HIF-1α synthesis (digoxin, rapamycin, and topotecan), inhibitors of HIF-1α protein stability (cyclosporine, guanylate cyclase activator YC-1, HSP90 inhibitor 17-AAG, and HDAC inhibitor LAQ824), inhibitors of DNA binding (doxorubicin and echinomycin), inhibitors of transactivation (proteasome inhibitor bortezomib and antifungal agent amphotericin B), and inhibitors of signal transduction (BCR–ABL inhibitor imatinib, cyclooxygenase inhibitor ibuprofen, EGFR inhibitors erlotinib and gefitinib, and HER2 inhibitor trastuzumab).[28] Unfortunately, all these drugs also affect other signaling pathways. Till date, no low-molecular-weight inhibitor selectively targeting HIF has been identified. It is expected that blocking HIF activation in stromal myelomonocytic cells would control the expression of several mitogenic, proinvasive, proangiogenic, and prometastatic genes.[129] As a consequence, tumor would be deprived of important environmental factors needed for its survival and progression.

Despite the generation of a large array of inhibitors, very few studies are available that examine their activity on immune cells, as they have been tested mainly on hypoxic cancer cells. Because HIF-1α-deficient myeloid cells have profound impairment in migration and cytotoxicity it is, however, likely that HIF inhibitors also modulate functions of infiltrating leukocytes.[62] How this contributes to the therapeutic effect of the drugs still remains elusive. A possible concern related to HIF inhibition is the essential role of phagocytes against infections, as HIF inhibition would interfere with innate immune functions in the event of opportunistic infections.

ACKNOWLEDGMENTS

This work was supported by Associazione Italiana Ricerca sul Cancro (AIRC), Italy; Fondazione Cariplo, Italy; and the Ministero Università Ricerca (MIUR), Italy.

REFERENCES

1. McDonald DM, Baluk P. Significance of blood vessel leakiness in cancer. *Cancer Res* 2002;**62**:5381–5.

2. Strehl C, Fangradt M, Fearon U, Gaber T, Buttgereit F, Veale DJ. Hypoxia: how does the monocyte-macrophage system respond to changes in oxygen availability? *J Leukoc Biol* 2014;**95**:233–41.

3. Jantsch J, Schodel J. Hypoxia and hypoxia-inducible factors in myeloid cell-driven host defense and tissue homeostasis. *Immunobiology* 2015;**220**:305–14.

4. Abbot NC, Beck JS, Carnochan FM, Gibbs JH, Harrison DK, James PB, et al. Effect of hyperoxia at 1 and 2 ATA on hypoxia and hypercapnia in human skin during experimental inflammation. *J Appl Physiol* 1985 1994;**77**:767–73.

5. Niinikoski J, Grislis G, Hunt TK. Respiratory gas tensions and collagen in infected wounds. *Ann Surg* 1972;**175**:588–93.

6. Raju R, Weiner M, Enquist IF. Quantitation of local acidosis and hypoxia produced by infection. *Am J Surg* 1976;**132**:64–6.

7. Vaupel P, Hockel M, Mayer A. Detection and characterization of tumor hypoxia using pO_2 histography. *Antioxid Redox Signal* 2007;**9**:1221–35.

8. Campbell EL, Bruyninckx WJ, Kelly CJ, Glover LE, McNamee EN, Bowers BE, et al. Transmigrating neutrophils shape the mucosal microenvironment through localized oxygen depletion to influence resolution of inflammation. *Immunity* 2014;**40**:66–77.

9. Karhausen J, Furuta GT, Tomaszewski JE, Johnson RS, Colgan SP, Haase VH. Epithelial hypoxiainducible factor-1 is protective in murine experimental colitis. *J Clin Invest* 2004;**114**:1098–106.

10. Wang XD, Wolfbeis OS. Optical methods for sensing and imaging oxygen: materials, spectroscopies and applications. *Chem Soc Rev* 2014;**43**:3666–761.

11. Hackett PH, Roach RC. High-altitude illness. *N Engl J Med* 2001;**345**:107–14.

12. Wen D, Zhang N, Shan B, Wang S. *Helicobacter pylori* infection may be implicated in the topography and geographic variation of upper gastrointestinal cancers in the Taihang Mountain high-risk region in northern China. *Helicobacter* 2010;**15**:416–21.

13. Doust JW. Differential tissue and organ anoxia in disease: the measurement of periarticular oxygen saturation levels in patients with arthritis. *Ann Rheum Dis* 1951;**10**:269–76.

14. Lund-Olesen K. Oxygen tension in synovial fluids. *Arthritis Rheum* 1970;**13**:769–76.

15. Stevens CR, Williams RB, Farrell AJ, Blake DR. Hypoxia and inflammatory synovitis: observations and speculation. *Ann Rheum Dis* 1991;**50**:124–32.

16. Treuhaft PS, DJ MC. Synovial fluid pH, lactate, oxygen and carbon dioxide partial pressure in various joint diseases. *Arthritis Rheum* 1971;**14**:475–84.

17. Bjornheden T, Levin M, Evaldsson M, Wiklund O. Evidence of hypoxic areas within the arterial wall *in vivo*. *Arterioscler Thromb Vasc Biol* 1999;**19**:870–6.

18. Sluimer JC, Gasc JM, van Wanroij JL, Kisters N, Groeneweg M, Sollewijn Gelpke MD, et al. Hypoxia, hypoxia-inducible transcription factor, and macrophages in human atherosclerotic plaques are correlated with intraplaque angiogenesis. *J Am Coll Cardiol* 2008;**51**:1258–65.

19. Biswas S, Roy S, Banerjee J, Hussain SR, Khanna S, Meenakshisundaram G, et al. Hypoxia inducible microRNA 210 attenuates keratinocyte proliferation and impairs closure in a murine model of ischemic wounds. *Proc Natl Acad Sci USA* 2010;**107**:6976–81.

20. Rankin EB, Giaccia AJ. The role of hypoxia-inducible factors in tumorigenesis. *Cell Death Differ* 2008;**15**:678–85.

21. Vaupel P, Mayer A. Hypoxia in cancer: significance and impact on clinical outcome. *Cancer Metastasis Rev* 2007;**26**:225–39.

22. Sullivan R, Graham CH. Hypoxia-driven selection of the metastatic phenotype. *Cancer Metastasis Rev* 2007;**26**:319–31.

23. Domej W, Oettl K, Renner W. Oxidative stress and free radicals in COPD – implications and relevance for treatment. *Int J Chron Obstruct Pulmon Dis* 2014;**9**:1207–24.

24. Brambilla G, Civitareale C, Ballerini A, Fiori M, Amadori M, Archetti LI, et al. Response to oxidative stress as a welfare parameter in swine. *Redox Rep* 2002;**7**:159–63.

25. Semenza GL. Hypoxia-inducible factors: mediators of cancer progression and targets for cancer therapy. *Trends Pharmacol Sci* 2012;**33**:207–14.

26. Rius J, Guma M, Schachtrup C, Akassoglou K, Zinkernagel AS, Nizet V, et al. NF-κB links innate immunity to the hypoxic response through transcriptional regulation of HIF-1α. *Nature* 2008;**453**:807–11.

27. Rahat MA, Bitterman H, Lahat N. Molecular mechanisms regulating macrophage response to hypoxia. *Front Immunol* 2011;**2**:45.

28. Semenza GL. Hypoxia-inducible factors in physiology and medicine. *Cell* 2012;**148**:399–408.

29. Biddlestone J, Bandarra D, Rocha S. The role of hypoxia in inflammatory disease (review). *Int J Mol Med* 2015;**35**:859–69.

30. Palazon A, Goldrath AW, Nizet V, Johnson RS. HIF transcription factors, inflammation, and immunity. *Immunity* 2014;**41**:518–28.

31. Chandel NS, McClintock DS, Feliciano CE, Wood TM, Melendez JA, Rodriguez AM, et al. Reactive oxygen species generated at mitochondrial complex III stabilize hypoxia-inducible factor-1α during hypoxia: a mechanism of O_2 sensing. *J Biol Chem* 2000;**275**:25118–30.

32. Dehne N, Brune B. HIF-1 in the inflammatory microenvironment. *Exp Cell Res* 2009;**315**:1791–7.

33. Kumar V, Gabrilovich DI. Hypoxia-inducible factors in regulation of immune responses in tumour microenvironment. *Immunology* 2014;**143**:512–9.

34. Warburg O. On respiratory impairment in cancer cells. *Science* 1956;**124**:269–70.

35. Mazurek S, Boschek CB, Hugo F, Eigenbrodt E. Pyruvate kinase type M2 and its role in tumor growth and spreading. *Semin Cancer Biol* 2005;**15**:300–8.

36. Beck-Schimmer B, Schimmer RC, Madjdpour C, Bonvini JM, Pasch T, Ward PA. Hypoxia mediates increased neutrophil and macrophage adhesiveness to alveolar epithelial cells. *Am J Respir Cell Mol Biol* 2001;**25**:780–7.

37. Bosco MC, Delfino S, Ferlito F, Puppo M, Gregorio A, Gambini C, et al. The hypoxic synovial environment regulates expression of vascular endothelial growth factor and osteopontin in juvenile idiopathic arthritis. *J Rheumatol* 2009;**36**:1318–29.

38. Kuhlicke J, Frick JS, Morote-Garcia JC, Rosenberger P, Eltzschig HK. Hypoxia inducible factor (HIF)-1 coordinates induction of Toll-like receptors TLR2 and TLR6 during hypoxia. *PLoS One* 2007;**2**:e1364.

39. Iyer NV, Kotch LE, Agani F, Leung SW, Laughner E, Wenger RH, et al. Cellular and developmental control of O_2 homeostasis by hypoxia-inducible factor 1 α. *Genes Dev* 1998;**12**:149–62.

40. Ryan HE, Lo J, Johnson RS. HIF-1 α is required for solid tumor formation and embryonic vascularization. *EMBO J* 1998;**17**:3005–15.

41. Peng J, Zhang L, Drysdale L, Fong GH. The transcription factor EPAS-1/hypoxia-inducible factor 2α plays an important role in vascular remodeling. *Proc Natl Acad Sci USA* 2000;**97**:8386–91.

42. Tian H, Hammer RE, Matsumoto AM, Russell DW, McKnight SL. The hypoxia-responsive transcription factor EPAS1 is essential for catecholamine homeostasis and protection against heart failure during embryonic development. *Genes Dev* 1998;**12**:3320–4.

43. Compernolle V, Brusselmans K, Acker T, Hoet P, Tjwa M, Beck H, et al. Loss of HIF-2α and inhibition of *VEGF* impair fetal lung maturation, whereas treatment with *VEGF* prevents fatal respiratory distress in premature mice. *Nat Med* 2002;**8**:702–10.

44. Scortegagna M, Ding K, Oktay Y, Gaur A, Thurmond F, Yan LJ, et al. Multiple organ pathology, metabolic abnormalities and impaired homeostasis of reactive oxygen species in EPAS1$^{-/-}$ mice. *Nat Genet* 2003;**35**:331–40.

45. Semenza GL. Targeting HIF-1 for cancer therapy. *Nat Rev Cancer* 2003;**3**:721–32.

46. Lofstedt T, Fredlund E, Holmquist-Mengelbier L, Pietras A, Ovenberger M, Poellinger L, et al. Hypoxia inducible factor-2α in cancer. *Cell Cycle* 2007;**6**:919–26.

47. Rapisarda A, Shoemaker RH, Melillo G. Antiangiogenic agents and HIF-1 inhibitors meet at the crossroads. *Cell Cycle* 2009;**8**:4040–3.

48. Swain L, Wottawa M, Hillemann A, Beneke A, Odagiri H, Terada K, et al. Prolyl-4-hydroxylase domain 3 (PHD3) is a critical terminator for cell survival of macrophages under stress conditions. *J Leukoc Biol* 2014;**96**:365–75.

49. Walmsley SR, Chilvers ER, Thompson AA, Vaughan K, Marriott HM, Parker LC, et al. Prolyl hydroxylase 3 (PHD3) is essential for hypoxic regulation of neutrophilic inflammation in humans and mice. *J Clin Invest* 2011;**121**:1053–63.

50. Escribese MM, Sierra-Filardi E, Nieto C, Samaniego R, Sanchez-Torres C, Matsuyama T, et al. The prolyl hydroxylase PHD3 identifies proinflammatory macrophages and its expression is regulated by activin A. *J Immunol* 2012;**189**:1946–54.

51. Kiss J, Mollenhauer M, Walmsley SR, Kirchberg J, Radhakrishnan P, Niemietz T, et al. Loss of the oxygen sensor PHD3 enhances the innate immune response to abdominal sepsis. *J Immunol* 2012;**189**:1955–65.

52. Tausendschon M, Dehne N, Brune B. Hypoxia causes epigenetic gene regulation in macrophages by attenuating Jumonji histone demethylase activity. *Cytokine* 2011;**53**:256–62.

53. Vallabhapurapu S, Karin M. Regulation and function of NF-κB transcription factors in the immune system. *Annu Rev Immunol* 2009;**27**:693–733.

54. Taylor CT, Cummins EP. The role of NF-κB in hypoxia-induced gene expression. *Ann N Y Acad Sci* 2009;**1177**:178–84.

55. Bonello S, Zahringer C, BelAiba RS, Djordjevic T, Hess J, Michiels C, et al. Reactive oxygen species activate the HIF-1α promoter via a functional NF-κB site. *Arterioscler Thromb Vasc Biol* 2007;**27**:755–61.

56. Chandel NS, Trzyna WC, McClintock DS, Schumacker PT. Role of oxidants in NF-κB activation and TNF-α gene transcription induced by hypoxia and endotoxin. *J Immunol* 2000;**165**:1013–21.

57. Takeda K, Ichiki T, Narabayashi E, Inanaga K, Miyazaki R, Hashimoto T, et al. Inhibition of prolyl hydroxylase domain-containing protein suppressed lipopolysaccharide-induced TNF-α expression. *Arterioscler Thromb Vasc Biol* 2009;**29**:2132–7.

58. Cummins EP, Berra E, Comerford KM, Ginouves A, Fitzgerald KT, Seeballuck F, et al. Prolyl hydroxylase-1 negatively regulates IκB kinase-β, giving insight into hypoxia-induced NF-κB activity. *Proc Natl Acad Sci USA* 2006;**103**:18154–9.

59. Patel SA, Simon MC. Biology of hypoxia-inducible factor-2α in development and disease. *Cell Death Differ* 2008;**15**:628–34.

60. van Uden P, Kenneth NS, Rocha S. Regulation of hypoxia-inducible factor-1α by NF-κB. *Biochem J* 2008;**412**:477–84.

61. O'Connell RM, Rao DS, Chaudhuri AA, Boldin MP, Taganov KD, Nicoll J, et al. Sustained expression of microRNA-155 in hematopoietic stem cells causes a myeloproliferative disorder. *J Exp Med* 2008;**205**:585–94.

62. Cramer T, Yamanishi Y, Clausen BE, Forster I, Pawlinski R, Mackman N, et al. HIF-1α is essential for myeloid cell-mediated inflammation. *Cell* 2003;**112**:645–57.

63. Peyssonnaux C, Cejudo-Martin P, Doedens A, Zinkernagel AS, Johnson RS, Nizet V. Cutting edge: essential role of hypoxia inducible factor-1α in development of lipopolysaccharide-induced sepsis. *J Immunol* 2007;**178**:7516–9.

64. Imtiyaz HZ, Williams EP, Hickey MM, Patel SA, Durham AC, Yuan LJ, et al. Hypoxia-inducible factor 2α regulates macrophage function in mouse models of acute and tumor inflammation. *J Clin Invest* 2010;**120**:2699–714.

65. Rymsa B, Wang JF, de Groot H. O_2^- release by activated Kupffer cells upon hypoxia-reoxygenation. *Am J Physiol* 1991;**261**:G602–7.

66. Daniliuc S, Bitterman H, Rahat MA, Kinarty A, Rosenzweig D, Lahat N. Hypoxia inactivates inducible nitric oxide synthase in mouse macrophages by disrupting its interaction with alpha-actinin 4. *J Immunol* 2003;**171**:3225–32.

67. Robinson MA, Baumgardner JE, Good VP, Otto CM. Physiological and hypoxic O_2 tensions rapidly regulate NO production by stimulated macrophages. *Am J Physiol Cell Physiol* 2008;**294**:C1079–87.

68. Schmidt SK, Ebel S, Keil E, Woite C, Ernst JF, Benzin AE, et al. Regulation of IDO activity by oxygen supply: inhibitory effects on antimicrobial and immunoregulatory functions. *PLoS One* 2013;**8**:e63301.

69. Peyssonnaux C, Datta V, Cramer T, Doedens A, Theodorakis EA, Gallo RL, et al. HIF-1α expression regulates the bactericidal capacity of phagocytes. *J Clin Invest* 2005;**115**:1806–15.

70. Nickel D, Busch M, Mayer D, Hagemann B, Knoll V, Stenger S. Hypoxia triggers the expression of human β defensin 2 and antimicrobial activity against *Mycobacterium tuberculosis* in human macrophages. *J Immunol* 2012;**188**:4001–7.

71. Owings RA, Boerma M, Wang J, Berbee M, Laderoute KR, Soderberg LS, et al. Selective deficiency of HIF-1α in myeloid cells influences secondary intention wound healing in mouse skin. *In Vivo* 2009;**23**:879–84.

72. Copple BL, Kaska S, Wentling C. Hypoxia-inducible factor activation in myeloid cells contributes to the development of liver fibrosis in cholestatic mice. *J Pharmacol Exp Ther* 2012;**341**:307–16.

73. Kobayashi H, Gilbert V, Liu Q, Kapitsinou PP, Unger TL, Rha J, et al. Myeloid cell-derived hypoxia-inducible factor attenuates inflammation in unilateral ureteral obstruction-induced kidney injury. *J Immunol* 2012;**188**:5106–15.

74. Sica A, Porta C, Morlacchi S, Banfi S, Strauss L, Rimoldi M, et al. Origin and functions of tumor-associated myeloid cells (TAMCs). *Cancer Microenviron* 2012;**5**:133–49.

75. Corzo CA, Condamine T, Lu L, Cotter MJ, Youn JI, Cheng P, et al. HIF-1α regulates function and differentiation of myeloid-derived suppressor cells in the tumor microenvironment. *J Exp Med* 2010;**207**:2439–53.

76. Liu G, Bi Y, Shen B, Yang H, Zhang Y, Wang X, et al. Sirt1 limits the function and fate of myeloid-derived suppressor cells in tumors by orchestrating HIF-1α-dependent glycolysis. *Cancer Res* 2014;**74**:727–37.

77. Noman MZ, Desantis G, Janji B, Hasmim M, Karray S, Dessen P, et al. PD-L1 is a novel direct target of HIF-1α, and its blockade under hypoxia enhanced MDSC-mediated T cell activation. *J Exp Med* 2014;**211**:781–90.

78. Cipolleschi MG, Dello Sbarba P, Olivotto M. The role of hypoxia in the maintenance of hematopoietic stem cells. *Blood* 1993;**82**:2031–7.

79. Roiniotis J, Dinh H, Masendycz P, Turner A, Elsegood CL, Scholz GM, et al. Hypoxia prolongs monocyte/macrophage survival and enhanced glycolysis is associated with their maturation under aerobic conditions. *J Immunol* 2009;**182**:7974–81.

80. Bosco MC, Puppo M, Santangelo C, Anfosso L, Pfeffer U, Fardin P, et al. Hypoxia modifies the transcriptome of primary human monocytes: modulation of novel immune-related genes and identification of CC-chemokine ligand 20 as a new hypoxia-inducible gene. *J Immunol* 2006;**177**:1941–55.

81. Burke B, Giannoudis A, Corke KP, Gill D, Wells M, Ziegler-Heitbrock L, et al. Hypoxia-induced gene expression in human macrophages: implications for ischemic tissues and hypoxia-regulated gene therapy. *Am J Pathol* 2003;**163**:1233–43.

82. Battaglia F, Delfino S, Merello E, Puppo M, Piva R, Varesio L, et al. Hypoxia transcriptionally induces macrophage-inflammatory protein-3alpha/CCL-20 in primary human mononuclear phagocytes through nuclear factor (NF)-κB. *J Leukoc Biol* 2008;**83**:648–62.

83. Schioppa T, Uranchimeg B, Saccani A, Biswas SK, Doni A, Rapisarda A, et al. Regulation of the chemokine receptor CXCR4 by hypoxia. *J Exp Med* 2003;**198**:1391–402.

84. Ceradini DJ, Kulkarni AR, Callaghan MJ, Tepper OM, Bastidas N, Kleinman ME, et al. Progenitor cell trafficking is regulated by hypoxic gradients through HIF-1 induction of SDF-1. *Nat Med* 2004;**10**:858–64.

85. Bosco MC, Reffo G, Puppo M, Varesio L. Hypoxia inhibits the expression of the CCR5 chemokine receptor in macrophages. *Cell Immunol* 2004;**228**:1–7.

86. Sica A, Bronte V. Altered macrophage differentiation and immune dysfunction in tumor development. *J Clin Invest* 2007;**117**:1155–66.

87. Sica A, Mantovani A. Macrophage plasticity and polarization: *in vivo* veritas. *J Clin Invest* 2012;**122**:787–95.

88. Werno C, Menrad H, Weigert A, Dehne N, Goerdt S, Schledzewski K, et al. Knockout of HIF-1α in tumor-associated macrophages enhances M2 polarization and attenuates their pro-angiogenic responses. *Carcinogenesis* 2010;**31**:1863–72.

89. Takeda N, O'Dea EL, Doedens A, Kim JW, Weidemann A, Stockmann C, et al. Differential activation and antagonistic function of HIF-α isoforms in macrophages are essential for NO homeostasis. *Genes Dev* 2010;**24**:491–501.

90. Shalova IN, Lim JY, Chittezhath M, Zinkernagel AS, Beasley F, Hernandez-Jimenez E, et al. Human monocytes undergo functional re-programming during sepsis mediated by hypoxia-inducible factor-1α. *Immunity* 2015;**42**:484–98.

91. Mantovani A, Sica A. Macrophages, innate immunity and cancer: balance, tolerance, and diversity. *Curr Opin Immunol* 2010;**22**:231–7.

92. Bingle L, Brown NJ, Lewis CE. The role of tumour-associated macrophages in tumour progression: implications for new anticancer therapies. *J Pathol* 2002;**196**:254–65.

93. Du R, Lu KV, Petritsch C, Liu P, Ganss R, Passegue E, et al. HIF-1α induces the recruitment of bone marrow-derived vascular modulatory cells to regulate tumor angiogenesis and invasion. *Cancer Cell* 2008;**13**:206–20.

94. Grimshaw MJ, Wilson JL, Balkwill FR. Endothelin-2 is a macrophage chemoattractant: implications for macrophage distribution in tumors. *Eur J Immunol* 2002;**32**:2393–400.

95. Casazza A, Laoui D, Wenes M, Rizzolio S, Bassani N, Mambretti M, et al. Impeding macrophage entry into hypoxic tumor areas by Sema3A/Nrp1 signaling blockade inhibits angiogenesis and restores antitumor immunity. *Cancer Cell* 2013;**24**:695–709.

96. Colegio OR, Chu NQ, Szabo AL, Chu T, Rhebergen AM, Jairam V, et al. Functional polarization of tumour-associated macrophages by tumour-derived lactic acid. *Nature* 2014;**513**:559–63.

97. Eubank TD, Roda JM, Liu H, O'Neil T, Marsh CB. Opposing roles for HIF-1α and HIF-2α in the regulation of angiogenesis by mononuclear phagocytes. *Blood* 2011;**117**:323–32.

98. De Palma M, Venneri MA, Galli R, Sergi Sergi L, Politi LS, Sampaolesi M, et al. Tie2 identifies a hematopoietic lineage of proangiogenic monocytes required for tumor vessel formation and a mesenchymal population of pericyte progenitors. *Cancer Cell* 2005;**8**:211–26.

99. Welford AF, Biziato D, Coffelt SB, Nucera S, Fisher M, Pucci F, et al. Tie2-expressing macrophages limit the therapeutic efficacy of the vascular-disrupting agent combretastatin A4 phosphate in mice. *J Clin Invest* 2011;**121**:1969–73.

100. Hempel SL, Monick MM, Hunninghake GW. Effect of hypoxia on release of IL-1 and TNF by human alveolar macrophages. *Am J Respir Cell Mol Biol* 1996;**14**:170–6.

101. Kim SY, Choi YJ, Joung SM, Lee BH, Jung YS, Lee JY. Hypoxic stress up-regulates the expression of Toll-like receptor 4 in macrophages via hypoxia-inducible factor. *Immunology* 2010;**129**:516–24.

102. Acosta-Iborra B, Elorza A, Olazabal IM, Martin-Cofreces NB, Martin-Puig S, Miro M, et al. Macrophage oxygen sensing modulates antigen presentation and phagocytic functions involving IFN-γ production through the HIF-1α transcription factor. *J Immunol* 2009;**182**:3155–64.

103. Tannahill GM, Curtis AM, Adamik J, Palsson-McDermott EM, McGettrick AF, Goel G, et al. Succinate is an inflammatory signal that induces IL-1β through HIF-1α. *Nature* 2013;**496**:238–42.

104. Bordon Y. Macrophages: innate memory training. *Nat Rev Immunol* 2014;**14**:713.

105. Cheng SC, Quintin J, Cramer RA, Shepardson KM, Saeed S, Kumar V, et al. mTOR- and HIF-1α-mediated aerobic glycolysis as metabolic basis for trained immunity. *Science* 2014;**345**:1250684.

106. Abtin A, Jain R, Mitchell AJ, Roediger B, Brzoska AJ, Tikoo S, et al. Perivascular macrophages mediate neutrophil recruitment during bacterial skin infection. *Nat Immunol* 2014;**15**:45–53.

107. Massberg S, Grahl L, Von Bruehl ML, Manukyan D, Pfeiler S, Goosmann C, et al. Reciprocal coupling of coagulation and innate immunity via neutrophil serine proteases. *Nat Med* 2010;**16**:887–96.

108. Hannah S, Mecklenburgh K, Rahman I, Bellingan GJ, Greening A, Haslett C, et al. Hypoxia prolongs neutrophil survival *in vitro*. *FEBS Lett* 1995;**372**:233–7.

109. Walmsley SR, Cowburn AS, Clatworthy MR, Morrell NW, Roper EC, Singleton V, et al. Neutrophils from patients with heterozygous germline mutations in the Von Hippel Lindau protein (pVHL) display delayed apoptosis and enhanced bacterial phagocytosis. *Blood* 2006;**108**:3176–8.

110. Thompson AA, Elks PM, Marriott HM, Eamsamarng S, Higgins KR, Lewis A, et al. Hypoxia-inducible factor 2α regulates key neutrophil functions in humans, mice, and zebrafish. *Blood* 2014;**123**:366–76.

111. Walmsley SR, Print C, Farahi N, Peyssonnaux C, Johnson RS, Cramer T, et al. Hypoxia-induced neutrophil survival is mediated by HIF-1α-dependent NF-κB activity. *J Exp Med* 2005;**201**:105–15.

112. Morote-Garcia JC, Napiwotzky D, Kohler D, Rosenberger P. Endothelial semaphorin 7A promotes neutrophil migration during hypoxia. *Proc Natl Acad Sci USA* 2012;**109**:14146–51.

113. McInturff AM, Cody MJ, Elliott EA, Glenn JW, Rowley JW, Rondina MT, et al. Mammalian target of rapamycin regulates neutrophil extracellular trap formation via induction of hypoxia-inducible factor 1α. *Blood* 2012;**120**:3118–25.

114. Crotty Alexander LE, Akong-Moore K, Feldstein S, Johansson P, Nguyen A, McEachern EK, et al. Myeloid cell HIF-1α regulates asthma airway resistance and eosinophil function. *J Mol Med (Berlin)* 2013;**91**:637–44.

115. Nissim Ben Efraim AH, Eliashar R, Levi-Schaffer F. Hypoxia modulates human eosinophil function. *Clin Mol Allergy* 2010;**8**:10.

116. Sumbayev VV, Yasinska I, Oniku AE, Streatfield CL, Gibbs BF. Involvement of hypoxia-inducible factor-1 in the inflammatory responses of human LAD2 mast cells and basophils. *PLoS One* 2012;**7**:e34259.

117. Jantsch J, Chakravortty D, Turza N, Prechtel AT, Buchholz B, Gerlach RG, et al. Hypoxia and hypoxia-inducible factor-1α modulate lipopolysaccharide-induced dendritic cell activation and function. *J Immunol* 2008;**180**:4697–705.

118. Kohler T, Reizis B, Johnson RS, Weighardt H, Forster I. Influence of hypoxia-inducible factor 1α on dendritic cell differentiation and migration. *Eur J Immunol* 2012;**42**:1226–36.

119. Spirig R, Djafarzadeh S, Regueira T, Shaw SG, Von Garnier C, Takala J, et al. Effects of TLR agonists on the hypoxia-regulated transcription factor HIF-1α and dendritic cell maturation under normoxic conditions. *PLoS One* 2010;**5**:e0010983.

120. Wobben R, Husecken Y, Lodewick C, Gibbert K, Fandrey J, Winning S. Role of hypoxia inducible factor-1α for interferon synthesis in mouse dendritic cells. *Biol Chem* 2013;**394**: 495–505.

121. Mancino A, Schioppa T, Larghi P, Pasqualini F, Nebuloni M, Chen IH, et al. Divergent effects of hypoxia on dendritic cell functions. *Blood* 2008;**112**:3723–34.

122. Bhandari T, Olson J, Johnson RS, Nizet V. HIF-1α influences myeloid cell antigen presentation and response to subcutaneous OVA vaccination. *J Mol Med (Berlin)* 2013;**91**:1199–205.

123. Bosco MC, Pierobon D, Blengio F, Raggi F, Vanni C, Gattorno M, et al. Hypoxia modulates the gene expression profile of immunoregulatory receptors in human mature dendritic cells: identification of TREM-1 as a novel hypoxic marker *in vitro* and *in vivo. Blood* 2011;**117**:2625–39.

124. Pierobon D, Bosco MC, Blengio F, Raggi F, Eva A, Filippi M, et al. Chronic hypoxia reprograms human immature dendritic cells by inducing a proinflammatory phenotype and TREM-1 expression. *Eur J Immunol* 2013;**43**:949–66.

125. Jantsch J, Wiese M, Schodel J, Castiglione K, Glasner J, Kolbe S, et al. Toll-like receptor activation and hypoxia use distinct signaling pathways to stabilize hypoxia-inducible factor 1alpha (HIF-1α) and result in differential HIF-1α-dependent gene expression. *J Leukoc Biol* 2011;**90**:551–62.

126. Naldini A, Morena E, Pucci A, Miglietta D, Riboldi E, Sozzani S, et al. Hypoxia affects dendritic cell survival: role of the hypoxia-inducible factor-1α and lipopolysaccharide. *J Cell Physiol* 2012;**227**:587–95.

127. Weigert A, Weichand B, Sekar D, Sha W, Hahn C, Mora J, et al. HIF-1α is a negative regulator of plasmacytoid DC development *in vitro* and *in vivo. Blood* 2012;**120**:3001–6.

128. Riboldi E, Zitelli F, Morlacchi, S, Porta C, Vezzoli I, Sica A. Study of the role of HIF-2 in dendritic cell maturation. Manuscript in preparation.

129. Sica A, Melillo G, Varesio L. Hypoxia: a double-edged sword of immunity. *J Mol Med (Berlin)* 2011;**89**:657–65.

130. Atkuri KR, Herzenberg LA, Niemi AK, Cowan T. Importance of culturing primary lymphocytes at physiological oxygen levels. *Proc Natl Acad Sci USA* 2007;**104**:4547–52.

131. Neumann AK, Yang J, Biju MP, Joseph SK, Johnson RS, Haase VH, et al. Hypoxia inducible factor 1 alpha regulates T cell receptor signal transduction. *Proc Natl Acad Sci USA* 2005;**102**:17071–6.

132. Lukashev D, Klebanov B, Kojima H, Grinberg A, Ohta A, Berenfeld L, et al. Cutting edge: hypoxia-inducible factor 1α and its activation-inducible short isoform I.1 negatively regulate functions of CD4+ and CD8+ T lymphocytes. *J Immunol* 2006;**177**:4962–5.

133. Thiel M, Caldwell CC, Kreth S, Kuboki S, Chen P, Smith P, et al. Targeted deletion of HIF-1α gene in T cells prevents their inhibition in hypoxic inflamed tissues and improves septic mice survival. *PLoS One* 2007;**2**:e853.

134. Dang EV, Barbi J, Yang HY, Jinasena D, Yu H, Zheng Y, et al. Control of T (h)17/T (reg) balance by hypoxia-inducible factor 1. *Cell* 2011;**146**:772–84.

135. Facciabene A, Peng X, Hagemann IS, Balint K, Barchetti A, Wang LP, et al. Tumour hypoxia promotes tolerance and angiogenesis via CCL28 and T (reg) cells. *Nature* 2011;**475**:226–30.

136. Glinka Y, Prud'homme GJ. Neuropilin-1 is a receptor for transforming growth factor β-1, activates its latent form, and promotes regulatory T cell activity. *J Leukoc Biol* 2008;**84**:302–10.

137. Sitkovsky M, Lukashev D. Regulation of immune cells by local-tissue oxygen tension: HIF1 α and adenosine receptors. *Nat Rev Immunol* 2005;**5**:712–21.

138. Sitkovsky MV, Kjaergaard J, Lukashev D, Ohta A. Hypoxia-adenosinergic immunosuppression: tumor protection by T regulatory cells and cancerous tissue hypoxia. *Clin Cancer Res* 2008;**14**:5947–52.

139. Doedens AL, Stockmann C, Rubinstein MP, Liao D, Zhang N, DeNardo DG, et al. Macrophage expression of hypoxia-inducible factor-1 α suppresses T-cell function and promotes tumor progression. *Cancer Res* 2010;**70**:7465–75.

140. Doedens AL, Phan AT, Stradner MH, Fujimoto JK, Nguyen JV, Yang E, et al. Hypoxia-inducible factors enhance the effector responses of CD8 (+) T cells to persistent antigen. *Nat Immunol* 2013;**14**:1173–82.

141. Kojima H, Gu H, Nomura S, Caldwell CC, Kobata T, Carmeliet P, et al. Abnormal B lymphocyte development and autoimmunity in hypoxia-inducible factor 1α-deficient chimeric mice. *Proc Natl Acad Sci USA* 2002;**99**:2170–4.

142. Goda N, Ryan HE, Khadivi B, McNulty W, Rickert RC, Johnson RS. Hypoxia-inducible factor 1α is essential for cell cycle arrest during hypoxia. *Mol Cell Biol* 2003;**23**:359–69.

143. Rhodes J. Comparative physiology of hypoxic pulmonary hypertension: historical clues from brisket disease. *J Appl Physiol* 2005;**98**:1092–100.

144. Glover GH, Newsom IE. Brisket disease (dropsy of high altitude). *Colorado Agriculture Experiment Station. 204 preliminary report* 1915;3–24.

145. El Kasmi KC, Pugliese SC, Riddle SR, Poth JM, Anderson AL, Frid MG, et al. Adventitial fibroblasts induce a distinct proinflammatory/profibrotic macrophage phenotype in pulmonary hypertension. *J Immunol* 2014;**193**:597–609.

146. Vergadi E, Chang MS, Lee C, Liang OD, Liu X, Fernandez-Gonzalez A, et al. Early macrophage recruitment and alternative activation are critical for the later development of hypoxia-induced pulmonary hypertension. *Circulation* 2011;**123**:1986–95.

147. Daley E, Emson C, Guignabert C, de Waal Malefyt R, Louten J, Kurup VP, et al. Pulmonary arterial remodeling induced by a Th2 immune response. *J Exp Med* 2008;**205**:361–72.

148. Teng X, Li D, Champion HC, Johns RA. Fizz1/RELMα, a novel hypoxia-induced mitogenic factor in lung with vasoconstrictive and angiogenic properties. *Circ Res* 2003;**92**:1065–7.

149. Veale D, Yanni G, Rogers S, Barnes L, Bresnihan B, Fitzgerald O. Reduced synovial membrane macrophage numbers, ELAM-1 expression, and lining layer hyperplasia in psoriatic arthritis as compared with rheumatoid arthritis. *Arthritis Rheum* 1993;**36**:893–900.

150. Mulherin D, Fitzgerald O, Bresnihan B. Clinical improvement and radiological deterioration in rheumatoid arthritis: evidence that the pathogenesis of synovial inflammation and articular erosion may differ. *Br J Rheumatol* 1996;**35**:1263–8.

151. Janusz MJ, Hare M. Cartilage degradation by cocultures of transformed macrophage and fibroblast cell lines. A model of metalloproteinase-mediated connective tissue degradation. *J Immunol* 1993;**150**:1922–31.

152. Bresnihan B, Pontifex E, Thurlings RM, Vinkenoog M, El-Gabalawy H, Fearon U, et al. Synovial tissue sublining CD68 expression is a biomarker of therapeutic response in rheumatoid arthritis clinical trials: consistency across centers. *J Rheumatol* 2009;**36**:1800–2.

153. Arnett TR, Gibbons DC, Utting JC, Orriss IR, Hoebertz A, Rosendaal M, et al. Hypoxia is a major stimulator of osteoclast formation and bone resorption. *J Cell Physiol* 2003; **196**:2–8.

154. Knowles HJ, Cleton-Jansen AM, Korsching E, Athanasou NA. Hypoxia-inducible factor regulates osteoclast-mediated bone resorption: role of angiopoietin-like 4. *FASEB J* 2010;**24**:4648–59.

155. Colgan SP, Eltzschig HK. Adenosine and hypoxia-inducible factor signaling in intestinal injury and recovery. *Annu Rev Physiol* 2012;**74**:153–75.

156. Neurath MF, Pettersson S, Meyer zum Buschenfelde KH, Strober W. Local administration of antisense phosphorothioate oligonucleotides to the p65 subunit of NF-κB abrogates established experimental colitis in mice. *Nat Med* 1996;**2**:998–1004.

157. Greten FR, Eckmann L, Greten TF, Park JM, Li ZW, Egan LJ, et al. IKKβ links inflammation and tumorigenesis in a mouse model of colitis-associated cancer. *Cell* 2004;**118**:285–96.

158. Zaph C, Troy AE, Taylor BC, Berman-Booty LD, Guild KJ, Du Y, et al. Epithelial-cell-intrinsic IKK-β expression regulates intestinal immune homeostasis. *Nature* 2007;**446**:552–6.

159. Shatrov VA, Sumbayev VV, Zhou J, Brune B. Oxidized low-density lipoprotein (oxLDL) triggers hypoxia-inducible factor-1α (HIF-1α) accumulation via redox-dependent mechanisms. *Blood* 2003;**101**:4847–9.

160. Vink A, Schoneveld AH, Lamers D, Houben AJ, van der Groep P, van Diest PJ, et al. HIF-1 α expression is associated with an atheromatous inflammatory plaque phenotype and upregulated in activated macrophages. *Atherosclerosis* 2007;**195**:e69–75.

161. Christoph M, Ibrahim K, Hesse K, Augstein A, Schmeisser A, Braun-Dullaeus RC, et al. Local inhibition of hypoxia-inducible factor reduces neointima formation after arterial injury in ApoE$^{-/-}$ mice. *Atherosclerosis* 2014;**233**:641–7.

162. Land WG. Emerging role of innate immunity in organ transplantation: part I: evolution of innate immunity and oxidative allograft injury. *Transplant Rev Orlando* 2012;**26**:60–72.

163. Kruger B, Krick S, Dhillon N, Lerner SM, Ames S, Bromberg JS, et al. Donor Toll-like receptor 4 contributes to ischemia and reperfusion injury following human kidney transplantation. *Proc Natl Acad Sci USA* 2009;**106**:3390–5.

164. Lambert JM, Lopez EF, Lindsey ML. Macrophage roles following myocardial infarction. *Int J Cardiol* 2008;**130**:147–58.

165. Jurgensen JS, Rosenberger C, Wiesener MS, Warnecke C, Horstrup JH, Grafe M, et al. Persistent induction of HIF-1α and -2α in cardiomyocytes and stromal cells of ischemic myocardium. *FASEB J* 2004;**18**:1415–7.

166. Weinstein JR, Koerner IP, Moller T. Microglia in ischemic brain injury. *Future Neurol* 2010;**5**:227–46.

167. Streit WJ. Microglia as neuroprotective, immunocompetent cells of the CNS. *Glia* 2002;**40**:133–9.

168. Lalancette-Hebert M, Gowing G, Simard A, Weng YC, Kriz J. Selective ablation of proliferating microglial cells exacerbates ischemic injury in the brain. *J Neurosci* 2007;**27**:2596–605.

169. Mor G, Abrahams VM. Potential role of macrophages as immunoregulators of pregnancy. *Reprod Biol Endocrinol* 2003;**1**:119.

170. Toussaint M, Fievez L, Drion PV, Cataldo D, Bureau F, Lekeux P, et al. Myeloid hypoxia-inducible factor 1α prevents airway allergy in mice through macrophage-mediated immunoregulation. *Mucosal Immunol* 2013;**6**:485–97.

171. Gabrilovich DI, Ostrand-Rosenberg S, Bronte V. Coordinated regulation of myeloid cells by tumours. *Nat Rev Immunol* 2012;**12**:253–68.

172. Hams E, Saunders SP, Cummins EP, O'Connor A, Tambuwala MT, Gallagher WM, et al. The hydroxylase inhibitor dimethyloxallyl glycine attenuates endotoxic shock via alternative activation of macrophages and IL-10 production by B1 cells. *Shock* 2011;**36**:295–302.

173. Elks PM, Brizee S, van der Vaart M, Walmsley SR, van Eeden FJ, Renshaw SA, et al. Hypoxia inducible factor signaling modulates susceptibility to mycobacterial infection via a nitric oxide dependent mechanism. *PLoS Pathog* 2013;**9**:e1003789.

174. Muthana M, Giannoudis A, Scott SD, Fang HY, Coffelt SB, Morrow FJ, et al. Use of macrophages to target therapeutic adenovirus to human prostate tumors. *Cancer Res* 2011;**71**:1805–15.

175. Murdoch C, Muthana M, Lewis CE. Hypoxia regulates macrophage functions in inflammation. *J Immunol* 2005;**175**:6257–63.

176. Mazzieri R, Pucci F, Moi D, Zonari E, Ranghetti A, Berti A, et al. Targeting the *Ang2/Tie2* axis inhibits tumor growth and metastasis by impairing angiogenesis and disabling rebounds of proangiogenic myeloid cells. *Cancer Cell* 2011;**19**:512–26.

177. Eltzschig HK, Bratton DL, Colgan SP. Targeting hypoxia signalling for the treatment of ischaemic and inflammatory diseases. *Nat Rev Drug Discov* 2014;**13**:852–69.

178. Takeda Y, Costa S, Delamarre E, Roncal C, Leite de Oliveira R, Squadrito ML, et al. Macrophage skewing by PHD2 haplodeficiency prevents ischaemia by inducing arteriogenesis. *Nature* 2011;**479**:122–6.

179. Scholz CC, Taylor CT. Targeting the HIF pathway in inflammation and immunity. *Curr Opin Pharmacol* 2013;**13**:646–53.

180. Cummins EP, Seeballuck F, Keely SJ, Mangan NE, Callanan JJ, Fallon PG, et al. The hydroxylase inhibitor dimethyloxalylglycine is protective in a murine model of colitis. *Gastroenterology* 2008;**134**:156–65.

181. Robinson A, Keely S, Karhausen J, Gerich ME, Furuta GT, Colgan SP. Mucosal protection by hypoxia-inducible factor prolyl hydroxylase inhibition. *Gastroenterology* 2008;**134**:145–55.

182. Fraisl P, Aragones J, Carmeliet P. Inhibition of oxygen sensors as a therapeutic strategy for ischaemic and inflammatory disease. *Nat Rev Drug Discov* 2009;**8**:139–52.

183. Melillo G. Targeting hypoxia cell signaling for cancer therapy. *Cancer Metastasis Rev* 2007;**26**:341–52.

Chapter 5

Metabolic Stress, Heat Shock Proteins, and Innate Immune Response

Nicola Lacetera

Department of Agriculture, Forests, Nature and Energy, University of Tuscia, Viterbo, Italy

INTRODUCTION

Metabolic stress may result from either lack or excess of nutrients and it has been recognized to occur in a number of living organisms, which range across yeast to mammals.[1] Even if metabolic stress in unicellular entities has been studied extensively and presents several analogies with that in pluricellular organisms,[2] its analysis is beyond the scope of this chapter.

Following a brief description of selected metabolic stress conditions of common interest for humans and intensively farmed livestock, this chapter will deal with the relationships between metabolic stress and innate immunity and in particular, will focus on the role played within this relationship by the heat-shock response (HSR) induced by metabolic stressors.

Among intensively managed livestock, special emphasis will be given to the periparturient period of present high yielding dairy cows. The interest for dairy cows around calving is based on epidemiological data indicating metabolic stress in early lactation, as a major factor underlying animal welfare and health problems, production losses, impaired fertility, and premature culling.[3] Furthermore, a number of analogies between metabolic, health, and immunological features of dairy cows and human beings authorize to candidate dairy cow as a promising large animal model.[4,5] The concepts illustrated in Chapter 9 complement and widen the scope of the chapter by Trevisi and coauthors in this same book.

METABOLIC STRESS CONDITIONS

In general terms, metabolic stress may be defined as a disequilibrium in the homeostasis of a living organism consequent to an anomalous utilization of nutrients.

The main cause of metabolic stress in multicellular organisms living under natural conditions is the availability of nutrients in the environment. This is subjected to seasonal and interannual variations and if limited in terms of quantity and/or quality may be responsible for metabolic stress due to lack of nutrients.[6] In animals living in the wild, the risk of metabolic stress due to excess of nutrients has to be considered between null and very limited.

On the contrary, in humans and domesticated animals, metabolic stress may be due to either deficiency or excess of nutrients, and it may depend on their availability in the environment, but more frequently on pathological or physiological conditions, which may alter nutrient intake, assimilation and/or correct utilization.[1–3]

A number of metabolic stress conditions of interest for human beings share common features with metabolic disorders of modern dairy cows and other farm animals (i.e., sows) under situations of intensive management.

The metabolic stress conditions this chapter deals with are linked primarily to energy and lipid metabolism, or to the balance between prooxidant and antioxidant factors.

In this context, a condition that deserves to be certainly considered is obesity. In human beings living in Western societies, it affects more than 35% of the adult population and is associated with multiple metabolic dysfunctions. These comprise dyslipidemia, insulin resistance, type 2 diabetes, fatty liver, and also a variable degree of oxidative stress.[6–9] In general terms, oxidative stress may be caused by increased production of reactive oxygen species (ROS), free radicals and/or a decrease in antioxidant defense, which leads to damages of biological macromolecules (i.e., lipids, proteins, and DNA) and disruption of normal metabolism and physiology.[10] Different mechanisms are implied in the oxidative stress induced by obesity.[11] Among them, mitochondrial and peroxisomal oxidation of glucose and fatty acids, and increases of proinflammatory cytokines release, which results in an increase of ROS and free radical concentrations. Additionally, in humans and dairy cows, obesity is also associated with a significant decline of the activity of antioxidant enzymes such as CuZn-superoxide dismutase (SOD), catalase (CAT), and glutathione peroxidase (GSH-Px), which may contribute to increasing the risk of oxidative stress in obese subjects.[9,12]

In modern dairy cows and sows, it is well documented that overconditioning before parturition is responsible for metabolic disturbances and it is one of the most important risk factors for these animals to develop health problems during lactation or to experience production losses and impaired fertility.[6,13] However, it should be stressed that in periparturient dairy cows and sows, obesity simply exacerbates a physiological tendency of all high yielding subjects to mobilize fat from the adipose tissue during early lactation.[14] Lipid mobilization after parturition is due to the high energy demand of milk synthesis, which is associated with a variable intensity of a status of negative energy balance. Therefore, weight loss and increase of plasma nonesterified fatty acids (NEFA) due to lipomobilization represent common findings in high yielding, early lactating dairy cows and sows. These processes have been studied extensively in dairy cows, where the intensity of lipomobilization around calving has also been associated with immunosuppression and reproductive failure.[15,16] Different studies documented that periparturient dairy cows also experience a variable degree of insulin resistance in peripheral tissues, hepatic lipidosis, and oxidative stress, the severity of which tends to be more pronounced in overconditioned animals.[17–19] With regard to the oxidative stress, fat cows with high body conditions score (BCS) before calving and with pronounced BCS losses during the periparturient period are more prone to undergo conditions of oxidative stress, as testified by higher plasma reactive oxygen metabolites (ROM), thiobarbituric acid-reactive substances (TBARS) and thiol groups (SH), and lower erythrocyte SH and SOD when compared with a thinner counterpart with lower BCS before calving and less pronounced BCS losses in the periparturient period.[19] Furthermore, one has to consider that enhanced oxidative stress may cause additional lipolysis in transition dairy cows, which can contribute to increasing concentrations of plasma NEFA.[20] Briefly, dairy cows are defined as transition dairy cows in the period from 3 weeks before calving to 3 weeks after calving.[21]

However, in humans and animals there are a number of additional factors, which may increase prooxidants, decrease antioxidants, or both and this may therefore be responsible for oxidative stress. Among these, a number of environmental pollutants (i.e., heavy metals), intense physical exercise, heat stress, exposure to mycotoxins, and deficiency of specific antioxidant nutrients.[22–25]

The association between either heat stress or exposure to mycotoxins and oxidative status, has been demonstrated in dairy cows.[24,25] A first series of studies on heat stress was relative to dairy cows in an advanced stage of lactation and it was pointed out that such a condition has no effect on the plasma concentration of vitamin E and β-carotene, on muscle content of TBARS,[26] or has a limited influence on plasma lipid soluble antioxidants (vitamin E and β-carotene) and plasma TBARS.[27] In a later study carried out in periparturient dairy cows, conditions of moderate heat stress were shown not to affect plasma markers of oxidative status and were associated with higher erythrocytes SOD, GSH-Px-E, SH, and TBARS, indicating a condition of oxidative stress.

Mycotoxins are secondary metabolites produced by molds and released in food as well as feed. They can cause several diseases (mycotoxicoses) in humans and animals after ingestion, skin contact, or inhalation.[28] Among them, aflatoxin B1 (AFB1) and fumonisin B1 (FB1) are a matter of concern due to their widespread contamination of cereal grain commodities, of corn in particular, and their adverse effects on human and animal health. An *in vitro* study carried out on peripheral blood mononuclear cells (PBMC) from dairy cows pointed out that one mechanism, through which mycotoxins can cause cytotoxicity is the induction of oxidative stress.[25] In particular, AFB1 and FB1 were shown to be responsible for a dose-dependent intracellular increase of malondialdehyde (MDA), which represents an end product of lipid peroxidation pathways and a reliable indicator of oxidative stress.

In conclusion of this section and in the light of what is being discussed next on the relationships between metabolic stress and immune functions, it has to be noted that metabolic stress elicits also a stress response, which increases glucocorticoid levels[29] and modulates innate and acquired immune responses. This aspect may be particularly relevant to periparturient dairy cows that are likely to experience also an immune suppression status associated with a high incidence of bacterial infections (namely, mastitis and metritis).[14]

METABOLIC STRESS AND INNATE IMMUNITY

Literature data referred to humans, laboratory, and domestic animals testify the existence of intricate and multidirectional relationships between metabolic status, inflammatory response, innate and adaptive immunity, and resistance to microbial infections.[14]

It is widely recognized that obesity in humans is accompanied by a low-grade inflammatory status characterized by a higher expression of proinflammatory cytokines.[30] A number of studies reported that also dairy cows around calving, display an overt systemic inflammatory response and this status can aggravate the metabolic stress of the early lactation period by increasing lipolysis, compromising liver functions, worsening insulin sensitivity, and aggravating oxidative stress.[3,31,32] Therefore, as anticipated earlier, it can be assumed that obese humans and high yielding periparturient dairy cows also share some features concerning activation/modulation of the innate immune system.

The metabolic implications of immune activation in dairy cows have received great attention, and it is now increasingly clear that an excessive/prolonged immune activation may alter metabolic status and nutrient requirements.[33] Important consequences of immune stimulation include production of the proinflammatory cytokines, activation of the acute phase response, fever, inappetence, amino acid resorption from muscle, and redirection of nutrients toward liver anabolism of acute phase proteins.[34] Therefore, it makes sense that under chronic activation of the immune system following an inflammatory state a reduction of productive and reproductive performances may take place in dairy cows. Different models have been used to test the effects of immune activation on nutrition and metabolism. One of these models is based on lipopolysaccharide (LPS) challenge. Using this model, it has been reported that immune activation is responsible for strong utilization of glutamine and threonine in sheep[35] and for dose-dependent changes of metabolic parameters linked to energy metabolism in dairy cows.[36] Results from studies based on administration of proinflammatory cytokines indicated that intravenous administration of TNF-α is responsible for a significant increase of plasma NEFA in dairy cows,[37] and very low physiological concentrations of TNF-α interfere with protein synthesis and muscle cell development, by inducing a state of insulin-like growth factor 1 receptor resistance in pigs.[38]

The innate immune system provides the first line of host defense against bacterial or viral infections and diseases. Cells involved in the innate immune responses include mast cells, neutrophils, monocytes, macrophages, dendritic cells, and natural killer cells. A well-known feature of innate immunity is the existence of defined sets of cellular sensors that mediate recognition of infectious agents to promote host defence.[32] Pathogenic microorganisms are promptly sensed by the immune cells through germline encoded pattern recognition receptors (PRRs). Thereafter, the activation of PRRs leads to either immediate phagocytosis and inactivation of the pathogens or the secretion of soluble mediators such as proinflammatory cytokines for the further recruitment of effector cells to the infection site.[39] Recent research has identified several families of such sensors that evolved to detect conserved microbial- or pathogen-associated molecular patterns (MAMPs or PAMPs). In addition, it has become progressively clear that the innate immune system also responds to danger signals known as danger-associated molecular patterns or DAMPs, as explained in detail in Chapter 1 by Gallucci. This model, initially proposed by Polly Matzinger in 1994,[40] provided an explanation for how apparently aseptic tissue injuries could result in the "sterile inflammation," which shared remarkably similar features with inflammation due to microbial infections. Examples of well-known danger molecules that can activate the inflammatory cascade are the high mobility group box 1 (HMGB1) protein, S100 protein, uric acid, heat shock proteins (HSPs), and others.[41,42] With regard to HSPs, it has been postulated that the release of HSP70 into the extracellular space after cellular stress may act as a danger signal to the innate immune system.[43] Extracellular HSP70 activates innate immunity by a CD14-dependent mechanism, and toll-like receptor (TLR) 4 is suggested to be involved in HSP70 signaling. Therefore, HSP70-induced signal transduction shares common features with endotoxin-induced signal transduction. However, evidence also suggests a role for a variety of other signals, which may arouse innate immunity after exposure to stressors.[44] These include catecholamines,[45,46] glucocorticoids,[47] and metabolites of commensal gut microbiota.[48] However, their significance under conditions of metabolic stress has not been investigated.

Activation of PRRs triggers downstream signaling cascades, and leads to the activation of transcription factors and production of proinflammatory cytokines.[7] The cytokines lead to a state of inflammation finalized to remove the cause of PRR activation and restore cell and tissue homeostasis. Cause/effect relationships and intimate mechanisms linking metabolic stress with the inflammatory response is a very active research field.[32] With regard to human or laboratory rodent studies, it has been demonstrated that two main signaling pathways monitor nutrient availability, control metabolic stress responses, and exert a central role in modulating innate immunity[31] – the mTOR- and eIF2α-dependent signal transduction cascades.[49,50] The most important regulators of mTOR- and eIF2α are cellular energy status (ATP/AMP ratio), amino acid availability, oxygen tension, and oxidative stress. However, other studies indicated that also binding of free fatty acids to TLR 4 is directly linked to the development of inflammation in states of hyperlipidemia, such as those that characterize obesity.[51] Such binding leads to a cascade of events resulting in the activation of the nuclear factor kappa-light-chain-enhancer of activated B cells (NF-κB) system and Jun N-terminal kinase, and to the subsequent induction of proinflammatory factors.[51] In the light of topics that will be discussed further, it has also been mentioned that the list of molecules that can function as alarm signals when released into the extracellular environment also includes HSPs.[44] Finally, it deserves to be mentioned that NOD-like receptors (NLR) protein also triggers the inflammasome reaction in response to the energy stress caused by metabolic inhibitors or nutrient deprivation.[44,52] In this case, the inflammasome assembly results in caspase-1 activation and cleavage of pro-IL-1b and pro-IL18 into the mature, biologically active, releasable forms. However, the list of newly described DAMPs, DAMP receptors, and relative pathways, is growing every year, and it seems clear that what has been described so far is only the tip of the iceberg and many more types of DAMPs are still waiting to be described.[53]

In addition to other potential triggering factors[54] and in line with conclusions referred to results from human and laboratory rodent studies, there is a general agreement that the increase of plasma NEFA and oxidative stress may also have a role in the inflammatory status of dairy cows around calving.[3] In particular, human and rodent studies demonstrated that lipid mobilization may alter endothelial and leukocyte function by affecting their inflammatory responses directly (lipotoxicity) and indirectly (fatty acids can modify intracellular signaling, induce oxidative stress, and alter lipid mediator biosynthesis).[55] Furthermore, a number of other studies carried out in sheep and cows, documented that NEFA may also affect mononuclear or polymorphonuclear leukocyte functions, and in particular the concentrations mimicking a high intensity of lipomobilization may be associated to immunosuppression.[14,15,56-59] The additional triggering factors that have been suggested to explain the inflammatory response taking place in cows around calving[54] include the massive infiltration of leukocyte in the mammary gland during late pregnancy to remove apoptotic cells and cell debris, the omental and subcutaneous adipose tissues production of interleukin (IL) 6 under regulation of glucocorticoids, states of clinical or subclinical ketosis, and so on. However, the inner mechanisms that integrate metabolic homeostasis with activation of the innate immune system have not been elucidated so far in dairy cows. Although numerous studies in the past decade have demonstrated that inflammatory mediators are elevated in the days after parturition even in cows that are apparently healthy, the main causes of the inflammatory state that characterize the periparturient period continue to be considered clinical or subclinical infections (i.e., metritis, mastitis, laminitis, etc.) or endotoxin absorption through the digestive system, uterus, or mammary gland. This interpretation has been discounted though by the demonstration in high yielding dairy cows of early signs of innate immune and inflammatory response in the last month of pregnancy, well before the occurrence of the aforementioned microbial infections.[60] Interestingly, a number of studies carried out in pigs indicated that early weaning causes a dramatic upregulation of inflammatory cytokine gene expression in proximal and distant tracts of the small intestine, which is linked to the combined metabolic, environmental, and emotional challenge at weaning, and aims to prevent weaning-associated health disorders.[61] These and other aspects relative to the inflammatory state of piglets at weaning, will be reviewed extensively in Chapter 8 by Razzuoli et al., in this book.

Irrespective of the same, the physiological significance of metabolically induced inflammatory response remains to be understood. This is likely to include both adaptive (i.e., energy mobilization, sickness behavior, etc.) and maladaptive (i.e., cytokine storm, exacerbated inflammatory disease, etc.) consequences.[41]

The analysis of how metabolic status may activate/modulate the immune system must also include results from studies demonstrating that glucose levels and fat depots may change energy allocation priorities among different physiological, biochemical, and behavioral processes.[6] In other words, under conditions of energy deficit, the balancing of energy allocation toward different biological processes may be responsible for energetic tradeoffs among physiological systems. In particular, one frequently observed energetic tradeoff occurs between the reproductive and immune systems. In this scenario under conditions of energy constraints, depending on glucose availability, and amount of fat depots, increased investment into one system results in decreased energy allocation to the other one with consequent impairment of the corresponding function.[62]

METABOLIC STRESS, OXIDATIVE STRESS, AND HEAT SHOCK PROTEINS

The HSPs were originally described for their roles as chaperones.[63] The principal HSPs range in molecular mass from about 15–110 kDa and are divided into groups based on size and function.[64] In this chapter, the primary focus will be on the ubiquitous HSP70 family proteins, which are the best known and conserved among HSPs.[65] In detail, two members of the HSP70 family, HSP73 and HSP72, share a high degree of sequence homology but differ in their expression pattern; HSP73 is expressed constitutively, while HSP72 is induced by stress and is the member mostly quoted in scientific papers. Even if it is now clear that all HSP families also encode constitutively expressed members, the heat shock genes (and the relevant protein family members) most extensively studied are those that are heat inducible.[66] Intracellular increase of HSPs, known as HSR, is triggered by several stressors, which include temperature shock, UV radiation, heavy metals, bacterial and parasitic infections, fever, growth factors, hormonal stimulation, tissue development, oxygen deprivation, pH extremes, and nutrient deprivation.[67] These cellular insults can cause protein denaturation and unfolding within the cells, leading to the formation of unwanted protein aggregates that can eventually kill the cells.[68] HSPs facilitate protein refolding, target misfolded proteins to the proteasome, and stabilize and transport partially folded proteins to different cellular compartments. Thus, with regard to their function as chaperones, HSPs substantially help to maintain normal cellular homeostasis in response to a variety of stressors. The induction of the HSR is mediated by the heat shock transcription factor 1 (HSF1). Under normal conditions HSF1 is kept in an inactive, monomeric form. A large variety of insults, such as heat shock and UV radiation, activate the trimerization and nuclear translocation of cytoplasmic HSF1 for binding with the HSR elements (HSE) and consequent transcription of HSP genes.[1,69]

In the last 10–15 years, a number of studies have demonstrated that metabolic and oxidative stress conditions have the potential to induce an HSR, and in some cases such a response may have an adaptive significance, and contribute to regulate the immune system.[1,65,70,71]

Literature data derived from a variety of experimental conditions suggest that caloric restriction, both hypo and hyperglycemia, and hyperlipidemia may differentially regulate HSPs expression in different species or body compartments.

In this context, a first series of studies focused on the role played by HSPs in the positive and well-known effects of caloric restriction on aging and lifespan of laboratory rodents.[72] Behind its effect on lifespan, chronic caloric restriction attenuated the age-related loss of HSP70 induction in rat hepatocytes in response to heat shock.[73] In another rat study, lifelong caloric restriction increased HSPs in soleus muscles and attenuated the reduction of HSPs expression associated with aging.[74] However, the ability of caloric restriction to help aging cells mount an HSR has still no proven correlation with its beneficial effect on lifespan. A further interesting aspect linking nutritional stressors with HSR pertains to the effects of hyperlipidic diets. In a mouse study, which provided important insights as to how fatty acids and HSPs affect immunity, it was reported that a diet rich in fatty acids induces the expression of HSPs of 70, 60, 27, and 25 kDa in splenic lymphocytes and makes these cells more susceptible to death by apoptosis.[70] Furthermore, the same study also revealed that predisposition of splenic lymphocytes to death by apoptosis is particularly marked when diet is rich of saturated fatty acids and that cells of animals fed with unsaturated fatty acid are instead more resistant.

Another interesting model that provides information on the relationship between metabolic stress and HSPs is that of physical exercise applied to laboratory animals and humans.[65] In one of the initial studies in this field, it was described that exhaustive treadmill running in rats increased synthesis of HSP70 in skeletal muscle, lymphocytes, and spleen.[75] Numerous subsequent studies carried out in laboratory animals confirmed that acute exercise may increase HSP70 levels in contracting skeletal muscle as well as in other critical organs such as the heart, kidney, and liver. However, they did not clarify whether the increase was due to temperature rise or to the concurrent action of other physiological stimuli.[65] In addition to the increase of body temperature, the main stressors associated with exercise and the potential to induce an HSR include metabolic disturbances, altered calcium fluxes, increased production of ROS, changed hormonal environment, and mechanical activation or deformation of tissues.[76] Human studies documented that exercise is associated with increase of serum concentration of HSP72[77,78] and reduced glycogen availability is associated with elevated HSP72 messenger ribonucleic acid and protein levels in contracting skeletal muscle.[79] A few years later, the same researchers demonstrated that reduced availability of glucose during exercise contribute to explain the HSR in humans. In particular, they observed that maintaining glucose availability during exercise by administering 250 mL of a 6.4% carbohydrate beverage attenuates the circulating HSP72–HSP60 response in healthy humans.[80] A direct indication that energy metabolites may trigger an HSR comes from a rat study indicating that intracellular ATP level acts as a regulator of the HSR in isolated perfused rat heart during ischemia and ischemia–reperfusion.[81] Briefly, a moderate reduction in ATP correlates with the activation of HSF1, whereas a severe depletion in ATP correlates with the attenuation in HSF1 activation, and the restoration of ATP leads to an even greater activation of HSF1. A number of studies also testified an important connection between diabetes and associated metabolic disturbances (i.e., hyperglycemia and insulin resistance) and the HSR.[1] With the exception of an elevation of HSF1, Hsp70, and Hsp90 in the pancreas of diabetic monkeys,[82] it is widely accepted that several cell types of monkey or human patients with type 2 diabetes have reduced gene expression of HSP72, which correlates with reduced insulin sensitivity.[1] Furthermore, it has also been reported that HSP72 is a potential target for therapeutic treatment of obesity-induced insulin resistance, in that an induced elevation could protect against obesity-induced hyperglycemia, hyperinsulinemia, glucose intolerance, and insulin resistance. In this regard, Morino et al.[83] demonstrated that heat shock-induced upregulation of intracellular HSP72 alleviates insulin resistance and improves fat metabolism in diabetes mouse models, in part by enhancing the insulin signaling pathway. Furthermore, it has been also reported that regardless of the means used to achieve an elevation in HSP72, this response protects against diet- or obesity-induced hyperglycemia, hyperinsulinemia, glucose intolerance, and insulin resistance.[84] However, a number of studies also described higher levels of extracellular HSP60 or HSP70 in people suffering from diabetes compared to healthy people and also indicated diabetes-associated metabolic disturbances (i.e., ketoacidosis, hyperglycemia, or oxidative stress) as direct inducers of the HSR.[85–87] In diabetic ketoacidosis, the increase of extracellular HSP72 could reflect the liver's heightened metabolic activity characteristic of this metabolic state, or be part of an acute stress response to hyperosmolality, acidosis, and/or oxidative stress.[85] However, the positive correlation between HSP72 levels and blood glucose suggested that under these conditions the HSR might also be linked to hyperglycemia. Interestingly, in a recent *in vitro* study with HeLa cells it was observed that hyperglycemic conditions and oxidative stress induced a higher expression of HSP60 and HSP70, suggesting that the increased serum levels of these molecular stress proteins observed in diabetic patients could be due also to uncontrolled hyperglycemia and oxidative stress.[88]

As already reported earlier, oxidative stress may surely contribute to explaining the HSR observed in conditions of metabolic stress.[76,84] However, several other factors associated with oxidative injuries have been shown to have the potential to trigger an HSR.[89] In this context, several groups have performed *in vitro* studies on the oxidation of mammalian HSF1 to explore whether it senses peroxides or whether its activation depends on the oxidant proteotoxic insult causing accumulation of damaged or misfolded proteins. If some studies indicate that direct redox regulation of HSF1 is possible, others suggest that direct oxidation may be a contributing factor but not a conserved mechanism of HSF1 activation.[90–92] Furthermore, it deserves to be noted that exposure of PBMC to heat induces an HSR, which protects cells from hydrogen peroxide-induced mitochondrial disturbance.[93] Heat-shock pretreatment decreases accumulation of intracellular superoxide and prevents the collapse of mitochondrial membrane potential and cytochrome c release from mitochondria during H_2O_2-induced oxidative stress.

The studies focusing on metabolic stress and expression or synthesis of HSPs in farm animals are very limited. The proteomic analysis of hypothalamic responses to energy restriction in dairy cows pointed out overexpression of the stress-induced phosphoprotein-1 (STI-1) together with upregulation of HSP70 and ubiquitin carboxy-terminal hydrolase L1 (UCHL1).[94] The roles of STI-1 in the formation of several HSPs, such as HSP70 and HSP90 (necessary for protein translocation across lysosomal membranes and subsequent degradation), and of protease UCHL1 (hydrolyzing esters, thioesters, and isopeptides to eliminate misfolded proteins either via proteasomal or lysosomal proteolysis) suggests that energy deprivation causes increased formation of misfolded or posttranslationally modified proteins that are counteracted by an augmented elimination via proteasomal or lysosomal proteolysis. Eitam et al.[95] reported that a 3-month, low-energy diet promoted a cell-specific HSR in lactating beef cattle with a significant increase of HSP90 but unchanged levels of HSP70 mRNA in white blood cells. The same study also revealed that the experimental conditions did reduce the expression of HSP70 in milk somatic cells that include neutrophils, macrophages, lymphocytes, eosinophils, and epithelial cells of the mammary gland.[96] With regard to farm animal species, a bit more information is available on the relationships between HSR and oxidative stress. Supplementation of late pregnant dairy cows with vitamin E improves the oxidative status and is also associated with lower concentrations of circulating HSP70.[97] In chicken, HSP70 is capable of protecting the intestinal mucosa from heat-stress injury by improving antioxidant capacity and inhibiting lipid peroxidation processes.[98] In a recent study, hepatocytes from chicken fed a selenium-deficient diet were shown to undergo oxidative stress as testified by increased intracellular concentrations of MDA and lower levels of glutathione and glutathione peroxidase.[99] At the same time, hepatocytes from selenium-deficient birds also showed increased gene and protein expression of some HSPs (namely, HSP60, 70, and 90 kDa).

The combination of profound changes in the endocrine status due to the passage from pregnancy to lactation, parturition itself, negative energy balance, metabolic and digestive disturbances, oxidative stress, inflammatory dysfunctions, environmental stress, infections (especially endometritis and mastitis), and a variable degree of immunosuppression[100,101] suggest that dairy cows around calving and in early lactation, may represent an interesting model for HSR studies. This hypothesis found a confirmation in a research work carried out to verify whether the periparturient and early lactation periods in dairy cows are associated with changes of intracellular and plasma HSP72, and to establish possible relationships between HSP72, and a set of metabolic or immunological parameters.[102] The cells considered in the study were PBMC. The study pointed out that intracellular and plasma concentrations of HSP72 increased significantly in the weeks following parturition (Figs 5.1 and 5.2). As anticipated earlier, a number of different physiological factors may contribute to explain these findings. One of these is parturition. Two different studies on sheep and women described an increase of HSP72 in the myometrium and in the amniotic fluid at the time of parturition.[103,104] Furthermore, the inflammatory and tissue remodeling processes taking place in the reproductive tract of dairy cows in the early postpartum period may also have a role.[105] However, in line with results from previous studies on the relationships between energy status and HSR, in the same study a postpartum decline of plasma glucose and BCS and an increase of plasma NEFA were also observed, which testify to the condition of negative energy balance. Furthermore, a significant positive correlation was found between plasma NEFA and intracellular HSP72 indicating that a higher concentration

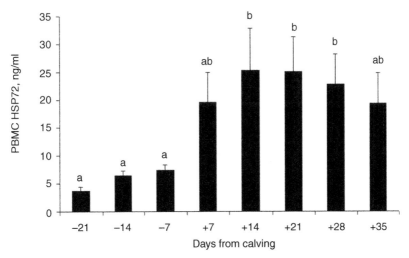

FIGURE 5.1   Concentrations of HSP 72 kDa molecular weight (HSP72) in PBMC isolated from periparturient high yielding dairy cows. Data are reported as least square means ± standard error. Different letters indicate significant differences between time points ($P < 0.05$). *(Modified from Ref. [102].)*

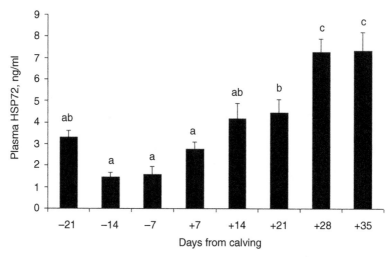

FIGURE 5.2   Concentrations of HSP 72 kDa molecular weight (HSP72) in plasma of peri-parturient high yielding dairy cows. Data are reported as least square means ± standard error. Different letters indicate significant differences between time points ($P < 0.05$). *(Modified from Ref. [102].)*

of plasma NEFA is associated with a higher HSP72 concentration in PBMC. Therefore, the negative energy balance and related changes of metabolic parameters is likely to contribute to the upregulation of HSP72 in the early lactation period. Additionally, it has to be reminded that periparturient dairy cows are likely to also undergo a certain degree of oxidative stress, which is probably a further factor contributing to upregulation of HSP72 around calving. What remains to be ascertained is whether such a response may be beneficial to animal health and performances.[93,101] Finally, as already reported earlier, the postcalving period is also characterized by moderate absorption of endotoxins, which may contribute to the development of the inflammatory status and increase of intracellular and circulating HSP72. In this regard, a number of studies carried out in different species demonstrated that bacterial endotoxins may represent strong HSR inducers and in some cases, this may be a part of the natural mechanisms of cell protection.[106,107]

HEAT-SHOCK PROTEINS AND INNATE IMMUNE RESPONSE

Recent studies have shown that HSPs interact with and regulate signaling intermediates involved in the activation/regulation of innate and adaptive immune responses.[108]

Even if the majority of HSPs have been recognized as immunomodulators, the high molecular weight HSPs of 60, 70, and 90 kDa have been studied more extensively and their role in activating/modulating the immune response has been described in more detail. In particular, knowledge reviewed in this chapter will be mostly referred to HSP70. Although it may be tempting to generalize the information on different HSPs, it has to be considered that this may lead to erroneous inferences, since the different HSP families do not show sequence or structure homologies. Also, they are encoded by different genes transcribed under the control of different transcription factors, not always activated in a coordinate manner.

Originally, HSPs were considered to be exclusively intracellular proteins that were passively released into cellular environments as a consequence of cellular injury or necrosis and, as such and as already mentioned earlier, they were considered to represent DAMPs.[42] In the last 10–15 years, it became evident that HSPs can be actively secreted into the extracellular milieu and that some of them (namely, HSP60, 70, and 90 kDa) are linked with the regulation of innate and/or acquired immune response. One of the first studies in this area indicated that human HSP70 could bind to and activate human monocytes, promoting the secretion of inflammatory cytokines, such as TNF-α, IL-1β, and IL-6.[109] Actually, literature data now indicate that HSPs are components of a complex network involved in the regulation and/or resolution of inflammatory events and whether they exert a pro- or anti-inflammatory action may depend primarily, but not exclusively, on the microenvironments these proteins dwell in.[110] More specifically, it has been frequently indicated that depending on their extra- or intracellular location and the type of immune cells, HSPs can exert an inflammatory immune activating signal for host defense or an anti-inflammatory immunosuppressive signal to prevent excessive inflammation.

The research on periparturient dairy cows already cited earlier describing changes of HSP72 and the relationships between these changes and metabolic and immunological parameters,[102] presented and discussed an interesting model to review and speculate the potential adaptive significance of HSP expression during a physiological phase critical for metabolic status, oxidative balance, immune system, and health maintenance. Besides changes of metabolic parameters and increase of intracellular and circulating HSP72, cows enrolled in that study presented relevant changes of immunological parameters consisting of a transient increase of plasma tumor necrosis (TNF)-α after calving, of a postcalving decrease of the percentage of PBMC expressing TLR-4, and of the ability of PBMC to proliferate *in vitro* in response to LPS stimulation. Furthermore, positive correlations were detected between the percentage of PBMC expressing TLR-4 and the LPS-driven proliferation of PBMC, whereas negative correlations were found between intra- and extracellular HSP72 and the proliferative response of PBMC to LPS. The increase of plasma TNF-α after parturition reflects the well-documented tendency of dairy cows to develop a certain degree of systemic inflammation in the first weeks after calving.[111,112] Instead, results of the correlation analyses are in line with those to other species,[42,113] and suggest that upregulation of HSP72 and decline of TLR-4-positive cells may play a role in the postcalving decrease of PBMC proliferation in response to LPS. Within this context and also in the light of what is going to be discussed next, it has been hypothesized that the postpartum decline of the PBMC proliferative response to LPS might be interpreted as an ancillary sign of hyporesponsiveness, compatible with a state of endotoxin tolerance.

As already repeatedly discussed earlier, numerous papers indicated that the inflammatory state of early lactating dairy cows may be at least partly attributed to Gram-negative bacterial endotoxins passing from the reproductive or digestive tracts or from the mammary gland to the general circulation.[114–116] Endotoxin tolerance was first reported in 1946[117] and it was defined as the abolition of the fever response of rabbits subjected to repeated daily injection of the same dose of a typhoid vaccine. Following studies carried out in different animal species confirmed that repeated exposure to endotoxins may be responsible for a progressive reduced responsiveness to further LPS challenges in terms of pyrogenic response, and also documented that this is also associated with lower inflammatory cytokine release.[118–122] In this regard, TNF-α is most probably the best marker of endotoxin tolerance as assessed by its dramatically reduced production following an LPS challenge in tolerized animals, in contrast to its fast and sharp peak in response to a first LPS injection.[121] Endotoxin tolerance has been suggested to represent a protective mechanism preventing excessive inflammatory conditions. However, it has also been indicated that a persisting hyporesponsiveness to LPS may cause immune suppression and, therefore, increased risk of infections.[122–126] This state shares common features with the state of immunologic hyporeactivity taking place in patients with sepsis, which has been termed inflammatory-induced immune suppression.[127] In this context, reduced levels of interferon have been described in animals pretreated with LPS and then challenged with Newcastle disease virus,[128] and a reduced leishmanicidal activity was observed after preexposure of macrophages to LPS.[129] Therefore, even if the endotoxin tolerance phenomenon has not been clearly recognized and described in early lactating dairy cows, some findings would actually confirm this tenet: the well-known translocation of bacterial endotoxin from periphery to general circulation that may account for a repeated exposure to LPS, the frequent and transient inflammatory state at the onset of lactation, the progressive decline of the ability of PBMC to respond to LPS, and the high incidence of infections in the early lactation period.[99,130] All of these conditions may account for an endotoxin tolerance-like condition in dairy cows in the early postcalving period. A diagrammatic representation of the possible relationships between metabolic and oxidative stress, inflammatory status (immune activation), HSR, immunosuppression, and infections in early lactating high yielding dairy cows is reported in Fig. 5.3.

Now, going back to the role of HSPs as regulators of immune functions, in the context of the postpartum inflammatory and immunosuppression state of dairy cows,[14,20,31] upregulation of PBMC and plasma HSP72 could prove to be of major importance in an adaptive view. In detail, intracellular HSPs might protect the host against an excessive amplification of the inflammatory response,[112,131] whereas circulating HSPs might sustain fundamental circuits of

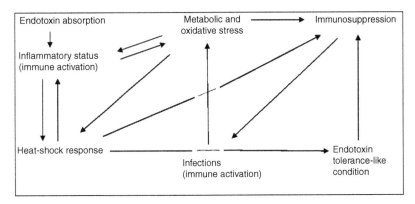

FIGURE 5.3   Diagrammatic representation of the possible relationships between metabolic and oxidative stress, inflammatory status (immune activation), heat shock response, immunosuppression, and infections in early lactating high yielding dairy cows. The diagram is based on results from several studies carried out in rodents, humans, or dairy cows and includes the hypothesis, not demonstrated, that an endotoxin tolerance-like condition may take place in dairy cows during the periparturient period. *(Modified from Ref. [14].)*

the immune response by optimizing antigen processing and presentation.[132–135] Furthermore, a few *in vitro* studies also suggested a direct involvement of HSP70 in the development of endotoxin tolerance. The first of these studies reported that preconditioning THP-1 cells with HSP70, at a concentration that does not activate NF-κB, induces tolerance to LPS.[43] Another study pointed out that endotoxin tolerance and heat shock appear to share a common immune suppressive effect, and that this effect may be linked to HSF-1-mediated competitive inhibition of NF-κB nuclear binding.[136]

In the last two decades, several findings have been accumulated on the anti-inflammatory role of intracellular HSPs. Induction of HSP72 *in vitro* by heat shock or HSP72 overexpression can reduce mortality in experimental models of septic shock and endotoxemia, and can regulate expression of several inflammatory genes.[137–141] In the course of infections, increased intracellular levels of HSP70 protect cells by inhibiting components of inflammatory signaling pathways, such as the NF-κB transcription factor.[142,143] Interestingly, in a mouse model, HSF-1 was shown to act as a negative regulator of TNF-α release in a condition of LPS-induced shock, and as a repressor of the transcription of both TNF-α and IL-1β.[144] In agreement with these findings, other authors suggested that the HSF1/HSP72 pathway may represent a constitutive anti-inflammatory system, protecting the organism from the deleterious effects of a prolonged and excessive activation of the inflammatory response. In this respect, HSF1 and HSP72 genes may be considered as anti-inflammatory genes, and their selective *in vivo* transactivation may lead to the remission of inflammation. Vice versa, inhibition of their expression may result in exacerbation of the inflammatory process.[145]

The analysis of literature data relative to the role of circulating HSPs on the innate immune response reveals conflicting results concerning anti- and proinflammatory effects under a large a variety of experimental conditions. In this regard, a distinction, which has to be made is between bacterial and eukaryotic HSPs.[146] If the ability of mammalian HSPs to stimulate the mammalian immune system is to a certain extent still controversial and under debate, convincing evidence has been accumulated that bacterial HSPs stimulate the innate immune system.[147,148] In the latter regard, the immunostimulating properties of HSPs have been exploited for the development of prophylactic vaccines against infectious diseases including tuberculosis, influenza, meningitis, and *Helicobacter pylori* infections. These attempts were and are still being made on HSP-based vaccines, in the form of pathogen-derived HSP–antigen complexes, or on recombinant HSPs combined with selected antigens *in vitro*.[149,150]

Focusing on eukaryotic HSPs and on the effects that endogenous HSPs may have on the innate immune system, it has been described that increased concentrations of circulating HSP70 stimulate an inflammatory response via a TLR2/TLR4/CD14-dependent mechanism that leads to NF-κB activation, and TNF-α, IL1-β, and IL-6 production.[133] Supporting an immunostimulating effect of HSPs, others reported that extracellular HSP70 binds to the lipid raft microdomain on the plasma membrane of macrophages and enhances their phagocytic ability.[151] This HSP70-mediated phagocytosis enhances the processing and presentation of internalized antigens to CD4T cells. In addition, HSP70 and HSP90 have been shown to be involved in the innate recognition of bacterial products and to be able to bind LPS and form a cluster with TLR4–MD2 within lipid raft to deliver LPS to the complex.[152] Contrarily, other studies indicated that extracellular HSP70 induces LPS tolerance and prevents the augmentation of proinflammatory cytokine levels that follow LPS stimulation.[43] The immunostimulating activity of HSP70 through TLR2 and TLR4 remains thus controversial, and it has been proposed that the proinflammatory activity of HSP70 described in the literature was linked to contaminating LPS.[153] Data from the HSP70 knockout mice suggest that extracellular HSP70 is important for the negative regulation of inflammatory mediators during systemic infection.[154] Furthermore, some authors considered that a proinflammatory role of extracellular HSP70 would be also difficult to reconcile with the anti-inflammatory role of intracellular HSP70 described earlier.[155] On the other hand, the same authors have demonstrated that the addition of HSP70 to TLR-activated monocytes downregulates secretion of TNF-α and IL-6 in response to LPS and that therefore extracellular HSP70 may also contribute to dampen the inflammatory response. Finally, HSPs expression or HSP-specific T cell responses have been positively associated with a better disease prognosis in several inflammatory conditions,[156,157] and their immunosuppressive action has been demonstrated in multiple rodent disease models.[158]

Therefore, if earlier studies have emphasized the proinflammatory nature of HSPs, later findings have suggested that such nature was likely to be due to endotoxin contamination of partially purified recombinant proteins used in the experiments.[153,159,160] On the other hand, evidence has been accumulated that strongly supports the concept of an immunosuppressive potential of HSP70 and authorizes their use in the therapy of inflammatory diseases.

CONCLUSIONS

Regardless of the species, metabolic stress conditions are connected bidirectionally with the innate immune system. The molecular mechanisms behind the activation of the innate immune response in humans and animals suffering from metabolic stress are numerous, and the physiological significance of such activation has not been fully understood, with adaptive and maladaptive consequences. Furthermore, immune activation has several metabolic implications and it is now clear that excessive/prolonged inflammatory conditions may alter metabolic status and nutrients requirement, which may be responsible for the reduction of productive and reproductive performances, metabolic diseases, immune suppression, and outbreaks of infections in farm animals. Metabolic stress conditions may be also associated with an HSR, and HSP may represent molecules at the interface between cellular stress and activation/modulation of the innate immune system. Although HSPs are only part of the response of pluricellular organisms to metabolic stress, the definition of their role may be definitely conducive to a better understanding of the profound impact of noninfectious stressors on functions and regulation of the innate immune system, and of the repercussions thereof on the animals' immune competence for environmental pathogens.

REFERENCES

1. Dancsó B, Spiró Z, Alper Arslan M, Tú Nguyen M, Papp D, Csermely P, et al. The heat shock connection of metabolic stress and dietary restriction. *Curr Pharmac Biotechnol* 2010;**11**:139–45.
2. Wellen KE, Thompson CB. Cellular metabolic stress: considering how cells respond to nutrient excess. *Mol Cell* 2010;**40**(2):323–32.
3. Sordillo LM, Mavangira V. The nexus between nutrient metabolism, oxidative stress and inflammation in transition cows. *Anim Prod Sci* 2014;**54**:1204–14.
4. Ceciliani F, Restelli L, Lecchi C. Proteomics in farm animals models of human diseases. *Proteomics Clin Appl* 2014;**8**:677–88.
5. De Koster J, Opsomer G. Are modern dairy cows suffering from modern diseases? *Vlaams Diergen Tijds* 2012;**81**:71–80.
6. Carlton ED, Cooper CL, Demas GE. Metabolic stressors and signals differentially affect energy allocation between reproduction and immune function. *Gen Comp Endocrinol* 2014;**208**:21–9.
7. Li HB, Jin C, Chen Y, Flavell RA. Inflammasome activation and metabolic disease progression. *Cytok Growth Fact Rev* 2014;**25**:699–706.
8. Gregor MF, Hotamisligil GS. Inflammatory mechanisms in obesity. *Ann Rev Immunol* 2011;**29**:415–45.

9. Fernández-Sánchez A, Madrigal-Santillán E, Bautista M, Esquivel-Soto J, Morales-González A, Esquivel-Chirino C, et al. Inflammation, oxidative stress, and obesity. *Int J Mol Sci* 2011;**12**:3117–32.

10. Trevisan M, Browne R, Ram M, Muti p, Freudenheim J, Carosella AN, et al. Correlates of markers of oxidative status in the general population. *Am J Epidemiol* 2001;**154**:348–56.

11. Marseglia L, Manti S, D'Angelo G, Nicotera A, Parisi E, Di Rosa G, et al. Oxidative stress in obesity: a critical component in human diseases. *Int J Mol Sci* 2015;**16**:378–400.

12. O'Boyle N, Corl CM, Gandy JC, Sordillo LM. Relationship of body condition score and oxidant stress to tumor necrosis factor expression in dairy cattle. *Vet Immunol Immunopathol* 2006;**113**:297–304.

13. Torres-Rovira L, Pallares P, Vigo E, Gonzalez-Añover P, Sanchez-Sanchez R, Mallo F, et al. Plasma leptin, ghrelin and indexes of glucose and lipid metabolism in relation to the appearance of post-weaning oestrus in Mediterranean obese sows (Iberian pig). *Reprod Domest Anim* 2011;**46**:558–60.

14. Lacetera N, Bernabucci U, Ronchi B. Interactions between energy and protein status, immunity and infections in farm animals. In: Crovetto GM, editor. *Energy and Protein Metabolism and Nutrition*. Wageningen Academic Publishers; 2010. p. 479–88 EAAP publ No. 127: Wageningen, The Netherlands.

15. Lacetera N, Scalia D, Bernabucci U, Ronchi B, Pirazzi D, Nardone A. Lymphocyte functions in overconditioned cows around parturition. *J Dairy Sci* 2005;**88**:2010–6.

16. Leroy JL, Vanholder T, Mateusen B, Christophe A, Opsomer G, de Kruif A, et al. Non-esterified fatty acids in follicular fluid of dairy cows and their effect on developmental capacity of bovine oocytes *in vitro*. *Reprod* 2005;**130**:485–95.

17. Leiva T, Cooke RF, Aboin AC, Drago FL, Gennari R, Vasconcelos JLM. Effects of excessive energy intake and supplementation with chromium propionate on insulin resistance parameters in nonlactating dairy cows. *J Anim Sci* 2014;**92**:775–82.

18. Bernabucci U, Basiricò L, Pirazzi D, Rueca F, Lacetera N, Lepri E, et al. Liver apolipoprotein B100 expression and secretion are down-regulated early postpartum in dairy cows. *Livest Sci* 2009;**125**:169–76.

19. Bernabucci U, Ronchi B, Lacetera N, Nardone A. Influence of body condition score on relationships between metabolic status and oxidative stress in periparturient dairy cows. *J Dairy Sci* 2005;**88**:2017–26.

20. Sordillo LM, Raphael W. Significance of metabolic stress, lipid mobilization, and inflammation on transition cow disorders. *Vet Clin N Am Food A* 2013;**29**:267–78.

21. Grummer RR. Impact of changes in organic nutrient metabolism on feeding the transition dairy cow. *J Anim Sci* 1995;**73**:2820–33.

22. Liu L, Tao R, Huang J, He X, Qu L, Jin Y, et al. Hepatic oxidative stress and inflammatory responses with cadmium exposure in male mice. *Environ Toxicol Pharmacol* 2015;**39**:229–36.

23. Fittipaldi S, Dimauro I, Mercatelli N, Caporossi D. Role of exercise-induced reactive oxygen species in the modulation of heat shock protein response. *Free Radical Res* 2014;**48**:52–70.

24. Bernabucci U, Ronchi B, Lacetera N, Nardone A. Markers of oxidative status in plasma and erythrocytes of transition dairy cows during the hot season. *J Dairy Sci* 2002;**85**:2173–9.

25. Bernabucci U, Colavecchia L, Danieli PP, Basiricò L, Lacetera N, Nardone A, et al. Aflatoxin B1 and fumonisin B1 affect the oxidative status of bovine peripheral blood mononuclear cells. *Toxycol In Vitro* 2011;**25**:684–91.

26. Trout JP, McDowell LR, Hansen PJ. Characteristics of the estrous cycle and antioxidant status of lactating Holstein cows exposed to heat stress. *J Dairy Sci* 1998;**81**:1244–50.

27. Calamari L, Maianti MG, Amendola F, Lombardi G. *On some aspects of the oxidative status and on antioxidants in blood of dairy cows during summer.* Proceedings 13th Associazione Scientifica Produzioni Animali Congress Piacenza, Italy 1999;**1**:449–51.

28. Smith JE, Solomons G, Lewis C, Anderson JG. The role of mycotoxins in human and animal nutrition and health. *Nat Toxins* 1995;**3**:187–92.

29. Hotamisligil GS. Inflammation and metabolic disorders. *Nature* 2006;**444**:860–7.

30. Karalis KP, Giannogonas P, Kodela E, Koutmani Y, Zoumakis M, Teli t. Mechanisms of obesity and related pathology: linking immune responses to metabolic stress. *FEBS J* 2009;**276**:5747–54.

31. Bertoni G, Trevisi E, Han X, Bionaz M. Effects of inflammatory conditions on liver activity in puerperium period and consequences for performance in dairy cows. *J Dairy Sci* 2008;**91**:3300–10.

32. Tsalikis J, Croitoru DO, Philpott DJ, Girardin SE. Nutrient sensing and metabolic stress pathways in innate immunity. *Cell Microbiol* 2013;**15**:1632–41.

33. Husband AJ, Bryden WL. Nutrition, stress and immune activation. *Proc Nutr Soc Austral* 1996;**20**:60–70.

34. Colditz IG. Effects of the immune system on metabolism: implications for production and disease resistance in livestock. *Liv Prod Sci* 2002;**75**:257–68.

35. Lobley GE, Hoskin SO, McNeil CJ. Glutamine in animal science and production. *J Nutr* 2001;**131**:2525S–31S.

36. Waldron MR, Nishida T, Nonnecke BJ, Overton TR. Effect of lipopolysaccharide on indices of peripheral and hepatic metabolism in lactating cows. *J Dairy Sci* 2003;**86**:3447–59.

37. Kushibiki S, Hodate K, Shingu H, Hayashi T, Touno E, Shinoda M, et al. Alterations in lipid metabolism induced by recombinant bovine tumor necrosis factor-α administration to dairy heifers. *J Anim Sci* 2002;**80**:2151–7.

38. Broussard SR, McCusker RH, Novakosfski JE, Strle K, Shen WH, Johnson RW, et al. Cytokine-hormone interactions: tumor necrosis factor α impairs biologic activity and downstream activation of signals of the insulin-like growth factor I receptor in myoblasts. *Endocrinology* 2003;**144**:2988–96.

39. Cheng SC, Joosten LAB, Netea MG. The interplay between central metabolism and innate immune responses. *Cytokine Growth Factor Rev* 2014;**25**:707–13.

40. Matzinger P. Tolerance, danger, and the extended family. *Annu Rev Immunol* 1994;**12**:991–1045.

41. Rosin DL, Okusa MD. Dangers within: DAMP responses to damage and cell death in kidney disease. *J Am Soc Nephrol* 2011;**22**:416–25.

42. Basu S, Binder RJ, Suto R, Anderson KM, Srivastava PK. Necrotic but not apoptotic cell death releases heat shock proteins, which deliver a partial maturation signal to dendritic cells and activate the NF-κB pathway. *Int Immunol* 2000;**12**:1539–46.

43. Aneja R, Odoms K, Dunsmore K, Shanley TP, Wong HR. Extracellular heat shock protein-70 induces endotoxin tolerance in THP-1 cells. *J Immunol* 2006;**177**:7184–92.

44. Fleshner M. Stress-evoked sterile inflammation, danger associated molecular patterns (DAMPs), microbial associated molecular patterns (MAMPs) and the inflammasome. *Brain Behav Immun* 2013;**27**:1–7.

45. Johnson JD, Campisi J, Sharkey CM, Kennedy SL, Nickerson M, Greenwood BN, et al. Catecholamines mediate stress-induced increases in peripheral and central inflammatory cytokines. *Neuroscience* 2005;**135**:1295–307.

46. Mazzeo RS, Donovan D, Fleshner M, Butterfield GE, Zamudio S, Wolfel EE, et al. Interleukin-6 response to exercise and high-altitude exposure: influence of α-adrenergic blockade. *J Appl Physiol* 2001;**91**:2143–9.

47. Frank MG, Thompson BM, Watkins LR, Maier SF. Glucocorticoids mediate stress-induced priming of microglial pro-inflammatory responses. *Brain Behav Immunol* 2012;**26**:337–45.

48. Maslanik T, Tannura K, Mahaffey L, Loughridge AB, Beninson L, Ursell L, et al. The commensal bacteria and MAMPs are necessary for stress-induced increases in IL-1β and IL18 but not IL-6, IL-10 or MCP-1. *PLoS One* 2012;7(12):e50636.

49. Wek RC, Jiang HY, Anthony TG. Coping with stress: eIF2 kinases and translational control. *Biochem Soc Trans* 2006;**34**:7–11.

50. Laplante M, Sabatini DM. mTOR signaling in growth control and disease. *Cell* 2012;**149**:274–93.

51. Song MJ, Kim KH, Yoon JM, Kim JB. Activation of Toll-like receptor 4 is associated with insulin resistance in adipocytes. *Biochem Biophys Res Commun* 2006;**346**:739–45.

52. Liao KC, Mogridge J. Activation of the Nlrp1b inflammasome by reduction of cytosolic ATP. *Infect Immun* 2013;**81**:570–9.

53. Schaefer L. Complexity of danger: the diverse nature of damage-associated molecular patterns. *J Biol Chem* 2014;**289**:35237–45.

54. Trevisi E, Amadori M, Cogrossi S, Razzuoli E, Bertoni G. Metabolic stress and inflammatory response in high-yielding, periparturient dairy cows. *Res Vet Sci* 2012;**93**:695–704.

55. Contreras GA, Sordillo LM. Lipid mobilization and inflammatory responses during the transition period of dairy cows. *Comp Immunol Microbiol Infect Dis* 2011;**34**:281–9.

56. Lacetera N, Bernabucci U, Ronchi B, Nardone A. Effects of subclinical pregnancy toxaemia on immune responses in sheep. *Am J Vet Res* 2001;**62**:1020–4.

57. Lacetera N, Franci O, Scalia D, Bernabucci U, Ronchi B, Nardone A. Effects of nonesterified fatty acids and β-hydroxybutyrate on functions of mononuclear cells obtained from ewes. *Am J Vet Res* 2002;**63**:414–8.

58. Lacetera N, Scalia D, Franci O, Bernabucci U, Ronchi B, Nardone A. Effects of nonesterified fatty acids on lymphocyte functions in dairy heifers. *J Dairy Sci* 2004;**87**:1012–4.

59. Scalia D, Lacetera N, Bernabucci U, Demeyere K, Duchateau L, Burvenich C. *In vitro* effects of non-esterified fatty acids on bovine neutrophils oxidative burst and viability. *J Dairy Sci* 2006;**89**:147–54.

60. Trevisi E, Amadori M, Cogrossi S, Razzuoli E, Bertoni G. Metabolic stress and inflammatory response in high-yielding, periparturient dairy cows. *Res Vet Sci* 2012;**93**:695–704.

61. Amadori M, Razzuoli E, Nassuato Ç. Issues and possible intervention strategies relating to early weaning of piglets. *CAB Rev* 2012;**7**:1–15.

62. Friggens NC, Disenhaus C, Petit HV. Nutritional sub-fertility in the dairy cow: towards improved reproductive management through a better biological understanding. *Animal* 2010;**4**:1197–213.

63. Hendrick JP, Hartl FU. Molecular chaperone functions of heat-shock proteins. *Ann Rev Biochem* 1993;**62**:349–84.

64. Schlesinger MJ. Heat shock proteins. *J Biol Chem* 1990;**265**:12111–4.

65. Kregel KC. Heat shock proteins: modifying factors in physiological stress responses and acquired thermotolerance. *J Appl Physiol* 2002;**92**:2177–86.

66. Kampinga HH, Hageman J, Vos MJ, Kubota H, Tanguay RM, Bruford EA, et al. Guidelines for the nomenclature of the human heat shock proteins. *Cell Stress Chaperon* 2009;**14**:105–11.

67. Lindquist S, Craig EA. The heat-shock proteins. *Ann Rev Genet* 1988;**22**:631–77.

68. Hightower LE. Heat shock, stress proteins, chaperones, and proteotoxicity. *Cell* 1991;**66**:191–7.

69. Asea A. Mechanisms of HSP72 release. *J Biosci* 2007;**32**:579–84.

70. Romano Carratelli C, Nuzzo I, Vitiello T, Galdiero E, Galdiero F. The effect of dietary lipid manipulation on murine splenic lymphocytes apoptosis and heat shock protein over expression. *FEMS Immunol Med Microbiol* 1999;**24**:19–25.

71. Moseley P. Stress proteins and the immune response. *Immunopharmacology* 2000;**48**:299–302.

72. Patel NV, Finch CE. The glucocorticoid paradox of caloric restriction in slowing brain aging. *Neurobiol Aging* 2002;**23**:707–17.

73. Heydari AR, Wu B, Takahashi R, Strong R, Richardson A. Expression of heat shock protein 70 is altered by age and diet at the level of transcription. *Mol Cell Biol* 1993;**13**:2909–18.

74. Selsbya JT, Judgea AR, Yimlamaia T, Leeuwenburghb C, Dodda SL. Life long calorie restriction increases heat shock proteins and proteasome activity in soleus muscles of Fisher 344 rats. *Exp Gerontol* 2005;**40**:37–42.

75. Locke M, Noble EG, Atkinson BG. Exercising mammals synthesize stress proteins. *Am J Physiol Cell Physiol* 1990;**258**:723–9.

76. Noble EG, Milne KJ, Melling CWJ. Heat shock proteins and exercise: a primer. *Appl Physiol Nutr Metab* 2008;**33**:1050–75.

77. Walsh RC, Koukoulas I, Garnham A, Moseley PL, Hargreaves M, Febbraio MA. Exercise increases serum HSP72 in humans. *Cell Stress Chaperon* 2001;**6**:386–93.

78. Febbraio MA, Ott P, Nielsen HB, Steensberg A, Keller C, Krustrup P, et al. Exercise induces hepatoplanchnic release of heat shock protein 72 in humans. *J Physiol* 2002;**544**:957–62.

79. Febbraio MA, Steensberg A, Walsh R, Koukoulas I, Van Hall G, Saltin B, et al. Reduced muscle glycogen availability elevates HSP72 in contracting human skeletal muscle. *J Physiol* 2002;**538**:911–7.

80. Febbraio MA, Mesa JL, Chung J, Steensberg A, Keller C, Nielsen HB, et al. Glucose ingestion attenuates the exercise-induced increase in circulating heat shock protein 72 and heat shock protein 60 in humans. *Cell Stress Chaperon* 2004;**9**:390–6.

81. Chang J, Knowlton AA, Xu F, Wasser JS. Activation of the heat shock response: relationship to energy metabolites. A 31P NMR study in rat hearts. *Am J Physiol Heart Circ Physiol* 2001;**280**:426–33.

82. Kavanagh K, Zhang L, Wagner JD. Tissue-specific regulation and expression of heat shock proteins in type 2 diabetic monkeys. *Cell Stress Chaperon* 2009;**14**:291–9.

83. Morino S, Kondo T, Sasaki K, Adachi H, Suico MA, Sekimoto E, et al. Mild electrical stimulation with heat shock ameliorates insulin resistance via enhanced insulin signalling. *PLoS ONE* 2008;e4068.

84. Chung J, Nguyen A-K, Henstridge DC, Holmes AG, Stanley Chan MH, Mesa JL, et al. HSP72 protects against obesity-induced insulin resistance. *PNAS* 2008;**105**:1739–44.

85. Oglesbee MJ, Herdmanb AV, Passmorec GG, Hoffman WH. Diabetic ketoacidosis increases extracellular levels of the major inducible 70-kDa heat shock protein. *Clin Biochem* 2005;**38**:900–4.

86. Nakhjavani M, Morteza A, Khajeali L, Esteghamati A, Khalilzadeh O, Asgarani F, et al. Increased serum HSP70 levels are associated with the duration of diabetes. *Cell Stress Chaperon* 2010;**15**:959–64.

87. Yuan J, Dunn P, Martinus RD. Detection of Hsp60 in saliva and serum from type 2 diabetic and non-diabetic control subjects. *Cell Stress Chaperon* 2011;**16**:689–93.

88. Hall L, Martinus RD. Hyperglycaemia and oxidative stress upregulate HSP60 & HSP70 expression in HeLa cells. *Springerplus* 2013;**2**:431–40.

89. Donati YRA, Slosman DO, POLLA BS. Oxidative injury and the heat shock response. *Biochem Pharmacol* 1990;**40**:2571–7.

90. West JD, Wang Y, Morano KA. Small molecule activators of the heat shock response: chemical properties, molecular targets, and therapeutic promise. *Chem Res Toxicol* 2012;**25**:2036–53.

91. Madamanchi NR, Li S, Patterson C, Runge MS. Reactive oxygen species regulate heat-shock protein 70 via the JAK/STAT pathway. *Arter Throm Vasc Biol* 2001;**21**:321–6.

92. Manalo DJ, Lin Z, Liu AY. Redox-dependent regulation of the conformation and function of human heat shock factor 1. *Biochem* 2002;**41**:2580–8.

93. Chiu H-Y, Tsao L-Y, Yang R-C. Heat-shock response protects peripheral blood mononuclear cells (PBMCs) from hydrogen peroxide-induced mitochondrial disturbance. *Cell Stress Chaperon* 2009;**14**:207–17.

94. Kuhla B, Kuhla S, Rudolph PE, Albrecht D, Metges CC. Proteomics analysis of hypothalamic response to energy restriction in dairy cows. *Proteomics* 2007;**7**:3602–17.

95. Eitam H, Brosh A, Orlov A, Izhakil SA. Caloric stress alters fat characteristics and HSP70 expression in somatic cells of lactating beef cows. *Cell Stress Chaperon* 2009;**14**:173–82.

96. Kehrli ME, Shuster DE. Factors affecting milk somatic cells and their role in health of the bovine mammary gland. *J Dairy Sci* 1994;**77**:619–27.

97. A.K. Heat shock protein 70, oxidative stress, and antioxidant status in periparturient crossbred cows supplemented with α-tocopherol acetate. *Trop Anim Health Prod* 2013;**45**:239–45.

98. Gu XH, Hao Y, Wang XL. Overexpression of heat shock protein 70 and its relationship to intestine under acute heat stress in broilers: 2. Intestinal oxidative stress. *Poult Sci* 2012;**91**:790–9.

99. Liu CP, Fu J, Xu FP, Wang XS, Li S. The role of heat shock proteins in oxidative stress damage induced by Se deficiency in chicken livers. *Biometals* 2015;**28**:163–73.

100. Mulligan FJ, Doherty ML. Production diseases of the transition cow. *Vet J* 2008;**176**:3–9.

101. Sordillo LM, Contreras GA, Aitken SL. Metabolic factors affecting the inflammatory response of periparturient dairy cows. *Anim Health Res Rev* 2009;**10**:53–63.

102. Catalani E, Amadori M, Vitali A, Bernabucci U, Nardone A, Lacetera N. The Hsp72 response in peri-parturient dairy cows: relationships with metabolic and immunological parameters. *Cell Stress Chaperon* 2010;**15**:781–90.

103. Wu WX, Derks JB, Zhang Q, Nathanielsz PW. Changes in heat shock protein-90 and -70 messenger ribonucleic acid in uterine tissues of the ewe in relation to parturition and regulation by estradiol and progesterone. *Endocrinol* 1996;**137**:5685–93.

104. Chaiworapongsa T, Erez O, Kusanovic JP, Vaisbuch E, Mazaki-Tovi S, Gotsch F, et al. Amniotic fluid heat shock protein 70 concentration in histologic chorioamnionitis, term and preterm parturition. *J Matern Fetal Neonatal Med* 2008;**21**:449–61.

105. Azawi OI. Postpartum uterine infection in cattle. *Anim Reprod Sci* 2008;**105**:187–208.

106. Miller L, Qureshi MA. Heat-shock protein synthesis in chicken macrophages: influence of *in vivo* and *in vitro* heat shock, lead acetate, and lipopolysaccharide. *Poult Sci* 1992;**71**:988–98.

107. Deitch EA, Beck SC, Cruz NC, De Maio A. Induction of heat shock gene expression in colonic epithelial cells after incubation with *Escherichia coli* or endotoxin. *Crit Care Med* 1995;**23**:1371–6.

108. Muralidharan S, Mandrekar P. Cellular stress response and innate immune signaling: integrating pathways in host defense and inflammation. *J Leukoc Biol* 2013;**94**:1167–84.

109. Asea A, Kabingu E, Stevenson MA, Calderwood SK. HSP70 peptide-bearing and peptide-negative preparations act as chaperokines. *Cell Stress Chaperon* 2000;**5**:425–31.

110. Pockley AG, Muthana M, Calderwood SK. The dual immunoregulatory roles of stress proteins. *Trends Biochem Sci* 2008;**33**:71–9.

111. Røntved CM, Andersen JB, Dernfalk J, Ingvartsen KL. Effects of diet energy density and milking frequency in early lactation on tumor necrosis factor-α responsiveness in dairy cows. *Vet Immunol Immunopathol* 2005;**104**:171–81.

112. Karcher EL, Beitz DC, Stabel JR. Modulation of cytokine gene expression and secretion during the peri-parturient period in dairy cows naturally infected with *Mycobacterium avium* subsp. *paratuberculosis*. *Vet Immunol Immunopathol* 2008;**123**:277–88.

113. Fan H, Cook JA. Molecular mechanisms of endotoxin tolerance. *J Endotoxin Res* 2004;**10**:71–84.

114. Dirksen G, Liebich H, Mayer H. Adaptive changes of the ruminal mucosa and functional and clinical significance. *Bov Pract* 1985;**20**:116–20.

115. Peter AT, Bosu WT, Gilbert RO. Absorption of *Escherichia coli* endotoxin (lipopolysaccharide) from the uteri of postpartum dairy cows. *Theriogenology* 1990;**33**:1011–4.

116. Plaizier JC, Krause DO, Gozho GN, McBride BW. Subacute ruminal acidosis in dairy cows, the physiological causes, incidence and consequences. *Vet J* 2008;**176**:21–31.

117. Beeson PB. Development of tolerance to typhoid bacterial pyrogen and its abolition by reticulo-endothelial blockade. *Proc Soc Exp Biol Med* 1946;**61**:248–50.

118. Hill AW, Shears AL, Hibbitt KG. Increased antibacterial activity against *Escherichia coli* in bovine serum after the induction of endotoxin tolerance. *Infect Immun* 1976;**14**:257–65.

119. Bieniek K, Szuster-Ciesielska A, Kamińska T, Kondracki M, Witek M, Kandefer-Szerszeń M. Tumor necrosis factor and interferon activity in the circulation of calves after repeated injection of low doses of lipopolysaccharide. *Vet Immunol Immunopathol* 1998;**62**:297–307.

120. Kahl S, Elsasser TH. Exogenous testosterone modulates tumor necrosis factor-α and acute phase protein responses to repeated endotoxin challenge in steers. *Domest Anim Endocrinol* 2006;**31**:301–11.

121. Cavaillon JM, Adib-Conquy M. Bench-to-bedside review: endotoxin tolerance as a model of leukocyte reprogramming in sepsis. *Crit Care* 2006;**10**:233–40.

122. Jacobsen S, Andersen PH, Aasted B. The cytokine response of circulating peripheral blood mononuclear cells is changed after intravenous injection of lipopolysaccharide in cattle. *Vet J* 2007;**174**:170–5.

123. Elsasser TH, Caperna TJ, Li CJ, Kahl S, Sartin JL. Critical control points in the impact of the proinflammatory immune response on growth and metabolism. *J Anim Sci* 2008;**86**:E105–125E.

124. Maas PJ, Colditz IG. Desensitization of the acute inflammatory response in skin and mammary gland of sheep. *Immunol* 1987;**61**:215–59.

125. Cavaillon JM, Adib-Conquy M, Cloëz-Tayarani I, Fitting C. Immunodepression in sepsis and SIRS assessed by *ex vivo* cytokine production is not a generalized phenomenon: a review. *J Endotoxin Res* 2001;**7**:85–93.

126. Opal SM. The host response to endotoxin, antilipopolysaccharide strategies, and the management of severe sepsis. *Int J Med Microbiol* 2007;**297**:365–77.

127. Cavaillon JM. The nonspecific nature of endotoxin tolerance. *Trends Microbiol* 1995;**3**:320–4.

128. Youngner JS, Stinebring WR. Interferon appearance stimulated by endotoxin bacteria or viruses in mice pre-treated with *Escherichia coli* endotoxin or infected with *Mycobacterium tuberculosis*. *Nature* 1965;**208**:456–8.

129. Severn A, Xu D, Doyle J, Leal LM, O'Donnell CA, Brett SJ, et al. Pre-exposure of murine macrophages to lipopolysaccharide inhibits the induction of nitric oxide synthase and reduces leishmanicidal activity. *Eur J Immunol* 1993;**23**:1711–4.

130. Pyörälä S. Mastitis in post-partum dairy cows. *Reprod Domest Anim* 2008;**43**:252–9.

131. Tang D, Kang R, Xiao W, Wang H, Calderwood SK, Xiao X. The anti-inflammatory effects of heat shock protein 72 involve inhibition of high-mobility-group box 1 release and proinflammatory function in macrophages. *J Immunol* 2007;**179**:1236–44.

132. Maridonneau-Parini J, Clerc J, Polla B. Heat shock inhibits NADPH oxidase in human neutrophils. *Biochem Biophys Res Commun* 1988;**154**:179–86.

133. Asea A, Kraeft SK, Kurt-Jones EA, Stevenson MA, Chen LB, Finberg RW, et al. HSP70 stimulates cytokine production through a CD14-dependant pathway, demonstrating its dual role as a chaperone and cytokine. *Nat Med* 2000;**6**:435–42.

134. Campisi J, Leem T, Fleshner M. Stress-induced extracellular HSP72 is a functionally significant danger signal to the immune system. *Cell Stress Chaperon* 2003;**8**:272–86.

135. Asea A. Stress proteins and initiation of immune response: chaperokine activity of HSP72. *Exerc Immunol Rev* 2005;**11**:34–45.

136. Song M, Pinsky MR, Kellum JA. Heat shock factor 1 inhibits nuclear factor-κB nuclear binding activity during endotoxin tolerance and heat shock. *J Crit Care* 2008;**23**:406–15.

137. Hotchkiss R, Nunnally I, Lindquist S, Taulien J, Perdrizet G, Karl I. Hyperthermia protects mice against the lethal effects of endotoxin. *Am J Physiol* 1993;**265**:R1447–57.

138. Van Molle W, Wielockx B, Mahieu T, Takada M, Taniguchi T, Sekikawa K, et al. HSP70 protects against TNF-induced lethal inflammatory shock. *Immunity* 2002;**16**:685–95.

139. Klosterhalfen B, Hauptmann S, Tietze L, Tons C, Winkeltau G, Kupper W, et al. The influence of heat shock protein 70 induction on hemodynamic variables in a porcine model of recurrent endotoxemia. *Shock* 1997;**7**:358–63.

140. Wang X, Zou Y, Wang Y, Li C, Chang Z. Differential regulation of interleukin-12 and interleukin-10 by heat shock response in murine peritoneal macrophages. *Biochem Biophys Res Commun* 2001;**287**:1041–4.

141. Shi Y, Tu Z, Tang D, Zhang H, Liu M, Wang K, et al. The inhibition of LPS induced production of inflammatory cytokines by HSP70 involves inactivation of the NF-κB pathway but not the MAPK pathways. *Shock* 2006;**26**:277–84.

142. Bruemmer-Smith S, Stuber F, Schroeder S. Protective functions of intracellular heat-shock protein (HSP) 70-expression in patients with severe sepsis. *Intensive Care Med* 2001;**27**:1835–41.

143. Chen H, Wu Y, Zhang Y, Jin L, Luo L, Xue B, et al. Hsp70 inhibits lipopolysaccharide-induced NF-κB activation by interacting with TRAF6 and inhibiting its ubiquitination. *FEBS Lett* 2006;**580**:3145–52.

144. Cahill CM, Waterman WR, Xie Y, Auron PE, Calderwood SK. Transcriptional repression of the prointerleukin 1beta gene by heat shock factor 1. *J Biol Chem* 1996;**271**:24874–9.

145. Ianaro A, Ialenti A, Maffia P, Pisano B, Di Rosa M. HSF1/hsp72 pathway as an endogenous anti-inflammatory system. *FEBS Lett* 2001;**499**:239–44.

146. Colaco CA, Bailey CR, Walker KB, Keeble J. Heat shock proteins: stimulators of innate and acquired immunity. *Biomed Res Int* 2013;**2013**:1–11.

147. Wang Y, Kelly CG, Singh M, McGowan EG, Carrara AS, Lesley A, et al. Bergmeier Stimulation of Th1-polarizing cytokines, C-C chemokines, maturation of dendritic cells, and adjuvant function by the peptide binding fragment of heat shock protein 70. *J Immunol* 2002;**169**:2422–9.

148. Lehner T, Wang Y, Whittall T, McGowan E, Kelly CG, Singh M. Functional domains of HSP70 stimulate generation of cytokines and chemokines, maturation of dendritic and adjuvanticity. *Biochem Soc Trans* 2004;**32**:629–32.

149. McNulty S, Colaco CA, Blandford LE, Bailey CR, Baschieri S, Todryk S. Heat-shock proteins as dendritic cell-targeting vaccines – getting warmer. *Immunol* 2013;**139**:407–15.

150. Chionh YT, Arulmuruganar A, Venditti E, Ng GZ, Han J-X, Entwisle C, et al. Heat shock protein complex vaccination induces protection against *Helicobacter pylori* without exogenous adjuvant. *Vaccine* 2014;**32**:2350–8.

151. Wang R, Kovalchin JT, Muhlenkamp P, Chandawarkar RY. Exogenous heat shock protein 70 binds macrophage lipid raft microdomain and stimulates phagocytosis, processing, and MHC-II presentation of antigens. *Blood* 2006;**107**:1636–42.

152. Lee1 CT, Repasky EA. Opposing roles for heat and heat shock proteins in macrophage functions during inflammation: a function of cell activation state? *Front Immunol* 2012;**3**:1–7 doi: 10.3389/fimmu.2012.00140.

153. Gao B, Tsan MF. Endotoxin contamination in recombinant human heat shock protein 70 (Hsp70) preparation is responsible for the induction of tumor necrosis factor α release by murine macrophages. *J Biol Chem* 2003;**278**:174–9.

154. Singleton KD, Wischmeyer PE. Effects of HSP70.1/3 gene knockout on acute respiratory distress syndrome and the inflammatory response following sepsis. *Am J Physiol Lung Cell Mol Physiol* 2006;**290**:L956–61.

155. Ferat-Osorio E, Sánchez-Anaya A, Gutiérrez-Mendoza M, Boscó-Gárate I, Wong-Baeza I, Pastelin-Palacios R, et al. Heat shock protein 70 down-regulates the production of toll-like receptor-induced pro-inflammatory cytokines by a heat shock factor-1/constitutive heat shock element-binding factor-dependent mechanism. *J Inflamm* 2014;**11**:1–12.

156. de Graeff-Meeder ER, van der Zee R, Rijkers GT, Schuurman HJ, Kuis W, Bijlsma JW, et al. Recognition of human 60 kD heat shock protein by mononuclear cells from patients with juvenile chronic arthritis. *Lancet* 1991;**337**:1368–72.

157. de Kleer IM, Kamphuis SM, Rijkers GT, Scholtens L, Gordon G, de Jager W, et al. The spontaneous remission of juvenile idiopathic arthritis is characterized by CD30+ T cells directed to human heat-shock protein 60 capable of producing the regulatory cytokine interleukin-10. *Arthritis Rheum* 2003;**48**:2001–10.

158. Borges TJ, Wieten L, van Herwijnen MJC, Broere F, van der Zee R, Bonorino C, et al. The anti-inflammatory mechanisms of Hsp70. *Front Immunol* 2012;**3**:1–12 doi: 10.3389/fimmu.2012.00095.

159. Bausinger H, Lipsker D, Ziylan U, Manie S, Briand JP, Cazenave JP, et al. Endotoxin-free heat-shock protein 70 fails to induce APC activation. *Eur J Immunol* 2002;**32**:3708–13.

160. Motta A, Schmitz C, Rodrigues L, Ribeiro F, Teixeira C, Detanico T, et al. *Mycobacterium tuberculosis* heat-shock protein 70 impairs maturation of dendritic cells from bone marrow precursors, induces interleukin-10 production and inhibits T-cell proliferation *in vitro*. *Immunology* 2007;**121**:462–72.

Chapter 6

Innate Immune Responses and Cancer Metastasis

Yoshiro Maru
Department of Pharmacology, Tokyo Women's Medical University, Shinjuku-ku, Tokyo, Japan

CLINICAL INFORMATION ON METASTASIS

An observation back in 1786 by surgeon John Hunter of pulmonary lesions about a metastatic manifestation from a tumorous disease in the femoral bone, which turned out to be a rare disease osteosarcoma, raised the curtain of metastatic diseases (Table 6.1). Immune cells originate from lymph nodes and bone marrow, and migrate through the whole body but actually accomplish their task at given sites. Tumor cells (seed) basically derive from the primary site, migrate through circulation, and cause metastasis at preferential sites (soil) as proposed by Stephan Paget in 1889. This resembles emboli that occlude vessels in a certain manner dependent on the physical properties including bloodstream flow and anatomical conditions.

A clinical example of lung cancer, which exhibited lymphangitis carcinomatosa in the lungs, has been shown here. When tumor cells make a massive entry into the vein, they often cause retrograde dissemination back into the lymphatic duct in the same organ. Lymphangitis carcinomatosa is one of the most difficult diseases to treat since the patients usually die of respiratory failure due to impaired gas exchange. In this case, however, the treatment was successful with gefitinib, a tyrosine kinase inhibitor against mutated forms of EGFR (epidermal growth factor receptor) in tumor cells (Fig. 6.1). The case indicates that metastasis partly depends on the trait of tumor cells by themselves. On the other hand, as it is usually the case that even advanced cancers always have some spared organs for metastasis, existence of tumor cells in circulation never guarantees metastasis in all organs, suggesting the need for cultivation of soil, namely, establishment of the microenvironment prior to the arrival of metastatic tumor cells. This is called the premetastatic microenvironment, which is the focus of this chapter.

TABLE 6.1 Time Course of Concepts

ca 460–370 BC	Hippocrates	Inflammation (Ref. [1])
1786	John Hunter	A concept of disease spreading to other organ (Ref. [2])
1865	Claude Bernard	An idea of milieu interior and homeostasis (Ref. [3])
1889	Stephan Paget	Seed and soil hypothesis (Ref. [4])
2006	Yoshiro Maru	TLR4 in metastatic niche (Ref. [5])
2009	Yoshiro Maru	Homeostatic inflammation in metastasis (Ref. [6])

The ideas of inflammation, tumor metastasis, homeostasis, and TLR4 in the context of metastasis were initially proposed as referenced.

ELEMENTS THAT CONSTITUTE METASTASIS

Definition and Understanding

The relationships among innate immunity, coagulation, angiogenesis, and inflammation are based on the concepts presented in this particular chapter. Inflammation has at least two essential features namely leukocyte mobilization and vascular permeability. The activated leukocytes, whether migrating or not, constitute the immune system, in which the first defense program without antibody production is operated by innate immunity. Angiogenesis is a new generation of vasculatures from the preexisting ones and is almost always accompanied by vascular permeability and endothelial cell (EC) growth, at least at certain time phases and sites. Deterioration of endothelial barrier against coagulation activates coagulation pathways involving coagulation factors and platelets, and is caused by intrinsic factors and/or damages such as external injuries and tissue necrosis. For example, pathologically increased vascular permeability even without hemorrhage (extravasation of red blood cells) often activates coagulation.

Currently, most of the accumulating evidence is based on tumor metastasis models of mice in which genetic engineering can be readily implemented. However, interspecies differences are often obstacles for interpretation of the results. For example, prostate cancer of spontaneous occurrence with osteoblastic bone metastasis is known only in humans and dogs, but canine prostate cancer cells are not dependent on androgens.[7] An old paper reported that 3.7 million pigs during the period 1965–1966 in slaughterhouses in the United Kingdom had only 14 metastatic lung tumors. Given that those pigs were supposed to be healthy for meat, the prevalence of metastatic lung tumor in pigs would be 0.38 per 100,000 subjects. An estimated US lung cancer prevalence of 0.1% was much higher than that in those pigs.[8] With regard to specific tumors, swine melanoma, for example, has preferential metastasis to lungs.[9]

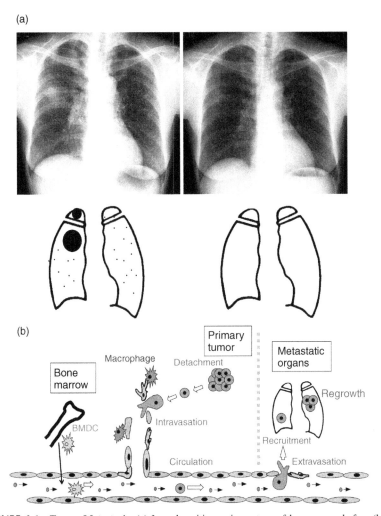

FIGURE 6.1   Tumor Metastasis. (a) Lymphangitis carcinomatosa of lung cancer before (left) and after (right) treatment with gefitinib. Not only the primary tumor in the right lung but also dissemination disappeared. (b) Metastatic progression of tumor cells consists of at least six steps, from detachment of tumor cells for the primary tumor to resettlement in distant organs such as lungs and regrowth. The tumor cell migration via circulation within the body is similar to mobilization of leukocytes from bone marrow (bone-marrow-derived cell, BMDC).

Metastasis is achieved by the interplay between tumor cells and host organs. Traits of tumor cells by themselves include genetic alterations of quality and/or quantity as represented by oncogenic mutations and behavioral characteristics such as stem-like properties. Hosts respond to those tumor cell traits mainly through angiogenesis and immunity in a manner dependent on unique microenvironmental features of the metastatic organs. Therefore, given that the current level of evidence is not enough to explain the mechanisms of metastasis in each organ, we can hardly generalize metastasis. Instead of doing so, here I focus on one model, that is, murine lung metastasis that has been confirmed by Maru and coworkers as well as by other groups, thereby proposing a mechanistic connection between innate immunity and metastasis.

Triangle

To prove the biological significance of the triangle consisting of coagulation, angiogenesis, and inflammation in tumor metastasis, knockout (KO) mouse models or functional inhibitions by antibody treatment are utilized to define necessary conditions. Here, experimental evidence on some of the well-known factors required for pulmonary metastasis have been shown by discussing the triangle, in which any two of the three corners have bidirectional interactions (Fig. 6.2).

As shown in Fig. 6.3, there are several experimental systems to evaluate lung metastasis. The simplest way is to implant tumor cells, either ectopically (e.g., subcutaneously) or orthotopically (as in the case of breast cancer cells into the mammary fat pads), and to let them accomplish spontaneous metastatic progression to several organs including the lungs. If implanted tumor cells never reach the lungs in a certain period of time, as judged by the genetic (e.g., neomycin-resistance gene that is integrated into the genome of the implanted tumor cells) or biological markers (integrated gene products emitting fluorescence for biodetection by imaging studies), the lungs can be in a premetastatic condition prior to the actual arrival of tumor cells.

Angiogenesis Promotes Coagulation and Induces Inflammation

The most potent angiogenic factor vascular endothelial growth factor (VEGF), which is produced by tumor cells and infiltrating macrophages in the primary tumor microenvironment, activates VEGFR2 to induce growth and migration of ECs (Fig. 6.2). This is regulated by VEGF anchoring to and detaching from the extracellular matrix through the action of matrix metalloproteases (MMPs) such as MMP9.[10] VEGFR1, which exists in either soluble or membrane-spanning form, shows 10-fold higher affinity to VEGF than VEGFR2, and serves as a decoy receptor for negative regulation. It should be noted that VEGF–VEGFR1 signaling induces cell migration of monocytes and macrophages that exceptionally express VEGFR1. EC-specific KO of VEGF revealed its homeostatic role in endothelial barrier formation since the KO mice displayed hemorrhage.[11] The homeostasis can also be disrupted by VEGF excess in the tumor microenvironment where tumor vessels are different from the physiological ones, such that they are tortuous, dilated, highly permeable, and mostly devoid of pericytes. To prevent vascular leakage by endothelial barrier disruption, a coagulation system is activated to eventually form fibrin, to protect against leakage.

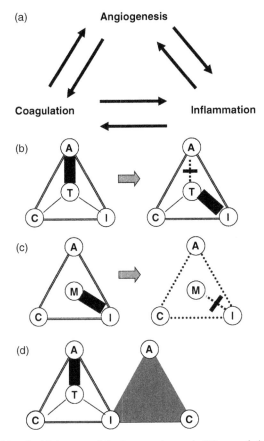

FIGURE 6.2   Triangle. (a) Any two of the three, angiogenesis (A), coagulation (C), and inflammation (I), have reciprocal interactions. (b) Tumor (T)-produced VEGF drives tumor angiogenesis. When tumor angiogenesis is abrogated by inhibitors of VEGFR2, immune cells are activated by necrotic tumor tissues, which persistently support the triangle stability giving resistance to anti-VEGF therapy. (c) Microbes (M) induce inflammation through pattern recognition receptors. However, total killing of the microbes can eliminate M-to-I signaling, which in turn destroys the stability of the triangle. (d) Inflammation can spread to other organs that still lack tumor cells where a new triangle may be established providing premetastatic soil prior to the arrival of metastasizing tumor cells.

If tumor cell growth exceeds the oxygen supply to tumor vessels in any sites at any time point during primary tumor progression, HIF-1 (hypoxia-inducible factor-1) is activated to upregulate not only VEGF but also a variety of chemokines including CXCL12 (also called SDF-1), PlGF (placenta growth factor), and G-CSF (granulocyte-colony stimulating factor) to establish an "inflamed state."[12] PlGF specifically binds and activates its own receptor VEGFR1. Leukocyte mobilization by those growth factors to the primary tumor under hypoxia matches the aforementioned definition of inflammation.

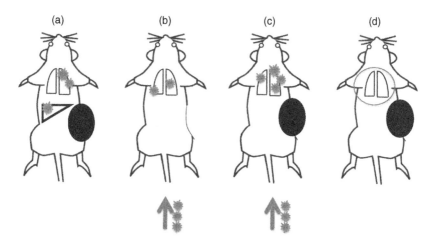

FIGURE 6.3 **Murine metastasis models.** (a) Implanted tumor cells disseminate to multiple organs such as lungs and liver. (b) Injection of labeled tumor cells through veins (usually the tail vein) into systemic circulation in tumor-nonbearing mice causes lung metastasis. (c) The same injection as c in tumor-bearing mice causes lung metastasis more efficiently than that in b. (d) A premetastatic lung condition, in which implanted tumor cells never reach the lungs.

With this fundamental information in mind, let us take a look at Table 6.2. In murine models, antibody against either VEGF or PlGF was shown to inhibit metastasis. Lentivirus-mediated knockdown of VEGFR1 in bone-marrow-derived myeloid cells (BMDCs) also inhibited lung metastasis. However, in clinical settings, anti-VEGF monotherapy has failed to meet the original expectation. Both VEGF-independent angiogenesis by, for example G-CSF (capable of inducing expression of angiogenic factor Bv8 in BMDC), and leukocyte mobilization by other chemokines confer resistance.[13] Sunitinib, a tyrosine kinase inhibitor of VEGFR2, also inhibits PDGFR essential for pericytes, resulting in further disruption of EC barrier.[14] Thus, although growth of the primary tumor and subsequent metastatic progression are dependent on VEGF abundantly supplied by the microenvironment, depletion of VEGF–VEGFR2 signaling may accelerate hypoxic and metabolically noxious conditions for the tumor cells that survived it. This potentiates their metastatic ability by changing tumor cell traits (due to hypoxia-induced ROS [reactive oxygen species] that may cause genetic alterations) and by aggravating inflammation in the microenvironment.[15]

Coagulation Promotes Angiogenesis and Inflammation

Plasticity of the EC barrier by fixing damages or stopping nonphysiological vascular leakages guarantees stability or homeostasis of vessels (Fig. 6.2). Thrombotic patchworks serve as a first-aid treatment. In the tumor microenvironment, expression of tissue factor (also called coagulation factor III) is elevated, which triggers the extrinsic pathway of coagulation cascade. On the other hand, the

TABLE 6.2 Necessary Conditions for Metastasis

Biology	Targets	Methods	Tumor cells	Systems	Primary	References
A-I	VEGF	Antibody	HM 7	B (liver) ↓	–	[16]
A-2	VEGFR1	TK-KO	B 16	B (lung) ↓	–	[17]
A-3	P1GF	Antibody	B 16	B (lung) ↓	–	[17]
A-4	VEGFR1	shRNA	B 16-m Cherry	B (lung) ↓	–	[18]
A-5	VEGFR2	Inhibitor	R P-Tag2	A (liver) ↑	←	[14]
A-6	Plasma Fn	KO	B 16, 3LL	B (lung) ↓	–	[19]
A-7	Neuropilin-2	Antibody	66c14 mammary carcinoma	A (lung) ↓	↑	[20]
A-8	EphA2	KO	LLC	B (lung) ↓	–	[21]
A-9	Angiopoietin-2	Antibody	4T1	B (lung) ↓	–	[22]
A-10	MMP-9	KO	17L3C-Luc	B (lung) ↓	–	[23]
A-11	MMP-13	KO	B 16F1-GFP	B (lung, liver) ↓	→	[24]
A-12	ADAM8	Antibody	MDA-MB-231	A (Lung, Brain) ↓	→	[25]
A-13	Tenascin-C	KO	RT2 insulinoma	A (lung ↓, liver→)	↑	[26]
A-14	Integrin α4	Knock-in (inactive)	PyMT-MMTV	A (lung, lymph node) ↓	→	[27]
A-15	Adrβ2/3	KO	PC3 Luc	A (lymph node) ↓	→	[28]
A-16	VCAM-1	Antibody	4T1	B (lung) ↓	–	[29]
C-1	III (tissue factor)	KO	EF (III-KO)	B (lung) ↓	–	[30]

(Continued)

TABLE 6.2 Necessary Conditions for Metastasis (cont.)

Biology	Targets	Methods	Tumor cells	Systems	Primary	References
C-2	III-V IIa	Antibody	CH0/TF (III)	B (lung) ↓	–	[31]
C-3	Plasminogen	KO	LLC, B I6	B (lung) →→	–	[32]
C-4	XIIIA	KO	LLCGFP	A, B (lung) ↓	↑	[33]
C-5	Xa	Inhibitor	LC 15S	B (lung, liver) ↓	–	[34]
C-6	II (thrombin)	Inhibitor	B 16	B (lung) ↓	–	[35]
C-7	I (fibrinogen)	KO	LLC, B 16	A, B (lung) ↓	↑	[32], [36]
P-I	Nf-E2	KO	B 16	B (lung) ↓	–	[37]
P-2	Par4	KO	B 16	B (lung) ↓	–	[37]
P-3	Parl or 2	KO	B 16	B (lung) →→	–	[37]
P-4	GPIb	KO	B 16	B (lung) ↓	–	[38]
P-5	GPIIb/IIIa	Inhibitor	LLC	B (lung) ↓	–	[39]
P-6	Gao1	KO	LLC-GFP	A, B (lung) ↓	↑	[40]
P-7	Platelet, gp44	Antibody	NL17	B (lung) ↓	–	[41]
P-8	Orai1	Inhibitor	MDAMB231	B (lung) ↓	–	[42]
P-9	P-selectin	KO, heparin	LS180	B (lung) ↓	–	[43]
I-1	TLR4	KO	LLC, 3LL	A,B,C (lung) ↓	→ (A), -(B)	[44]
I-2	TNFα	KO	LLC	B (lung) ↓	–	[45]
I-3	TLR2	KO	LLC-D sRed, LLC	B (lung) ↓, A (lung, liver, adrenal) ↓	→ (A), -(B)	[45]
I-4	COX	Inhibitor	410.4	A, B (lung) ↓	→	[46]

I-5	HGF	HGF antagonist	B 16F10, LLC	B (lung) ↓	—	[47]
I-6	HGF	HGF antagonist	MC 38	B (liver) ↓	—	[48]
I-7	TQFβ	Inhibitor, neutralizing Ab	4T1, MDA-MB-231	A (lung) ↓	→	[49]
I-8	TGFβ	TGFβR inhibitor	MDA-MB-231	A, B (lung, bone) ↓	↓ (A),–(B)	[50]
I-9	G-CSF	Neutralizing Ab	4T1, MDA-MB-231, PyMT	A (lung) ↓	↑	[51]
I-10	MMP-8	KO	B 16F10, LLC	A, B (lung) ↑	↑	[52]
I-11	MMP-13	KO	E0771	A (lung) ↑	↑	[53]
I-12	AhR	KO	B 16F10	B (lung) ↓	—	[54]
I-13	Hsp70	KO	PymT	A (lung) ↓	→	[55]
I-14	EP4	Inhibitor	66.1	B (lung) ↓	—	[56]
I-15	ADAM12	KO	PyMT-driven mammary adenocarcinoma	A (lung) ↓	→	[57]
I-16	Clots	KO	TC-1, B 16F10	A B (lung) ↓	→	[58]
I-17	TLR 7	KO	LLC	B (lung) ↓	—	[59]
I-18	Periostin	KO	MMTV/PyMT	A (lung) ↓	↑	[60]
I-19	MD-2	KO	E0771	B (lung) ↓	—	[61]
I-20	CCL5	Inhibitor	MC38, LS180	B (lung) ↓	—	[62]
I-21	SAA3	Antibody	LLC	C (lung) ↓	—	[44]
I-22	CXCR4	KO +/–	B 16	B (lung) ↓	—	[63]
I-23	TAM receptor	Inhibitor	B 16F10, 4T1	A (liver) ↓, B (lung) ↓	↑	[58]
T-1	ADAM15	shRNA	PC-3	B (Bone, Lung) ↓	—	[64]

(Continued)

TABLE 6.2 Necessary Conditions for Metastasis (cont.)

Biology	Targets	Methods	Tumor cells	Systems	Primary	References
T-2	EGFR	EGFR inhibitor	SUM 149	A (lung) ↓	↓	[65]
T-3	AhR	shRNA	MDAMB231	B (lung) ↓	–	[66]
T-4	Plasma Hsp90a	Antibody	B 16/F10, MDA-MB-231	A (lymph nodes, lung) liver ↓	↑	[67]
T-5	ZEB1	shRNA	HCT116	A (liver) ↓	↑	[68]
T-6	Fra1	shRNA	MDA-MB-231	B (lung) ↓	–	[69]
T-7	BACH1	shRNA	MDA-MB-231	B (Bone) ↓	–	[70]
T-8	Cathepsin S	shRNA	MDA-MB-231-TK-GFP-Luc	A (Brain) ↓	↑	[71]
T-9	ELF5	Overexpression	4T1, MDA-MHB-231	A, B (lung) ↓	–(B), → (A)	[72]
T-10	CoCo	shRNA	MDA-MB-231	B (lung) ↓	–	[73]
T-11	CEBPδ	KO	MMTV-Neu mammary tumor	A (lung) ↓	←	[74]
T-12	LOX	shRNA	MDA-MB-231	A (lung) ↓	ND	[75]
T-13	CXCL1	shRNA	LS174T	B (liver) ↓	–	[76]

Well-known factors in the host arm including angiogenesis (A), platelet (P), coagulation (C), and inflammation (I), as well as in the tumor cell arm (T) are targeted by antibody, shRNAs, genetic KO, or pharmacological inhibition. The influences on the primary tumor and metastasis as evaluated by experimental methods in Fig. 6.3 are shown. It cannot be distinguished perfectly whether a given factor is related to A or T. For example, VEGF is produced from both macrophages of host origin and tumor cells. Anti-VEGF antibody inhibits liver metastasis of HM7 colon cancer cells after splenic-portal injection without establishing the primary tumor (A-1). Needless to say, VEGF of both origins is inhibited. On the other hand, embryonic fibroblasts (EF) (C-1) derived from tissue factor (coagulation factor III)-KO mice were transformed by an oncogene and subjected to the type B metastasis assay. An effect on the III-stimulated activation of host coagulation system was negative in lung metastasis. While B16 melanoma cells displayed poor lung metastasis in AhR-KO mice (I-12), an shRNA-mediated knockdown of AhR in MDA-MB-231 tumor cells (T-3) inhibited their lung metastasis after intravenous injection without the primary tumor. TK-KO (A-2), tyrosine kinase KO; Fn (A-6), fibronectin.

intrinsic pathway is activated by contact with negatively charged substances such as phospholipids on the surface of and pyrophosphates released from activated platelets by a variety of signals such as collagen. These are cross-linked with each other by fibrinogen via GPIIb/IIIa and with exposed collagen fibers by GPIa/IIa- or GPIb-mediated vWF (von Willebrand factor). In both pathways activated thrombin (coagulation factor II) eventually converts fibrinogen to fibrin. Generally, a clot is blood cells embedded within fibrin, that is, blood minus serum (remember that serum is devoid of clotting factors such as fibrinogen after blood is allowed to clot and they are consumed) (clot = cells + fibrin = blood − serum, plasma = serum + clotting factors), and includes fibronectin that can make a complex with fibrin. In addition to platelet dense bodies containing 5-HT, ADP, and pyrophosphates, platelet α granules contain a variety of bioactive peptides including vWF, fibrinogen, coagulation factor V, VEGF, and PDGF. Activated platelets sustain increased Ca levels through the Ca channel called Orai1. Thus, even VEGF alone released from activated platelets potentially induces angiogenic and chemotactic responses.

An old study showed the evidence that elimination of platelets by an antiidiotype monoclonal antibody against its surface molecule suppressed lung metastasis of colon cancer cells.[41] Coagulation factors are not necessarily required for metastasis. Both genetic KO of fibrinogen and pharmacological inhibition of thrombin gave only partially negative influences on metastasis in a time-dependent fashion. Genetic inhibition of coagulation factor X showed both partial inhibition (Table 6.2) and enhancement (our laboratory, unpublished results) of metastasis in a manner dependent on experimental contexts. As described earlier platelet tethering is partly mediated by the GPIb–vWF interaction. While lung metastasis by melanoma cells was reduced in GPIb-KO mice,[38] it was enhanced in vWF-KO,[77] suggesting the complicated participation of coagulation system in lung metastasis.

To further complicate the story, pharmacological targets in platelets are also found in tumor and stromal cells including EC, fibroblasts, and immune cells. The widely used antiplatelet drug aspirin irreversibly inhibits COX-2 through which both proaggregatory TXA2 (thromboxane A2) and PGE2 (prostaglandin E2) are synthesized. Primary tumor growth was diminished with less angiogenesis in the background of COX-2-KO since one of its products PGE2 appears to induce VEGF expression through transcription factor AP-1.[78] Pharmacological or genetic inhibition of PGE2 receptors, such as EP3 and EP4, resulted in reduced tumor progression.[79] Decreased number of BMDC and concomitant reduction in CXCL12–CXCR4 expression were observed in primary tumor in the background of EP4-KO.[80] A Ca channel blocker verapamil gave similar inhibition.[42,81]

Inflammation Participates in Both Angiogenesis and Coagulation

The most understandable example is bacterial endotoxin-induced biological response (Fig. 6.2). Endotoxin consists of lipopolysaccharide (LPS) in the bacterial wall. LPS induces endothelial hyperpermeability and leukocyte mobilization through its receptor TLR4 on ECs and leukocytes, respectively. Activation of TLR4 is mediated by direct binding of LPS to its coreceptor called MD-2, which induces dimerization of TLR4 with subsequent intracellular signaling to ultimately activate transcription factor NFκB whose target genes include inflammatory cytokines such as IL-6 and IL-1. To be accurate, the receptor for LPS is the TLR4/MD-2 complex. Here in this chapter, the complex is thereafter simply referred to as TLR4 unless otherwise indicated. C-reactive protein (CRP) is a clinically useful and reliable biomarker of inflammation and is synthesized in the liver in response to those cytokines.

Here I briefly comment on an alleged notion in innate immunity. In addition to the cellular arm of the innate immune system as represented by macrophages, the humoral arm includes complements and pentraxins. Each arm has sensing and effector functions. While CRP belongs to a short pentraxin family, a long family includes pentraxin 3 (PTX3). CRP is an acute-phase homopentamer protein and is a ligand for FcγRII (CD32) on phagocytes that recognizes the Fc portion of IgG (note: while FcγRII is a single polypeptide chain, FcγRI, for example, has a coreceptor called γ chain homodimer, FcRγ. Do not get confused.). For example, antiplatelet autoantibody of IgG type binds platelets causing oxidation of the membrane where phosphorylcholine residues are exposed, thus enabling CRP to make an attachment. Thus, platelet-bound CRP is recognized by FcγR on macrophages with subsequent phagocytosis. Infection therefore aggravates autoimmune thrombocytopenia.[82] Moreover, CRP stimulates migration of myeloid cells, induces expression of CCL2 in ECs, and activates the classical pathway of complement by binding to C1q. Multiple myeloma cells often express FcγRII conferring chemoresistance on them.[83] Recent evidence showed that PTX3-KO deinhibited factor H-regulated complement activation resulting in C5a accumulation with subsequent induction of CCL2 expression.[84] Administration of anti-CCL2 blocking antibody completely reversed 3-MC-induced sarcoma development in PTX3-KO mice. This indicates that PTX3 plays a homeostatic role in inflammation by mitigating the overshoot of CCL2 via complement.

CRP and LPS promote tissue factor (coagulation factor III) production.[85] Conversely, coagulation is likely to aggravate inflammation. LPS-induced expression patterns of inflammatory cytokines including IL-1, IL-4, VEGF, MIP-1, and IFNγ are similar to each other between KO mice of receptor Par1 (receptor for thrombin) and S1P3 (receptor 3 for S1P (sphingosine-1-phosphate)). This suggests one mechanism of the aggravation may be coupling of coagulation with S1P receptor signaling, which is abundant in the nongranule compartment of platelets. Evidence of a bridging function of S1P between coagulation and angiogenesis has been provided. Postnatal loss of function of S1P1 by mouse engineering showed that S1P plays a vessel-stabilizing role. EC-specific deletion of S1P1 resulted in enhanced vascular permeability. Interestingly, phosphorylated status of VE-cadherin in lung ECs was increased twofold, suggesting junctional destabilization.[86]

IL-6 induces VEGF expression in ECs for angiogenesis. VEGF and LPS augment production of NO via eNOS and iNOS, respectively, which in turn binds its soluble receptor guanylyl cyclase (sGC) to generate cGMP. PKG, cGMP-dependent protein kinase, activates the Erk1/2 pathway to induce vascular hyperpermeability. VEGFR2 signaling activates Akt, which phosphorylates eNOS to release caveolin-1-mediated suppression of eNOS activity. In eNOS-KO mice, vascular permeability in the primary tumor was diminished with concomitant reduction in tumor size.[87] Conversely, vascular permeability is increased in caveolin-1-KO mice.

In premetastatic lungs that are supposed to lack tumor cells (discussed here), vascular permeability is increased by a variety of factors including CCL2, S100A8, and SAA3 (serum amyloid A3), and fibrin deposits were observed as a final product of activated coagulation.[61,88]

LUNG HOMEOSTASIS

Interphase

The fundamentals of lung inflammation are determined by the interphase between air and circulation. Bacterial infection through the airway eventually causes leukocyte mobilization on the circulation side by stimulation from the epithelial side with interstitial space in between, where macrophages and fibroblasts are presumed to play a connecting role (Fig. 6.4).

Since the goal of this article is to convince readers of the premetastatic roles of endogenous TLR4 ligands, let us suppose that an authentic exogenous TLR4 ligand LPS represents bacterial infection in the lungs. One of the sensory epithelial cells for LPS is club cells, previously called Clara cells, which are specifically located in the terminal bronchioles.[89] They express TLR4 and stimulation of club cells by LPS induces enormous production of SAA3, an acute-phase reactant protein highly potent in vascular permeability and cell migration. Since SAA3 is an endogenous ligand for TLR4 (see section on premetastasis), LPS can trigger autoamplification of SAA3 in murine club cells.[90] Generally, it is believed that club cells play a biological role in the metabolism of xenobiotics.

To mitigate overstimulation of TLR4 in club cells to maintain epithelial homeostasis, there is a mechanism for LPS tolerance. The first exposure of LPS is known to induce resistance to a second exposure. TLR4 induces activation of aryl hydrocarbon receptor (AhR) in club cells whose ligands include dioxin of environmental origin as well as endogenous kynurenine, a product of tryptophan catabolism by indoleamine 2,3-dioxygenase 1 (IDO1), which is also induced by TLR4 activation.[91] AhR-KO failed to confer LPS tolerance on the mice and therefore they are more sensitive to LPS. Another possible mechanism of mitigation is that SAA3 may serve as a partial agonist for LPS.[44] While SAA3 competes for TLR4 against LPS in the presence of LPS, SAA3 just autoamplifies itself via TLR4 in the absence of LPS.

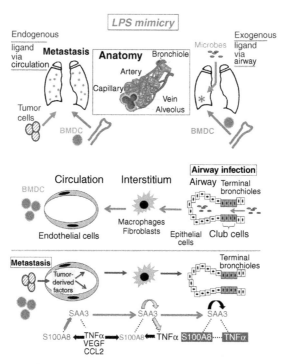

FIGURE 6.4 Bidirectional paracrine signaling in lungs. Lungs have an interphase between circulation and airway. Exogenously borne microbes through the airway induce mobilization of BMDCs to the lungs. The triggering mechanism may involve microbe-originated LPS, which activates TLR4 in club cells in terminal bronchioles. The paracrine signaling goes in the direction to the circulation side. Expression of endogenous ligands, such as S100A8 and SAA3 in ECs in premetastatic lungs, is induced by primary tumor-derived growth factors, such as CCL2, from the circulation side and the paracrine signaling goes in an opposite direction from the circulation to the airway side to result in amplification of SAA3 in club cells. Therefore, premetastatic lungs mimic pulmonary infection.

LPS-induced expression of TNF-α and IL-1β in epithelial cells stimulates macrophages in the interstitial space to secrete chemokines such as CXCL1, CXCL2, and CCL2. KO mice of individual receptors for them, CXCR2 and CCR2, displayed reduced number of leukocytes, neutrophils, and monocytes, respectively, in alveolar spaces.[92]

Cell Mobilization

As stated earlier, TLR4 activation results in the production of a variety of growth factors capable of mobilizing leukocytes from bone marrow to lungs. Here, the mode of cell migration has been briefly discussed. In general, directional cues for migrating cells are given by concentration gradients of soluble factors such as PDGF (this is called chemotaxis), attached factors as found in a linear gradient of extracellular matrix like fibronectin (called haptotaxis), and mechanical stiffness that is sensed by dynamic actin in the cytoskeleton (durotaxis). Leukocytes are also known to migrate toward laser-irradiated dead cells for their phagocytosis. This special form is called necrotaxis.[93] It is also known in euglena cells that their lysis by heat gives a repellent stimulus to intact euglena cells to show negative necrotaxis. A fibroblastic cell line derived from Ink4a/Arf-KO mice, in which an almost perfect and stable absence of Arp2/3 was established, showed defects in cell spreading and haptotaxis, whereas PDGF-dependent chemotaxis was not affected,[94] indicating separate mechanisms for the two modes of cell migration.

Although leukocytes involved in the establishment of premetastatic microenvironment mainly undergo chemotaxis and haptotaxis, evidence is accumulating to show metastatic progression of tumor cells in clusters. This is called collective cell migration or plithotaxis.[95] To further complicate the cell migration system *in vivo*, mobilized leukocytes do not necessarily extravasate to the tissue of interest. In a renal injury model, they just stay within the lumen of vessels by patrolling until local signal activation by TLR7 recruits them to the ECs to cause their necrosis. This homeostatic level of leukocyte mobilization and patrolling without extravasation is called negative chemotactism.[96]

Even without clinically apparent inflammation such as pneumonia, it can safely be said that lungs are subjected to constant assaults by environmental chemicals and air-borne LPS or microbes although alveolar space is basically sterile. These physiological levels of inflammation are not likely to cause lung diseases as manifested in clinical settings and our idea of homeostatic inflammation includes both this subclinical settings and danger signals (see section on Homeostatic Inflammation and Therapeutic Targeting).

In addition to leukocytes, resident epithelial cells in the lungs are also supplied from bone marrow. Club cells are thought to produce an anti-inflammatory substance called club cell secretory protein (CCSP). Roughly 2% of bone marrow cells are CCSP-positive, and acute lung injury by naphthalene, which causes specific apoptosis of Club cells, mobilizes those CCSP-positive club progenitor cells to the lungs.[97] Our laboratory also found that bone marrow cells of GFP mice migrate to the lungs to become club cells.[90]

Therefore, it is likely that cells of mesenchymal and epithelial origin or fate can participate in the tissue architecture of the lungs. The possible mechanisms of travel of tumor cells to the lungs have been discussed in the further sections. Two examples have been reported here about documented cell mobilization phenomenon of cells of epithelial fate in the body. The Harold Varmus laboratory reported the injection of dissociated mammary gland cells, in which expression of oncogenes Myc and K-RasD12 could be induced in a tetracycline-inducible manner and a theoretically untransformed phenotype could be obtained prior to induction. These cells showed pulmonary dissemination and a long stay in the lungs until their transformation to form metastatic foci after switching on the activation of the oncogenes.[98] Timothy C. Wang and coworkers showed that GFP-labeled immune cells from bone marrow, which infiltrated into postapoptotic gastric mucosa caused by *Helicobacter felis* infection, were eventually transformed to adenocarcinoma cells.[99]

Mimicry

Given that those cell movements within the body can take place under sterile conditions, that is, without direct evidence of infection, at least two ideas can be proposed. When the destination of cell mobilization is the frontline that is exposed to microbial invasion, that is, for example, *Helicobacter pylori* in the stomach and *Hemophilus influenza* in the lungs, production of endogenous substances whose functions can mimic those of the microbes may cause similar biological consequences. They are called endogenous TLR4 ligands, such as SAA3, to be discussed in the following sections. Second, in the absence of any local triggering mechanisms for generation of the endogenous ligands in the destination, the destination needs to be stimulated in an endocrine manner from the circulation side as exemplified by growth factors, produced by the primary tumor distantly located from the destination. Thus, we can assume that the interphase between circulation and airway in the case of lungs, may use the same paracrine system but the signaling sequence goes in an opposite direction (Fig. 6.4).

In the case of sepsis by Gram-negative bacteria, pathogenic concentration levels of LPS are in circulation from the beginning. In physiological conditions, lymph flow from lungs represents fluid filtration from the pulmonary vessels and lymph protein content is not altered. In an old experiment with sheep awake, in which SAA3 is evolutionarily conserved, intravenous injection of *Pseudomonas aeruginosa* induced increased transvascular fluid and protein movement in a prolonged period of time. This steady state was completely reversible and returned to the baseline in 24–72 h.[100] When LPS from *Escherichia coli* was injected in sheep intra-amniotically either as a single injection or repeatedly prior to preterm delivery, increased SAA3 expression in the lung epithelial cells by the single injection, was blunted after the subsequent injections, suggesting again LPS tolerance as monitored by SAA3 expression.[101]

As stated at the beginning of this section, SAA3 may serve as a TLR4 agonist in sterile conditions (LPS absence) resulting in its persistent expression in a premetastatic microenvironment.

PREMETASTASIS

An Idea of Premetastasis

The well-known German philosopher Martin Heidegger described in his masterpiece Sein und Zeit in 1927 that "Die Gewesenheit entspringt der Zukunft" (the character of having been arises from the future). I have no intention of saying that premetastasis is a philosophy. The premetastatic microenvironment is just a concept prior to the actual arrival of tumor cells in there, but physical evidence has been accumulating to demonstrate that primary tumors cultivate distant organs as soil in an endocrine manner ahead of tumor cells as seeds reach those destinations. In our experimental system of premetastasis, tumor cells are labeled by genetic integration of the neomycin-resistant gene for tracing them within the implanted body and its copy number per lung lobe below a certain level as calculated by sensitive qPCR analysis is defined as premetastasis.[5] This condition reproducibly takes place when we implant a given number of tumor cells either ectopically or orthotopically and let them grow for a certain period of time (Fig. 6.3). Depending on the types of tumor cell lines, some of them metastasize to the lungs long after this premetastatic period. During the premetastatic period, the gene expression profile of the lungs changes as compared to that of intact lungs and myeloid cells are mobilized from bone marrow to the lungs.

Isolated Lung Perfusion

Before plunging onto lung premetastasis, I will discuss a locoregional therapy for lung metastasis, that is, isolated lung perfusion (ILuP) plus or minus lung metastasectomy. The illustration of these cases can conveniently introduce the concepts of premetastasis.

An old medical literature with 5206 cases of lung metastasectomy tells us that median survival time (MST) of complete resection was 35 months as compared to 15 months after incomplete resection.[102] The situation after resection of the metastatic lung tumors is similar to that of primary tumor. In IluP with high-dose chemotherapy, both of the cannulated lung artery and veins are under extracorporeal circuit. To avoid lung damages on both sides by bilateral perfusion, bilateral metastasis needs perfusion in a staged manner. This is followed by metastasectomy (Fig. 6.5). In a phase I clinical trial of ILuP with melphalan for 30 min in 23 patients mostly of renal and colon cancer, overall MST was 84 months (95% confidence interval: 41–128).[103] This trial in humans raises a number of fundamental issues:

1. Lung metastasis is recognized by clinical imaging and therefore treated. The treated lungs are a combined microenvironment of premetastasis and post-metastasis. In addition to tumor cells, what else is affected? For example, recruited myeloid cells should also be influenced by ILuP.
2. High-dose chemotherapy can be feasible only in a locoregional manner due to systemic side effects and what medical doctors need to do is to target just an organ(s) of metastasis critical for prognosis. Since the peak concentration and area under the curve of melphalan, which causes DNA damage by alkylation, were 250- and 10-fold higher than those in systemic circulation, respectively,[104] micrometastatic tumor cells that are invisible in the clinical

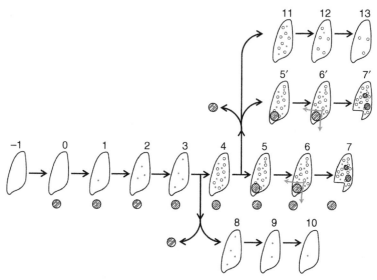

FIGURE 6.5   ILuP and metastasectomy. The lungs of tumor-bearing mice, or patients are called premetastatic lungs, if they are theoretically devoid of tumor cells disseminated from the primary tumor (0) and are different from those without the primary tumor (−1). CSC-like population of tumor cells in the primary tumor are prone to disseminate to the lungs as indicated by black dots [red in the web version] and their number expands during tumor progression.[1–3] Removal of primary tumor at 3 could weaken the premetastatic soil thereby reducing their number.[8–10] If not removed, each population may grow to form tumor cell clusters called micrometastasis but still beyond detection by clinical imaging studies as shown by white circles. Some of them may develop to clinically recognizable metastatic lung tumors[5] from micrometastasis, resection of which by metastasectomy without that of the primary tumor[6] may leave its ability to maintain premetastatic soil, and other clinically detectable metastatic outgrowth in the lungs may take place.[7] Depending on the timing of the primary tumor resection and its trait (e.g., if the primary tumor expresses an inhibitory angiogenic factor such as thrombospondin-1), its removal could unleash the regrowth of micrometastatic tumors. The consequence may be the same as in 5–7 (5′–7′) or decrease of micrometastatic lesions[11–13] in addition to CSC as shown in 8–9. ILuP at 11 or 6′ is feasible.

setting should be targeted under the high dose. The cancer stem cells (CSC) are more prone to lung metastasis as demonstrated in the CD90+ CD24+ CSC in MMTV-PyMT mouse breast cancer model.[60] For example, 5-FU and oxaliplatin counter-selected CD26+ CSC-like population of tumor cells from colon cancer patients *in vitro* and *in vivo* in SCID mice.[105] Although they show resistance to cytotoxic drugs, is elimination of CSC possible under a high dose or other sort of cytotoxic agents as evidenced by the effectiveness of cytotoxic farnesyltransferase inhibitor BMS-214662 in chronic myeloid leukemia stem cells?[106]

3. One phase I clinical trial used TNF-α in ILuP in 15 patients and showed only three patients with a short-term partial response.[107] Is TNF-α useful or harmful?

Molecular Biology of Premetastatic Lungs

By means of cDNA microarray analysis of lungs between tumor-bearing and nonbearing mice, we discovered upregulation of chemokines S100A8 and SAA3 in the top 50 genes.[5] Subsequently, we demonstrated that both are endogenous ligands for TLR4 that has been believed to be a molecular sensor for extrinsic pathogens recognizing LPS. Precisely, LPS, S100A8, and SAA3 bind MD-2 (myeloid differentiation protein-2), the coreceptor of TLR4, on the plasma membrane.[108,109] Upregulation of the endogenous ligands S100A8 and SAA3 attracts TLR4-expressing BMDC. In other words, bone marrow misrecognizes those endogenous ligands as LPS derived from lung infection and mobilizes the myeloid cells there to battle against the phantom microbes. In fact, serum concentrations of S100A8 and SAA3 increase during the premetastatic period.[6,110] The recruited myeloid cells in the lungs establish a metastatic niche for metastasizing tumor cells since blocking the myeloid cell mobilization into the lungs by neutralizing antibody against S100A8 or SAA3, or individual genetic KO of TLR4 or MD-2, or the TLR4 inhibitor eritoran capable of binding to MD-2, all of them not only resulted in reduction in the number of myeloid cells recruited in the lungs but also in inhibition of lung metastasis.[5,44,61,109] Therefore, myeloid cell recruitment at least via TLR4 signaling through S100A8–SAA3 in the lungs is a prerequisite for metastasis. This would serve as an answer to question one raised earlier.

I remind readers of the definition of inflammation in this article, that is, vascular permeability in addition to leukocyte mobilization (see section on Elements that Constitute Metastasis). S100A8 and SAA3 are potent permeability factors causing pulmonary vascular permeability to a level comparable to that induced by LPS and VEGF.[61] As I stated earlier, vascular leakage activates the coagulation system with perivascular fibrin deposits. A comparative analysis of lungs of patients who died of cancer and by accident without any cancers revealed that significantly increased expression of S100A8 and CCR2, the receptor for CCL2, was observed in the lungs of tumor-bearing patients.[61]

Although other groups have also shown necessary conditions induced by innate immune responses for lung metastasis, they do not always underlie premetastatic lungs. For example, David Lyden's group showed that undefined tumor-derived factors upregulated fibronectin and CXCL12 in the lungs of tumor-bearing mice, which in turn attracted BMDCs that expressed the respective receptors, VLA-4 (very late antigen-4, CD49d/CD29) integrin and CXCR4 in addition to VEGFR1.[111] Michael Karin reported that versican, a proteoglycan in the extracellular matrix, is produced from primary tumor, it binds and stimulates TLR2 in BMDC, which results in the secretion of TNF-α causing multiple organ metastasis.[45] In this system, genetic KO of TNF-α but not IL-6 abrogated metastatic progression of tumor cells. Given that TNF-α infusion in a phase I clinical trial of ILuP was almost ineffective, S100A8 and SAA3 can induce expression of TNF-α and IL-6 and that anti-TNF-α and anti-IL-6 therapy have been effective in rheumatoid arthritis (RA), there should be distinct and overlapping events between the inflammation-like state in lung metastasis and autoinflammatory disorders as exemplified by RA. This information would be useful to think of how to answer questions two and three discussed earlier. Pharmacological targeting of CSC is still underway.

Then what factor(s) originated from the primary tumor is responsible for upregulation of those chemokines in the premetastatic lungs? We demonstrated that VEGF, TNF-α, and CCL2 are the major factors working in an endocrine fashion that are produced in the primary tumor and activate the paracrine system in the lungs involving S100A8 and SAA3 (Fig. 6.4). VEGF and TNFα in the serum are necessary and sufficient for the pulmonary S100A8 induction in organ culture experiments, and they showed combinatory effects. Anti-TNF-α neutralizing antibody could also inhibit S100A8 induction in tumor-bearing mice.[5] By utilizing individual KO mice of CCL2 and CCR2, we have also shown that CCL2 was necessary and sufficient to induce S100A8 and SAA3 expression in the lung areas with enhanced vascular permeability.[61] S100A8 purified from mammalian cells stimulated microvascular ECs isolated from lungs to induce SAA3 expression. Synthetic SAA3 peptides were capable of inducing expression of TNF-α, IL-6, and SAA3 but not CCL2 in macrophages (Fig. 6.4).[108]

Defective Conservation of SAA3

Currently, much evidence is based on murine experiments. However, experimental results with higher large mammals may provide us with precious information valuable for clinical trials in humans. I have already reported in this article canine prostate cancer, swine metastatic lung tumor, and LPS-induced SAA3 expression in sheep. SAA proteins have four isoforms named SAA1 through SAA4. Here I focus on SAA3 since it is a good example to discuss partial conservation in evolution. SAA3 in humans and chimpanzee has been believed to be a pseudogene in the previous literature[112] and the predicted protein sequences retain only the first alpha helix out of five helices owing to a single base insertion in exon 2 generating unique 12 amino acids in the carboxyl-terminus (Fig. 6.6). We have discovered that chimeric SAA2-SAA3 mRNAs actively transcribed in human lung cancer cells with low but appreciable amounts of the translated proteins.[113] Interestingly, most of the 43–57 sequences in murine SAA3, which is the most potent portion in cell migration *in vitro*, are missing in the chimeric SAA2–SAA3 protein,[108] and the chimeric protein changes its receptor from the TLR4/MD-2 complex to LOX-1, a receptor for oxidized LDL in ECs. A synthetic human SAA3 peptide of 44-mer containing the unique 12 amino acids, which failed to bind TLR4/MD-2 complex, stimulated cell migration in a human monocytic cell line U937 cells endogenously expressing LOX-1 (A. Deguchi and Y. Maru, unpublished results). Although this suggests the conservation of biological effects even under the evolutionary change of ligand–receptor system, precise biological roles of SAA2–SAA3–LOX-1 still remain to be elucidated.

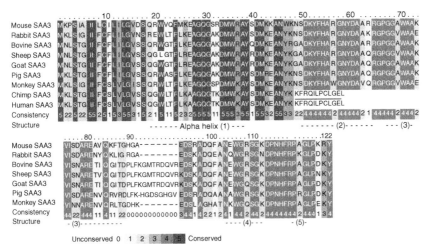

FIGURE 6.6 Evolution of SAA3 proteins. SAA3 protein sequences except for those of chimpanzee (Chimp) and human, are fully conserved in 56% of amino acid residues. In chimpanzee and human, the SAA3 gene is believed to be a pseudogene. Their amino acid alignments are deduced from the corresponding genomic sequences that contain one base insertion generating a frame shift and truncated protein if expressed.

While SAA1 and SAA2 are the major circulating monomeric isoforms in many species that are produced in the liver and bound to HDL, SAA3 is the dominant form in circulation in pigs after infection and SAA1 may be a pseudogene.[114,115] Given the systemic nature of swine SAA3 not present in the HDL-rich serum but in the soluble fraction as multimers, it may display similar behaviors to SAA3 in other species except human and chimpanzee under premetastatic conditions.

HOMEOSTATIC INFLAMMATION AND THERAPEUTIC TARGETING

In the danger hypothesis proposed by Polly Matzinger, the immune system is activated not by nonself but by damaged cells. What is recognized by immune cells includes substances that are self in physiological conditions but are transformed to nonself by cellular mislocalization or conformational changes. For example, nucleosomal protein HMGB1 (high mobility group box 1) is released from damaged or necrotic cells to the extracellular space, where it never exists in normal settings and activates TLR4 in pathological circumstances (Fig. 6.7).

Recent evidence shows that HMGB1 is released under activation of inflammasome in a manner dependent on double stranded RNA-dependent protein kinase (PKR), which may accompany macrophage pyroptosis.[116] HMGB1 is also one of the more than 20 proposed endogenous ligands for TLR4. Inflammasone is neither activated as monitored by caspase-1 activation (M. Takita

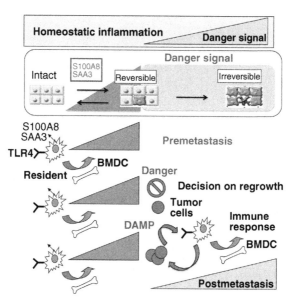

FIGURE 6.7 **Homeostatic inflammation includes danger signal.** Danger signal is transmitted from damaged cells. The release substances could be converted from self to nonself. In premetastatic lungs, expression of S100A8 is induced in ECs with subsequent activation of the paracrine system involving SAA3 amplification as shown in Figure 6.4. Toward S100A8 and SAA3 abundantly expressed in the lungs, TLR4-expressing BMDCs are recruited. During the recruitment, tumor cells expressing TLR4 develop metastatic lesions releasing danger-associated molecular patterns (DAMP) such as HMGB1, which in turn activates the immune system. This is the danger signal in postmetastatic lungs.

and Y. Maru, unpublished results),[117] nor is HMGB1 upregulated in premetastatic lungs. However, its expression levels increase after treatment with naphthalene, capable of inducing apoptosis specifically in club cells in the presence or absence of primary tumor.[90] However, S100A8 and SAA3 are distinct from HMGB1 in that they are actively secreted to the extracellular space without cellular damages or cell death even in physiological condition. Their roles in normal settings should be elucidated in individual KO mice.

SAA3 is abundantly expressed in adipose tissues in obese mice and engaged in the recruitment of myeloid cells by working in concert with CCL2. SAA3-KO exhibited resistance to obesogenic diet in female but not male mice, which is accompanied by diminished hepatic expression of SAA1 and SAA2,[118] indicating an essential role of SAA3 in adipose tissue remodeling at least in female mice. This sexual dimorphism suggests the presence of male specific and efficient compensation mechanisms by CCL2 in myeloid cell recruitment in adipose tissues.

SAA3-KO mice showed no prominent phenotypes in metastasis experiments in our hands (T. Tomita and Y. Maru, unpublished results). In addition, given that SAA3 may be autoamplified in club cells and AhR can confer tolerance to

TLR4 signaling by LPS (see section on Lung Homeostasis), it can be assumed that the AhR-KO background could abolish the AhR-mediated resistance enhancing SAA3 amplification and subsequent lung metastasis. However, lung metastasis by intravenous injection of tumor cells in tumor-nonbearing mice was abolished in AhR-KO mice. Since this phenomenon took place irrespective of expression and activation levels of AhR in tumor cells by themselves,[54] and AhR is constantly activated in aggressive tumors in general,[119] precise contribution of AhR in premetastatic soil still remains to be elucidated. Since S100A8-KO mice are embryonic lethal, we are currently trying to establish conditional S100A8-KO mice to uncover the homeostatic role of S100A8.

Antibodies can be raised against DNA in autoimmune diseases. In the primary tumor microenvironment, tumor cells are always exposed to relative deficiency in oxygen and nutrition and therefore occasionally damaged. In combination with cytokine production, the tumor tissue is inflammatory. Under these conditions, antitumorigenic M1 type macrophages are educated to make a conversion to M2 type resulting in the expression of a set of protumorigenic genes in support of tumor progression. I believe that this process is irreversible as long as tumor cells are present, which was nicely described by Harold F. Dvorak as wounds that do not heal.[120]

On the other hand, there exist no tumor cells at least theoretically in premetastatic lungs. Myeloid cells, such as those doubly Gr1- and CD11b-positive, are increased in number but there is clear evidence to show neither the phenotypic shift of macrophages to M2 nor damaged cells releasing the transformed self. However, active secretion of S100A8 and SAA3 takes place in tumor-bearing mice, both of which activate TLR4 in lung cells as well as in bone marrow. Removal of the primary tumor from the tumor-bearing mice could reverse the increased number of Gr1+ CD11b+ cells and the upregulated S100A8–SAA3 expression in the premetastatic lungs (T. Tomita and Y. Maru, unpublished results). And the true danger, which is the tumor cells metastasizing to the lungs, comes after this reversible process (Fig. 6.7).

Needless to say, the premetastatic microenvironment at least theoretically lacks any single tumor cell. However, when we think of therapeutic strategies against metastasis from the standpoint of the premetastatic microenvironment without tumor cells, good lessons derive from the studies of primary tumors. What is the difference between the two microenvironments in addition to the presence or absence of tumor cells? One of the clear differences is that the primary tumor microenvironment has macrophages (tumor-associated macrophage = TAM) and fibroblasts (carcinoma-associated fibroblast = CAF) that are closely associated with tumor cells. CAFs are positive in α-SMA (smooth muscle actin) and vimentin, originated from resident fibroblasts and/or bone-marrow-derived mesenchymal cells and secrete CXCL12 and TGFβ capable of inducing expression of CXCR4, the receptor for CXCL12, in tumor cells, inducing growth advantages in tumor cells. TAMs are of M2 type and differentiated from resident macrophages and/or BMDCs. Reciprocal activation between

EGFR-positive tumor cells secreting CSF-1 and CSF-1R-expressing macrophages producing EGF has been proposed a long time ago by Jeffery Pollard.[121]

In premetastatic lungs we have failed to detect macrophage populations shifted toward M1 or M2. What is similar between the two microenvironments is the CCL2-dependent recruitment of myeloid cells. Hyperpermeability regions in the premetastatic lungs of tumor-bearing mice are enriched in cells with higher expression levels of CCR2 and G-CSFR, with respect to low permeability regions.[61]

Anti-CCL2 neutralizing antibody therapy can abrogate the influx of myeloid cells into not only primary tumors without changing their growth, but also into premetastatic lungs, resulting in reduced numbers of circulating tumor cells (CTC) and lung metastases. Although the antibody carlumab is currently under use in clinical trials, it was shown by murine experiments with breast cancer cells such as 4T1 that anti-CCL2 therapy for 14 days, followed by its discontinuation for 10 days, (during which the antibody is cleared out of circulation) induced rebound expression of CCL2 and IL-6 proteins in the lungs, which was accompanied by increase in pulmonary myeloid cells, CTC, and metastatic foci.[122] The aggravation of metastasis could be prevented by administration of a CSF1R inhibitor or an anti-IL-6 antibody after cessation of the anti-CCL2 therapy. The ability of IL-6 to induce VEGF in myeloid cells may underlie the overshoot. The CSF1R inhibition depleted lung macrophages that are obligate partners for future metastasizing tumor cells from the primary site as in the case of primary tumor cells. In RCAS-hPDGFB/nestin-Tv-a;Cdkn2a−/− transgenic mice of a human glioblastoma multiform model, administration of the brain permeable CSF-1R inhibitor BLZ945, which showed 10,000-fold less affinity for PDGFR-α and therefore could not efficiently inhibit pericytes, decreased numbers of microglia in normal brain but not of TAM due to glioma-derived survival factors such as GM-CSF, IFNγ, and CXCL10.[123] However, it shifted the M2 type of macrophages back to M1 thereby inhibiting their protumorigenic activity.

Given that both tumor cells and macrophages are the main source of VEGF, cessation of anti-CCL2 therapy is supposed to induce angiogenic activation in the lungs, which prepares a metastatic microenvironment suitable for growth of metastasizing tumor cells.

Upregulation of G-CSFR in the hyperpermeability regions in tumor-bearing mice may also serve as a good soil for G-CSF-producing tumor cells to achieve metastatic growth.[61] G-CSF induces expression of Bv8 in myeloid cells, which is capable of inducing VEGF-independent angiogenesis and myeloid cell mobilization.[124] This is indeed one of the mechanisms of resistance against anti-VEGF therapy. The source of G-CSF includes tumor cells transformed by the Ras-MEK pathway[125] and host CAF through NFκB and Erk signaling. Resistance to anti-VEGF therapy could be overcome in IL-17R-KO (precisely, IL-17A binds to a heterodimer of IL-17RA and IL-17RC, and here IL-17R-KO means KO of IL-17RC) or G-CSFR-KO. Also, IL-17A from tumor-infiltrating Th17 cells induces G-CSF in CAF.[126]

Thus, the premetastatic microenvironment is always ready to respond to VEGF-dependent and -independent angiogenic activation, as well as to establish tumor cell–stromal cell obligate interactions immediately after tumor cell arrival. To prevent metastatic growth, it is reasonable to abrogate signaling by CSF-1R, IL-6R, and G-CSFR during the period when primary tumor cells start to disseminate.

Then what is the relationship between endogenous TLR4 ligands and those growth factors? By utilizing KO mice and stimulation experiments in organ culture of lungs, we have shown that CCL2–CCR2 signaling is necessary and sufficient for the expression of S100A8 and SAA3 in the lungs of tumor-bearing mice.[61] Therefore, if anti-CCL2 therapy needs caution as described earlier, anti-S100A8 antibody therapy or anti-TLR4/MD-2 strategy, such as eritoran, may be useful. We have shown that targeting S100A8 resulted in the inhibition of primary tumor growth and metastasis,[109] which was accompanied by decreased numbers of not only TAM in the primary tumor but also of Gr1+ CD11b+ BMDC in the premetastatic lungs. Given that an obligatory relationship between tumor cells and TAM that are converted from recruited myeloid cells can upregulate endogenous TLR4 ligands not only in the primary tumor (through primary tumor-derived chemokines such as CCL2 and VEGF in a paracrine manner), but also in the premetastatic lungs through the same chemokines in an endocrine manner, it is ideal to inhibit both by endogenous ligand inhibitors.

Gr1+ CD11b+ cells in tumor-bearing mice appear to acquire their T cell-suppressing functions (myeloid-derived suppressor cells, MDSC) through arginase-1 and iNOS in a manner dependent on their localization in the body.[127] A series of adoptive transfer experiments utilizing congenic mice revealed that Gr1+ CD11b+ cells from the spleen with less suppressor functions exhibited strong suppressive activities as early as 4 h after their transfer to the tumor microenvironment where hypoxia was shown to be responsible for the conversion. Spleen, blood, and tumor of tumor-bearing, but not of nontumor-bearing, mice have lower numbers of MDSCs in the genetic background of IL-17R-KO than wild-type mice with reduced expression levels of Arginase-1, MMP9, and S100A8/S100A9,[128] suggesting that IL-17 is necessary for MDSC development. Therefore, IL-17 and S100A8 would be reasonable targets to prevent lung metastasis. There is no hypoxic soil in premetastatic lungs of tumor-bearing mice and clear evidence must still be obtained to support that BMDCs in premetastatic lungs have suppressor functions.

REFERENCES

1. Jones WHS. *Hippocrates collected works I*. Cambridge Harvard University Press; 2006. Retrieved September 28, 2006.
2. Sweetnam R. Osteosarcoma. *Ann R Coll Surg Engl* 1969;**44**:38–58.
3. Claude B. *Introduction a l' etude de la medecine experimentale*. Paris: Bailliere et Fils; 1865 107–112.

4. Paget S. The distribution of secondary growths in cancer of the breast. *Lancet* 1889;**133**:571–3.

5. Hiratsuka S, Watanabe A, Aburatani H, Maru Y. Tumour-mediated upregulation of chemoattractants and recruitment of myeloid cells predetermines lung metastasis. *Nat Cell Biol* 2006;**8**:1369–75.

6. Maru Y. A concept of homeostatic inflammation provided by endogenous TLR4 agonists that function before and after danger signal for metastasis. *Antiinflamm Antiallergy Agents Med Chem* 2009;**8**:337–47.

7. Simmons JK, Elshafae SM, Keller ET, McCauley LK, Rosol TJ. Review of animal models of prostate cancer bone metastasis. *Vet Sci* 2014;**1**:16–39.

8. National Cancer Institute Browse the SEER Cancer Statistics Review 1975–2011. <http://seer.cancer.gov/csr/1975_2011/browse_csr.php?sectionSEL=15&pageSEL=sect_15_table.27.html#content>

9. Oxenhandler RW, Adelstein EH, Haigh JP, Hook Jr RR, Clark Jr WH. Malignant melanoma in the Sinclair miniature swine: an autopsy study of 60 cases. *Am J Pathol* 1979;**96**:707–20.

10. Chen TT, Luque A, Lee S, Anderson SM, Segura T, Iruela-Arispe ML. Anchorage of VEGF to the extracellular matrix conveys differential signaling responses to endothelial cells. *J Cell Biol* 2010;**188**:595–609.

11. Lee S, Chen TT, Barber CL, Jordan MC, Murdock J, Desai S, et al. Autocrine VEGF signaling is required for vascular homeostasis. *Cell* 2007;**130**:691–703.

12. Loges S, Mazzone M, Hohensinner P, Carmeliet P. Silencing or fueling metastasis with VEGF inhibitors: antiangiogenesis revisited. *Cancer Cell* 2009;**15**:167–70.

13. Ferrara N. Pathways mediating VEGF-independent tumor angiogenesis. *Cytokine Growth Factor Rev* 2010;**21**:21–6.

14. Paez-Ribes M, Allen E, Hudock J, Takeda T, Okuyama H, Vinals F, et al. Antiangiogenic therapy elicits malignant progression of tumors to increased local invasion and distant metastasis. *Cancer Cell* 2009;**15**:220–31.

15. Gao P, Zhang H, Dinavahi R, Li F, Xiang Y, Raman V, et al. HIF-dependent antitumorigenic effect of antioxidants *in vivo*. *Cancer Cell* 2007;**12**:230–8.

16. Warren RS, Yuan H, Matli MR, Gillett NA, Ferrara N. Regulation by vascular endothelial growth factor of human colon cancer tumorigenesis in a mouse model of experimental liver metastasis. *J Clin Invest* 1995;**95**:1789–97.

17. Bais C, Wu X, Yao J, Yang S, Crawford Y, McCutcheon K, et al. PlGF blockade does not inhibit angiogenesis during primary tumor growth. *Cell* 2010;**141**:166–77.

18. Dawson MR, Duda DG, Fukumura D, Jain RK. VEGFR1-activity-independent metastasis formation. *Nature* 2009;**461**:E4.

19. Malik G, Knowles LM, Dhir R, Xu S, Yang S, Ruoslahti E, et al. Plasma fibronectin promotes lung metastasis by contributions to fibrin clots and tumor cell invasion. *Cancer Res* 2010;**70**:4327–34.

20. Caunt M, Mak J, Liang WC, Stawicki S, Pan Q, Tong RK, et al. Blocking neuropilin-2 function inhibits tumor cell metastasis. *Cancer Cell* 2008;**13**:331–42.

21. Ieguchi K, Tomita T, Omori T, Komatsu A, Deguchi A, Masuda J, et al. ADAM12-cleaved ephrin-A1 contributes to lung metastasis. *Oncogene* 2014;**33**:2179–90.

22. Keskin D, Kim J, Cooke VG, Wu CC, Sugimoto H, Gu C, et al. Targeting vascular pericytes in hypoxic tumors increases lung metastasis via angiopoietin-2. *Cell Rep* 2015;**10**:1066–81.

23. Martin MD, Carter KJ, Jean-Philippe SR, Chang M, Mobashery S, Thiolloy S, et al. Effect of ablation or inhibition of stromal matrix metalloproteinase-9 on lung metastasis in a breast cancer model is dependent on genetic background. *Cancer Res* 2008;**68**:6251–9.

24. Zigrino P, Kuhn I, Bauerle T, Zamek J, Fox JW, Neumann S, et al. Stromal expression of MMP-13 is required for melanoma invasion and metastasis. *J Invest Dermatol* 2009;**129**:2686–26893.

25. Romagnoli M, Mineva ND, Polmear M, Conrad C, Srinivasan S, Loussouarn D, et al. ADAM8 expression in invasive breast cancer promotes tumor dissemination and metastasis. *EMBO Mol Med* 2014;**6**:278–94.

26. Saupe F, Schwenzer A, Jia Y, Gasser I, Spenle C, Langlois B, et al. Tenascin-C downregulates wnt inhibitor dickkopf-1, promoting tumorigenesis in a neuroendocrine tumor model. *Cell Rep* 2013;**5**:482–92.

27. Garmy-Susini B, Avraamides CJ, Desgrosellier JS, Schmid MC, Foubert P, Ellies LG, et al. PI3Kα activates integrin α4β1 to establish a metastatic niche in lymph nodes. *Proc Natl Acad Sci USA* 2013;**110**:9042–7.

28. Magnon C, Hall SJ, Lin J, Xue X, Gerber L, Freedland SJ, et al. Autonomic nerve development contributes to prostate cancer progression. *Science* 2013;**341**:1236361.

29. Ferjancic S, Gil-Bernabe AM, Hill SA, Allen PD, Richardson P, Sparey T, et al. VCAM-1 and VAP-1 recruit myeloid cells that promote pulmonary metastasis in mice. *Blood* 2013;**121**:3289–97.

30. Palumbo JS, Talmage KE, Massari JV, La Jeunesse CM, Flick MJ, Kombrinck KW, et al. Tumor cell-associated tissue factor and circulating hemostatic factors cooperate to increase metastatic potential through natural killer cell-dependent and -independent mechanisms. *Blood* 2007;**110**:133–41.

31. Mueller BM, Ruf W. Requirement for binding of catalytically active factor VIIa in tissue factor-dependent experimental metastasis. *J Clin Invest* 1998;**101**:1372–8.

32. Palumbo JS, Kombrinck KW, Drew AF, Grimes TS, Kiser JH, Degen JL, et al. Fibrinogen is an important determinant of the metastatic potential of circulating tumor cells. *Blood* 2000;**96**:3302–9.

33. Palumbo JS, Barney KA, Blevins EA, Shaw MA, Mishra A, Flick MJ, et al. Factor XIII transglutaminase supports hematogenous tumor cell metastasis through a mechanism dependent on natural killer cell function. *J Thromb Haemost* 2008;**6**:812–9.

34. Banke IJ, Arlt MJ, Mueller MM, Sperl S, Stemberger A, Sturzebecher J, et al. Effective inhibition of experimental metastasis and prolongation of survival in mice by a potent factor Xa-specific synthetic serine protease inhibitor with weak anticoagulant activity. *Thromb Haemost* 2005;**94**:1084–93.

35. Esumi N, Fan D, Fidler IJ. Inhibition of murine melanoma experimental metastasis by recombinant desulfatohirudin, a highly specific thrombin inhibitor. *Cancer Res* 1991;**51**:4549–56.

36. Palumbo JS, Potter JM, Kaplan LS, Talmage K, Jackson DG, Degen JL. Spontaneous hematogenous and lymphatic metastasis, but not primary tumor growth or angiogenesis, is diminished in fibrinogen-deficient mice. *Cancer Res* 2002;**62**:6966–72.

37. Camerer E, Qazi AA, Duong DN, Cornelissen I, Advincula R, Coughlin SR. Platelets, protease-activated receptors, and fibrinogen in hematogenous metastasis. *Blood* 2004;**104**:397–401.

38. Jain S, Zuka M, Liu J, Russell S, Dent J, Guerrero JA, et al. Platelet glycoprotein Ib α supports experimental lung metastasis. *Proc Natl Acad Sci USA* 2007;**104**:9024–8.

39. Amirkhosravi A, Mousa SA, Amaya M, Blaydes S, Desai H, Meyer T, et al. Inhibition of tumor cell-induced platelet aggregation and lung metastasis by the oral GpIIb/IIIa antagonist XV454. *Thromb Haemost* 2003;**90**:549–54.

40. Palumbo JS, Talmage KE, Massari JV, La Jeunesse CM, Flick MJ, Kombrinck KW, et al. Platelets and fibrin(ogen) increase metastatic potential by impeding natural killer cell-mediated elimination of tumor cells. *Blood* 2005;**105**:178–85.

41. Kato Y, Fujita N, Yano H, Tsuruo T. Suppression of experimental lung colonization of mouse colon adenocarcinoma 26 *in vivo* by an anti-idiotype monoclonal antibody recognizing a platelet surface molecule. *Cancer Res* 1997;**57**:3040–5.

42. Yang S, Zhang JJ, Huang XY. Orai1 and STIM1 are critical for breast tumor cell migration and metastasis. *Cancer Cell* 2009;**15**:124–34.

43. Borsig L, Wong R, Feramisco J, Nadeau DR, Varki NM, Varki A. Heparin and cancer revisited: mechanistic connections involving platelets, P-selectin, carcinoma mucins, and tumor metastasis. *Proc Natl Acad Sci USA* 2001;**98**:3352–7.

44. Hiratsuka S, Watanabe A, Sakurai Y, Akashi-Takamura S, Ishibashi S, Miyake K, et al. The S100A8-serum amyloid A3-TLR4 paracrine cascade establishes a pre-metastatic phase. *Nat Cell Biol* 2008;**10**:1349–55.

45. Kim S, Takahashi H, Lin WW, Descargues P, Grivennikov S, Kim Y, et al. Carcinoma-produced factors activate myeloid cells through TLR2 to stimulate metastasis. *Nature* 2009;**457**:102–6.

46. Kundu N, Walser TC, Ma X, Fulton AM. Cyclooxygenase inhibitors modulate NK activities that control metastatic disease. *Cancer Immunol Immunother* 2005;**54**:981–7.

47. Kishi Y, Kuba K, Nakamura T, Wen J, Suzuki Y, Mizuno S, et al. Systemic NK4 gene therapy inhibits tumor growth and metastasis of melanoma and lung carcinoma in syngeneic mouse tumor models. *Cancer Sci* 2009;**100**:1351–8.

48. Wen J, Matsumoto K, Taniura N, Tomioka D, Nakamura T. Hepatic gene expression of NK4, an HGF-antagonist/angiogenesis inhibitor, suppresses liver metastasis and invasive growth of colon cancer in mice. *Cancer Gene Ther* 2004;**11**:419–30.

49. Liu J, Liao S, Diop-Frimpong B, Chen W, Goel S, Naxerova K, et al. TGF-β blockade improves the distribution and efficacy of therapeutics in breast carcinoma by normalizing the tumor stroma. *Proc Natl Acad Sci USA* 2012;**109**:16618–23.

50. Bandyopadhyay A, Agyin JK, Wang L, Tang Y, Lei X, Story BM, et al. Inhibition of pulmonary and skeletal metastasis by a transforming growth factor-β type I receptor kinase inhibitor. *Cancer Res* 2006;**66**:6714–21.

51. Kowanetz M, Wu X, Lee J, Tan M, Hagenbeek T, Qu X, et al. Granulocyte-colony stimulating factor promotes lung metastasis through mobilization of Ly6G+Ly6C+ granulocytes. *Proc Natl Acad Sci USA* 2010;**107**:21248–55.

52. Gutierrez-Fernandez A, Fueyo A, Folgueras AR, Garabaya C, Pennington CJ, Pilgrim S, et al. Matrix metalloproteinase-8 functions as a metastasis suppressor through modulation of tumor cell adhesion and invasion. *Cancer Res* 2008;**68**:2755–63.

53. Perry SW, Schueckler JM, Burke K, Arcuri GL, Brown EB. Stromal matrix metalloprotease-13 knockout alters Collagen I structure at the tumor-host interface and increases lung metastasis of C57BL/6 syngeneic E0771 mammary tumor cells. *BMC Cancer* 2013;**13**:411.

54. Contador-Troca M, Alvarez-Barrientos A, Barrasa E, Rico-Leo EM, Catalina-Fernandez I, Menacho-Marquez M, et al. The dioxin receptor has tumor suppressor activity in melanoma growth and metastasis. *Carcinogenesis* 2013;**34**:2683–93.

55. Gong J, Weng D, Eguchi T, Murshid A, Sherman MY, Song B, et al. Targeting the hsp70 gene delays mammary tumor initiation and inhibits tumor cell metastasis. *Oncogene* 2015;1–12.

56. Ma X, Kundu N, Rifat S, Walser T, Fulton AM. Prostaglandin E receptor EP4 antagonism inhibits breast cancer metastasis. *Cancer Res* 2006;**66**:2923–7.

57. Frohlich C, Nehammer C, Albrechtsen R, Kronqvist P, Kveiborg M, Sehara-Fujisawa A, et al. ADAM12 produced by tumor cells rather than stromal cells accelerates breast tumor progression. *Mol Cancer Res* 2011;**9**:1449–61.

58. Paolino M, Choidas A, Wallner S, Pranjic B, Uribesalgo I, Loeser S, et al. The E3 ligase Cbl-b and TAM receptors regulate cancer metastasis via natural killer cells. *Nature* 2014;**507**:508–12.

59. Fabbri M, Paone A, Calore F, Galli R, Gaudio E, Santhanam R, et al. MicroRNAs bind to Toll-like receptors to induce prometastatic inflammatory response. *Proc Natl Acad Sci USA* 2012;**109**:E2110–6.

60. Malanchi I, Santamaria-Martinez A, Susanto E, Peng H, Lehr HA, Delaloye JF, et al. Interactions between cancer stem cells and their niche govern metastatic colonization. *Nature* 2012;**481**:85–9.

61. Hiratsuka S, Ishibashi S, Tomita T, Watanabe A, Akashi-Takamura S, Murakami M, et al. Primary tumours modulate innate immune signalling to create pre-metastatic vascular hyper-permeability foci. *Nature communications* 2013;**4**:1853.

62. Laubli H, Spanaus KS, Borsig L. Selectin-mediated activation of endothelial cells induces expression of CCL5 and promotes metastasis through recruitment of monocytes. *Blood* 2009;**114**:4583–91.

63. D'Alterio C, Barbieri A, Portella L, Palma G, Polimeno M, Riccio A, et al. Inhibition of stromal CXCR4 impairs development of lung metastases. *Cancer Immunol Immunother* 2012;**61**:1713–20.

64. Najy AJ, Day KC, Day ML. ADAM15 supports prostate cancer metastasis by modulating tumor cell-endothelial cell interaction. *Cancer Res* 2008;**68**:1092–9.

65. Zhang D, LaFortune TA, Krishnamurthy S, Esteva FJ, Cristofanilli M, Liu P, et al. Epidermal growth factor receptor tyrosine kinase inhibitor reverses mesenchymal to epithelial phenotype and inhibits metastasis in inflammatory breast cancer. *Clin Cancer Res* 2009;**15**:6639–48.

66. Goode GD, Ballard BR, Manning HC, Freeman ML, Kang Y, Eltom SE. Knockdown of aberrantly upregulated aryl hydrocarbon receptor reduces tumor growth and metastasis of MDA-MB-231 human breast cancer cell line. *Int J Cancer* 2013;**133**:2769–80.

67. Wang X, Song X, Zhuo W, Fu Y, Shi H, Liang Y, et al. The regulatory mechanism of Hsp90α secretion and its function in tumor malignancy. *Proc Natl Acad Sci USA* 2009;**106**:21288–93.

68. Spaderna S, Schmalhofer O, Wahlbuhl M, Dimmler A, Bauer K, Sultan A, et al. The transcriptional repressor ZEB1 promotes metastasis and loss of cell polarity in cancer. *Cancer Res* 2008;**68**:537–44.

69. Desmet CJ, Gallenne T, Prieur A, Reyal F, Visser NL, Wittner BS, et al. Identification of a pharmacologically tractable Fra-1/ADORA2B axis promoting breast cancer metastasis. *Proc Natl Acad Sci USA* 2013;**110**:5139–44.

70. Liang Y, Wu H, Lei R, Chong RA, Wei Y, Lu X, et al. Transcriptional network analysis identifies BACH1 as a master regulator of breast cancer bone metastasis. *J Biol Chem* 2012;**287**:33533–44.

71. Sevenich L, Bowman RL, Mason SD, Quail DF, Rapaport F, Elie BT, et al. Analysis of tumour- and stroma-supplied proteolytic networks reveals a brain-metastasis-promoting role for cathepsin S. *Nat Cell Biol* 2014;**16**:876–88.

72. Chakrabarti R, Hwang J, Andres Blanco M, Wei Y, Lukacisin M, Romano RA, et al. Elf5 inhibits the epithelial-mesenchymal transition in mammary gland development and breast cancer metastasis by transcriptionally repressing Snail2. *Nat Cell Biol* 2012;**14**:1212–22.

73. Gao H, Chakraborty G, Lee-Lim AP, Mo Q, Decker M, Vonica A, et al. The BMP inhibitor CoCo reactivates breast cancer cells at lung metastatic sites. *Cell* 2012;**150**:764–79.

74. Balamurugan K, Wang JM, Tsai HH, Sharan S, Anver M, Leighty R, et al. The tumour suppressor C/EBPδ inhibits FBXW7 expression and promotes mammary tumour metastasis. *EMBO J* 2010;**29**:4106–17.

75. Erler JT, Bennewith KL, Cox TR, Lang G, Bird D, Koong A, et al. Hypoxia-induced lysyl oxidase is a critical mediator of bone marrow cell recruitment to form the premetastatic niche. *Cancer Cell* 2009;**15**:35–44.

76. Bandapalli OR, Ehrmann F, Ehemann V, Gaida M, Macher-Goeppinger S, Wente M, et al. Down-regulation of CXCL1 inhibits tumor growth in colorectal liver metastasis. *Cytokine* 2012;**57**:46–53.
77. Terraube V, Pendu R, Baruch D, Gebbink MF, Meyer D, Lenting PJ, et al. Increased metastatic potential of tumor cells in von Willebrand factor-deficient mice. *J Thromb Haemost* 2006;**4**:519–26.
78. Williams CS, Tsujii M, Reese J, Dey SK, DuBois RN. Host cyclooxygenase-2 modulates carcinoma growth. *J Clin Invest* 2000;**105**:1589–94.
79. Ogawa F, Amano H, Eshima K, Ito Y, Matsui Y, Hosono K, et al. Prostanoid induces premetastatic niche in regional lymph nodes. *J Clin Invest* 2014;**124**:4882–94.
80. Katoh H, Hosono K, Ito Y, Suzuki T, Ogawa Y, Kubo H, et al. COX-2 and prostaglandin EP3/EP4 signaling regulate the tumor stromal proangiogenic microenvironment via CXCL12-CXCR4 chemokine systems. *Am J Pathol* 2010;**176**:1469–83.
81. Tsuruo T, Iida H, Makishima F, Yamori T, Kawabata H, Tsukagoshi S, et al. Inhibition of spontaneous and experimental tumor metastasis by the calcium antagonist verapamil. *Cancer Chemother Pharmacol* 1985;**14**:30–3.
82. Kapur R, Heitink-Polle KM, Porcelijn L, Bentlage AE, Bruin MC, Visser R, et al. C-reactive protein enhances IgG-mediated phagocyte responses and thrombocytopenia. *Blood* 2015;**125**:1793–802.
83. Yang J, Wezeman M, Zhang X, Lin P, Wang M, Qian J, et al. Human C-reactive protein binds activating Fcγ receptors and protects myeloma tumor cells from apoptosis. *Cancer Cell* 2007;**12**:252–65.
84. Bonavita E, Gentile S, Rubino M, Maina V, Papait R, Kunderfranco P, et al. PTX3 is an extrinsic oncosuppressor regulating complement-dependent inflammation in cancer. *Cell* 2015;**160**:700–14.
85. Cermak J, Key NS, Bach RR, Balla J, Jacob HS, Vercellotti GM. C-reactive protein induces human peripheral blood monocytes to synthesize tissue factor. *Blood* 1993;**82**:513–20.
86. Jung B, Obinata H, Galvani S, Mendelson K, Ding BS, Skoura A, et al. Flow-regulated endothelial S1P receptor-1 signaling sustains vascular development. *Dev Cell* 2012;**23**:600–10.
87. Gratton JP, Lin MI, Yu J, Weiss ED, Jiang ZL, Fairchild TA, et al. Selective inhibition of tumor microvascular permeability by cavtratin blocks tumor progression in mice. *Cancer Cell* 2003;**4**:31–9.
88. Huang Y, Song N, Ding Y, Yuan S, Li X, Cai H, et al. Pulmonary vascular destabilization in the premetastatic phase facilitates lung metastasis. *Cancer Res* 2009;**69**:7529–37.
89. Irwin RS, Augustyn N, French CT, Rice J, Tedeschi V, Welch SJ. Spread the word about the journal in 2013: from citation manipulation to invalidation of patient-reported outcomes measures to renaming the Clara cell to new journal features. *Chest* 2013;**143**:1–4.
90. Tomita T, Sakurai Y, Ishibashi S, Maru Y. Imbalance of Clara cell-mediated homeostatic inflammation is involved in lung metastasis. *Oncogene* 2011;**30**:3429–39.
91. Bessede A, Gargaro M, Pallotta MT, Matino D, Servillo G, Brunacci C, et al. Aryl hydrocarbon receptor control of a disease tolerance defence pathway. *Nature* 2014;**511**:184–90.
92. Maus UA, Wellmann S, Hampl C, Kuziel WA, Srivastava M, Mack M, et al. CCR2-positive monocytes recruited to inflamed lungs downregulate local CCL2 chemokine levels. *Am J Physiol Lung Cell Mol Physiol* 2005;**288**:L350–8.
93. Hu CL, Barnes FS. A theory of necrotaxis. *Biophys J* 1970;**10**:958–69.
94. Wu C, Asokan SB, Berginski ME, Haynes EM, Sharpless NE, Griffith JD, et al. Arp2/3 is critical for lamellipodia and response to extracellular matrix cues but is dispensable for chemotaxis. *Cell* 2012;**148**:973–87.

95. Trepat X, Fredberg JJ. Plithotaxis and emergent dynamics in collective cellular migration. *Trends Cell Biol* 2011;**21**:638–46.

96. Carlin LM, Stamatiades EG, Auffray C, Hanna RN, Glover L, Vizcay-Barrena G, et al. Nr4a1-dependent Ly6C(low) monocytes monitor endothelial cells and orchestrate their disposal. *Cell* 2013;**153**:362–75.

97. Wong AP, Keating A, Lu WY, Duchesneau P, Wang X, Sacher A, et al. Identification of a bone marrow-derived epithelial-like population capable of repopulating injured mouse airway epithelium. *J Clin Invest* 2009;**119**:336–48.

98. Podsypanina K, Du YC, Jechlinger M, Beverly LJ, Hambardzumyan D, Varmus H. Seeding and propagation of untransformed mouse mammary cells in the lung. *Science* 2008;**321**:1841–4.

99. Houghton J, Stoicov C, Nomura S, Rogers AB, Carlson J, Li H, et al. Gastric cancer originating from bone marrow-derived cells. *Science* 2004;**306**:1568–71.

100. Brigham KL, Woolverton WC, Blake LH, Staub NC. Increased sheep lung vascular permeability caused by pseudomonas bacteremia. *J Clin Invest* 1974;**54**:792–804.

101. Kallapur SG, Jobe AH, Ball MK, Nitsos I, Moss TJ, Hillman NH, et al. Pulmonary and systemic endotoxin tolerance in preterm fetal sheep exposed to chorioamnionitis. *J Immunol* 2007;**179**:8491–9.

102. Pastorino U, Buyse M, Friedel G, Ginsberg RJ, Girard P, Goldstraw P, et al. Long-term results of lung metastasectomy: prognostic analyses based on 5206 cases. *J Thorac Cardiovasc Surg* 1997;**113**:37–49.

103. Den Hengst WA, Van Putte BP, Hendriks JM, Stockman B, van Boven WJ, Weyler J, et al. Long-term survival of a phase I clinical trial of isolated lung perfusion with melphalan for resectable lung metastases. *Eur J Cardiothorac Surg* 2010;**38**:621–7.

104. Van Schil PE, Furrer M, Friedel G. Locoregional therapy. *J Thorac Oncol* 2010;**5**:S151–4.

105. Pang R, Law WL, Chu AC, Poon JT, Lam CS, Chow AK, et al. A subpopulation of CD26+ cancer stem cells with metastatic capacity in human colorectal cancer. *Cell Stem Cell* 2010;**6**:603–15.

106. Copland M, Pellicano F, Richmond L, Allan EK, Hamilton A, Lee FY, et al. BMS-214662 potently induces apoptosis of chronic myeloid leukemia stem and progenitor cells and synergizes with tyrosine kinase inhibitors. *Blood* 2008;**111**:2843–53.

107. Pass HI, Mew DJ, Kranda KC, Temeck BK, Donington JS, Rosenberg SA. Isolated lung perfusion with tumor necrosis factor for pulmonary metastases. *Ann Thorac Surg* 1996;**61**:1609–17.

108. Deguchi A, Tomita T, Omori T, Komatsu A, Ohto U, Takahashi S, et al. Serum amyloid A3 binds MD-2 to activate p38 and NF-κB pathways in a MyD88-dependent manner. *J Immunol* 2013;**191**:1856–64.

109. Deguchi A, Tomita T, Ohto U, Takemura K, Kitao A, Akashi-Takamura S, et al. Eritoran inhibits S100A8-mediated TLR4/MD-2 activation and tumor growth by changing the immune microenvironment. *Oncogene* 2015; doi:10.1038/onc.2015.211.

110. Maru Y. Premetastatic milieu explained by TLR4 agonist-mediated homeostatic inflammation. *Cell Mol Immunol* 2010;**7**:94–9.

111. Kaplan RN, Riba RD, Zacharoulis S, Bramley AH, Vincent L, Costa C, et al. VEGFR1-positive haematopoietic bone marrow progenitors initiate the pre-metastatic niche. *Nature* 2005;**438**:820–7.

112. Sjoholm K, Palming J, Olofsson LE, Gummesson A, Svensson PA, Lystig TC, et al. A microarray search for genes predominantly expressed in human omental adipocytes: adipose tissue as a major production site of serum amyloid A. *J Clin Endocrinol Metab* 2005;**90**:2233–9.

113. Tomita T, Ieguchi K, Sawamura T, Maru Y. Human serum amyloid A3 (SAA3) protein, expressed as a fusion protein with SAA2, binds the oxidized low density lipoprotein receptor. *PLoS One* 2015;**10**:e0118835.

114. Soler L, Luyten T, Stinckens A, Buys N, Ceron JJ, Niewold TA. Serum amyloid A3 (SAA3), not SAA1 appears to be the major acute phase SAA isoform in the pig. *Vet Immunol Immunopathol* 2011;**141**:109–15.

115. Olsen HG, Skovgaard K, Nielsen OL, Leifsson PS, Jensen HE, Iburg T, et al. Organization and biology of the porcine serum amyloid A (SAA) gene cluster: isoform specific responses to bacterial infection. *PLoS One* 2013;**8**:e76695.

116. Lu B, Nakamura T, Inouye K, Li J, Tang Y, Lundback P, et al. Novel role of PKR in inflammasome activation and HMGB1 release. *Nature* 2012;**488**:670–4.

117. Liu T, Yamaguchi Y, Shirasaki Y, Shikada K, Yamagishi M, Hoshino K, et al. Single-cell imaging of caspase-1 dynamics reveals an all-or-none inflammasome signaling response. *Cell Rep* 2014;**8**:974–82.

118. den Hartigh LJ, Wang S, Goodspeed L, Ding Y, Averill M, Subramanian S, et al. Deletion of serum amyloid A3 improves high fat high sucrose diet-induced adipose tissue inflammation and hyperlipidemia in female mice. *PLoS One* 2014;**9**:e108564.

119. Murray IA, Patterson AD, Perdew GH. Aryl hydrocarbon receptor ligands in cancer: friend and foe. *Nat Rev Cancer* 2014;**14**:801–14.

120. Dvorak HF. Tumors: wounds that do not heal. Similarities between tumor stroma generation and wound healing. *N Engl J Med* 1986;**315**:1650–9.

121. Condeelis J, Pollard JW. Macrophages: obligate partners for tumor cell migration, invasion, and metastasis. *Cell* 2006;**124**:263–6.

122. Bonapace L, Coissieux MM, Wyckoff J, Mertz KD, Varga Z, Junt T, et al. Cessation of CCL2 inhibition accelerates breast cancer metastasis by promoting angiogenesis. *Nature* 2014;**515**:130–3.

123. Pyonteck SM, Akkari L, Schuhmacher AJ, Bowman RL, Sevenich L, Quail DF, et al. CSF-1R inhibition alters macrophage polarization and blocks glioma progression. *Nat Med* 2013;**19**:1264–72.

124. Shojaei F, Wu X, Zhong C, Yu L, Liang XH, Yao J, et al. Bv8 regulates myeloid-cell-dependent tumour angiogenesis. *Nature* 2007;**450**:825–31.

125. Phan VT, Wu X, Cheng JH, Sheng RX, Chung AS, Zhuang G, et al. Oncogenic RAS pathway activation promotes resistance to anti-VEGF therapy through G-CSF-induced neutrophil recruitment. *Proc Natl Acad Sci USA* 2013;**110**:6079–84.

126. Chung AS, Wu X, Zhuang G, Ngu H, Kasman I, Zhang J, et al. An interleukin-17-mediated paracrine network promotes tumor resistance to anti-angiogenic therapy. *Nat Med* 2013;**19**:1114–23.

127. Corzo CA, Condamine T, Lu L, Cotter MJ, Youn JI, Cheng P, et al. HIF-1alpha regulates function and differentiation of myeloid-derived suppressor cells in the tumor microenvironment. *J Exp Med* 2010;**207**:2439–53.

128. He D, Li H, Yusuf N, Elmets CA, Li J, Mountz JD, et al. IL-17 promotes tumor development through the induction of tumor promoting microenvironments at tumor sites and myeloid-derived suppressor cells. *J Immunol* 2010;**184**:2281–8.

Chapter 7

Innate Immune Response and Psychotic Disorders

Jaana Suvisaari, Outi Mantere
Department of Health, Mental Health Unit, National Institute for Health and Welfare, Helsinki, Finland

INTRODUCTION

Activation of the immune system is often associated with symptoms resembling those seen in mental disorders, such as fatigue, loss of appetite, depressed or irritable mood, and sleep disorders.[1] Conversely, high-dose cytokine treatments with, for example, interferons, commonly cause psychiatric symptoms, ranging from mood disturbance to psychosis and delirium.[2] Neurotropic viruses preferentially infect neurons and can cause severe, sometimes fatal brain inflammation, encephalitis, which in most cases includes psychiatric symptoms.[3] Autoimmune diseases are risk factors of major mental disorders.[4–6] The mechanisms linking dysregulated immune system to major mental disorders have been studied intensively in the recent years.

Inflammation represents an adaptive response to any condition perceived as potentially dangerous to the host, which aims at removal of the danger, induction of tissue repair, and restoration of tissue homeostasis.[7] Conceptually, inflammation can be viewed as a four-stage process, including a triggering system (the danger), a sensor mechanism (danger receptors), the transmission of signal and the production of mediators, and the activation of cellular effectors.[7] A primary inflammatory response called innate immunity, is set in motion by a wide variety of infectious and noninfectious stimuli, from exogenous or endogenous sources.[7]

There is a reciprocal regulation of immune response and central nervous system (CNS) function, as also reported in the preface to this book.[8] CNS is involved in sensing and regulating peripheral inflammation.[9] The brain receives signals indicating inflammation through several routes, including specialized cells in the brain vasculature, choroid plexus and circumventricular organs, through toll-like receptors (TLR), and cytokine receptors in the brain.[9] In addition, peripheral afferent nerves elicit neural reflexes, which regulate the immune response. For example, the "inflammatory reflex" of the vagus nerve, which includes a sensory arm in the afferent vagus and a motor arm in the efferent vagus nerve, has been shown to regulate T cells, which in turn produce acetylcholine required to control innate immune responses.[10] The mechanisms through which the CNS can regulate the peripheral immune system include stress responses by the hypothalamic–pituitary–adrenal (HPA) axis and responses mediated by the sympathetic nervous system.[8] Even more important for the repercussions on psychiatric diseases may be the multiple roles of microglia, the tissue-resident macrophages in the CNS.

Microglia are the effectors and regulators of CNS homeostasis, and their dysfunction contributes to many neurodegenerative diseases.[11] Microglia originate from hematopoietic stem cells in the yolk sac, from which they migrate toward the developing CNS. In addition to microglia, the brain also contains macrophages in the outer boundaries of the brain, such as choroid plexus and the meninges. Microglia monitor their environment constantly and respond to even minor changes.[12] While they are the first-line defense against pathogens in the CNS, they also monitor the functional state of synapses, eliminate defunct synapses, and control synaptogenesis.[12] Thus, in the absence of inflammation, they have a neurosupportive role.[12]

Cytokines are important messenger molecules of the immune system. They are peptide molecules that are mainly produced by cells of the immune system but also by other cell types. Although their main role is exerted in the coordination of the immune system, they have been shown to be important for neural development and function, paralleling the role of microglia.[13] For example, tumor necrosis factor (TNF)-α and IL-1β are involved in homeostatic synaptic plasticity by increasing excitatory and decreasing inhibitory synaptic strength.[14] They contribute to the temporal regulation of neurogenesis and gliogenesis, progenitor migration, proliferation and axon pathfinding, and development of microglia during the fetal development.[13] Some cytokines, such as IL-1β, TNF-α, and INF-γ, have stressor-like effects on the CNS, including changes in tryptophan metabolism, HPA axis, and brain-derived neurotrophic factor (BDNF) expression.[1,15]

Neurogenesis refers to the process by which new neurons are generated from neural stem cells. In the adult brain, neurogenesis occurs in the subventricular zone of the lateral ventricles and in the hippocampus, and neurons formed in the subventricular zone migrate toward the striatum to develop into mature neurons.[16] Cytokines have an important regulatory role in all processes related to neurogenesis.[16] For example, IL-1α and IL-4 promote neurogenesis, whereas IL-1β and TNF-α decrease neurogenesis and increase gliogenesis.[16]

One common feature in severe mental disorders is stress and activation of the HPA axis, one of the primary neural systems governing the stress response. The stress response of the HPA axis involves activation of the corticotropin-releasing hormone (CRH) neurons in the paraventricular nucleus of the hypothalamus, which causes the release of CRH into pituitary circulation. CRH stimulates secretion of adrenocorticotrophic hormone (ATCH) from the pituitary gland into the bloodstream, which in turn stimulates the adrenal gland to secrete glucocorticoids, mainly cortisol, which is the main stress hormone of the body acting in several tissues. Cortisol, in turn, inhibits CRH production in the hypothalamus and pituitary gland in a negative feedback loop to control the stress response. Dysregulation of the HPA axis is a common feature in many psychiatric disorders. For example, in the early stages of psychotic disorders, basal cortisol level is elevated, and administration of exogenous glucocorticoid does not lead to suppression of cortisol secretion.[17] The same abnormality has been seen in depressive disorders.[18] Glucocorticoids exert immunomodulatory functions by acting on every immune cell type.[19] In acute stress, activation of the glucocorticoid receptors in leukocytes by cortisol, results in suppression of proinflammatory gene networks, antiviral gene programs, and induction of anti-inflammatory genes.[8] In chronic stress, glucocorticoid receptors become desensitized to elevated glucocorticoid levels in the circulation, resulting in a significant reduction in glucocorticoid-mediated transcription, which explains why the anti-inflammatory response diminishes.[8] Glucocorticoid receptors are abundant in the microglia, and depending on the nature and chronicity of the stressor, glucocorticoids can drive the microglia toward tissue maintenance/repair or damage.[19]

The other arm of stress response mediated by the sympathetic nervous system stimulates proinflammatory genes.[8]

Cytokines, especially INF-γ, stimulate the conversion of tryptophan into kynurenine via the kynurenine (KYNA) pathway.[20] This has several consequences. While the conversion of tryptophan into serotonin is reduced, kynurenine is also an antagonist of glutamate receptors.[20] It inhibits all three ionotropic excitatory glutamate receptors (NMDA, kainate, and AMPA). Disturbance in glutaminergic transmission in turn, is one of the hallmarks of psychotic disorders. Activation of the KYNA pathway may be one factor linking inflammation to psychiatric disorders.[20,21] However, kynurenine produced from tryptophan is also a ligand of the aryl hydrocarbon receptor (AhR), a ligand-operated transcription factor, which is essential for endotoxin tolerance.[22] Endotoxin tolerance is a regulatory, anti-inflammatory response that aims to reduce the negative impact of infection on the host fitness.[22]

Oxidative stress plays a crucial role in the development and perpetuation of inflammation. Oxidants affect all stages of the inflammatory response, including the release from damaged tissues of molecules acting as endogenous danger signals, their sensing by innate immune receptors from the Toll- and NOD-like receptor families, induction of an assembly of multiprotein inflammatory complexes called the inflammasomes in the tissues, and the activation of signaling pathways initiating the adaptive cellular response to such signals.[7,23] Lowered or impaired antioxidant defenses is one potential mechanism involved in a delayed emergence of anomalies driven by developmental alterations of schizophrenia.[24,25] Excessive reactive oxygen species (ROS) production in psychiatric patients is caused by cumulative effects of genetic factors, for example a mitochondrial dysfunction,[25] severe psychological stress and environmental factors (excessive food intake, physical inactivity, smoking), but also, for example, nutrition, alcohol consumption, and infectious diseases.[25,26] Major targets of oxidative stress are proteins, lipids, and DNA. Oxidative stress can affect prefrontal cortex function and cause cell damage or death via several mechanisms.[24-26] Furthermore, many synaptic proteins include regulatory redox sites; for example, NMDA receptors become hypofunctional following oxidation. Indeed, redox and glutamatergic systems are intimately dependent.[27]

PSYCHOTIC DISORDERS: NEURODEVELOPMENTAL DISORDERS WITH A NEUROPROGRESSIVE COMPONENT

Psychotic disorders are severe mental disorders, which have reality distortion as their core feature. Psychotic symptoms include delusions, hallucinations, disorganized speech, and bizarre or catatonic behavior. Their lifetime prevalence in the adult population is 3–4%, the most common being schizophrenia with about 1.0–1.5% lifetime prevalence.[28,29] Their onset peaks in late adolescence and early adulthood.[29] Psychotic disorders are commonly divided into nonaffective, schizophrenia-like psychoses, and affective psychoses. Affective psychoses comprise bipolar I and II disorders with psychotic features, and major depressive disorder with psychotic features. However, the symptoms of different psychotic disorders overlap.[30] They can be grouped into five main categories: (1) delusions and hallucinations, which are called positive symptoms; (2) lack of motivation, reduction in spontaneous speech, and social withdrawal, which are called negative symptoms; (3) cognitive difficulties, such as difficulties in memory, attention, and executive functioning – the cognitive-symptom dimension; (4) affective symptoms, that is, depressive and manic symptoms; and (5) disorganization, which includes disorganized speech and bizarre behavior. The symptom profile of different patients varies considerably even within the same diagnostic category, and the longitudinal course of psychotic disorders is variable. Most commonly, acute psychotic episodes are followed by periods when patients have residual symptoms, such as negative symptoms and cognitive difficulties. Full remission between episodes is common in affective psychoses but rare in schizophrenia. It is also possible to have only one psychotic episode in a lifetime, but these acute and transient psychotic disorders are rare.[28]

Psychotic disorders are complex, multifactorial disorders caused by a combination of genetic and environmental risk factors. Estimates of heritability for schizophrenia and bipolar I disorder, the most common psychotic disorders, vary from 65% to over 80%,[31-33] suggesting that the genetic contribution to the risk of these disorders is substantial. Environmental risk factors can be grouped into biological, such as prenatal infections and insults, psychosocial, such as traumatic experiences, and lifestyle-related, such as cannabis use.

The current consensus is that schizophrenia has a neurodevelopmental component, although it is uncertain whether this also applies to late-onset cases.

Disturbances of brain development begin prenatally, and environmental insults further affect postnatal brain maturation during childhood and adolescence.[34] The contribution of neurodevelopmental factors in other psychotic disorders is not that well established. For example, the decline in cognitive functioning has been found in adolescents who later developed schizophrenia and other nonaffective psychoses but not in adolescents who later developed bipolar disorders.[35] Nevertheless, the genetic risk variants of schizophrenia and affective psychoses converge into the same biological pathways involving histone methylation processes and multiple immune and neuronal signaling pathways,[36] suggesting that their etiological mechanisms are at least partly shared. Patients with clinical high risk state, that is, with distressing psychotic symptoms, have subtle brain structural changes, for example, smaller gray matter volume in some frontal and temporal areas than healthy controls, and some of these predict the onset of psychotic disorder.[37] Furthermore, structural brain changes, for example, thinning of cortical gray matter, progress from clinical high risk state to the onset of psychosis and during the first years of illness,[38,39] suggesting that there is also a neurodegenerative component in the illness. A recent study of patients with clinical high-risk symptoms found that elevation in an aggregate measure of serum levels of proinflammatory cytokines, an index described in detail by Cannon et al., predicted steeper gray matter loss in frontal cortical areas, particularly in high-risk patients who transitioned to psychosis during follow up.[38] This suggests that inflammation may be involved in neurodegenerative changes occurring in psychotic disorders.

In the further sections, we review studies on the possible role of innate immunity in the pathophysiology of psychotic disorders in different stages of illness. We consider possible confounding factors, which may explain innate immune responses in psychotic disorders, and review trials of anti-inflammatory drugs as adjunctive medication in psychotic disorders.

PRE- AND PERINATAL EXPOSURES

Several prenatal exposures increase the risk of schizophrenia, including maternal infections, obstetric complications, low birth weight, starvation, and severe traumatic events.[40–44] It has been suggested that a common mechanism behind these exposures is the activation of maternal immune responses, which could harm the developing fetal CNS.[40] Indeed, there is supporting evidence on the elevated levels of interleukin (IL)-8, TNF-α, complement factor C1q, and C-reactive protein (CRP) during pregnancy in mothers of offsprings who developed schizophrenia.[45–48] Animal studies have also shown that prenatal exposure to influenza virus infection or immunostimulating antigens, such as (polyriboinosinic-polyribocytidilic acid (polyI:C)) or bacterial lipopolysaccharides (LPS) causes changes in the brain development, behavior, and gene expression in the offspring.[49] These changes resemble those seen in animal models of schizophrenia and tend to be more severe if the exposure occurs early in fetal development.[49]

In contrast, newborns, who as adults are diagnosed with schizophrenia, do not have evidence of immune activation. Gardner et al. investigated the newborn serum concentrations of nine acute-phase proteins in 196 individuals with a verified register-based diagnosis of nonaffective psychosis and 502 controls matched on age, sex, and hospital of birth, and found that higher concentrations of three acute-phase proteins – tissue plasminogen activator, serum amyloid P, and procalcitonin – were protective against developing nonaffective psychosis.[50] An even larger Danish study of newborn serum samples found no significant difference between the level of 17 inflammatory markers (including IL-1β, IL-6, IL-8, IL-12, IL-18, interferon (IFN)-γ, transforming growth factor (TGF)-β, and CRP) in people who later developed schizophrenia and in age-matched controls.[51] These studies suggest that schizophrenia is not associated with an activation of the newborn immune system.

CHILDHOOD AND ADOLESCENCE EXPOSURES

Childhood infections seem to be risk factors of psychotic and mood disorders; especially hospital-treated bacterial infections and viral CNS infections are associated with increased risk of schizophrenia and other psychotic disorders.[4,52–54] These may reflect adverse effects of severe infections on the developing brain, or increased susceptibility to severe microbial infections. Supporting the hypothesis that inflammation may be harmful to the developing brain, higher level of IL-6 at the age of 9 years has been associated with increased risk of mood disorders and psychotic-like experiences at the age of 18 years.[55] However, patients with schizophrenia and bipolar disorder have increased risk of infections, such as influenza and pneumonia, after the onset of psychotic disorder, suggesting that one feature related to these disorders might be an increased susceptibility to infections.[56,57]

Inflammation could be the underlying mechanism as to how some childhood and adolescent exposures increase the risk of psychotic disorders. For example, childhood maltreatment is associated with increased risk of psychotic disorders and with elevated CRP and other proinflammatory markers later in life.[58,59] In line with this, CRP levels were increased in patients with first-episode psychosis with a history of childhood maltreatment but not in those who did not have a history of trauma.[60]

Different exposures may also have synergistic effects. This was elegantly shown in an animal study where mice were first exposed to prenatal immune activation, which was induced by polyI:C.[61] Later, the offspring were exposed to variable and unpredictable stress during peripubertal development. While both stressors had independent effects on brain development, a synergistic effect of prenatal immune activation and peripubertal stress were seen in sensorimotor gating deficiency, as assessed by the paradigm of prepulse inhibition of the acoustic startle reflex, as well as in behavioral hypersensitivity to psychotomimetic drugs, which are deficits seen in genetic mouse models of schizophrenia.

Furthermore, combined prenatal immune activation and peripubertal stress led to a 2.5–threefold increase in hippocampal and prefrontal expression of markers characteristic of activated microglia and elevation of proinflammatory cytokines in the respective brain areas.[61]

GENETIC EVIDENCE OF THE CONTRIBUTION OF IMMUNOLOGICAL FACTORS TO PSYCHOTIC DISORDERS

Large genome-wide association study (GWAS) consortiums have consistently identified the human leukocyte antigen (HLA) locus in chromosome 6 as the genetic region most significantly associated with schizophrenia,[62] although no individual HLA allele has been definitely identified as a risk factor for schizophrenia. In addition, when the credible sets of causal genetic variants were mapped onto sequences with epigenetic markers characteristic of active enhancers in different tissues and cell types, schizophrenia associations were strongly enriched at enhancers that are active in cells and tissues of the immune system, particularly cells of the adaptive immune system.[60] A further analysis of this dataset with other psychiatric GWAS consortia revealed that immune pathways are important in several psychiatric disorders.[36] As in the schizophrenia GWAS analysis, these immune pathways were particularly associated with adaptive immunity.

Velocardiofacial syndrome or 22q11.2 deletion syndrome is the strongest known risk factor for psychotic disorders: over 40% develop psychotic disorders in adulthood.[63] Interestingly, the syndrome also causes thymic hypoplasia in over 80% of the cases, which in turn causes multiple abnormalities in different T cell populations, particularly in regulatory T cells.[64] The genes within the 22q11.2 deletion region that are responsible for elevated psychosis risk have not been identified, and the possible role of a dysfunctional immune system in causing psychosis risk has not been investigated.

Numerous studies on individual genes or gene pathways related to the immune system in schizophrenia have been conducted and are not reviewed here. Currently, genes related to the immune system are among the most investigated putative risk genes of psychotic disorders.

INNATE IMMUNITY DISTURBANCES IN PEOPLE WITH PSYCHOTIC DISORDERS

Acute-phase proteins are proteins whose plasma concentration increases or decreases at least 25% during inflammatory disorders.[65] The most widely studied of these is CRP. People with schizophrenia and other nonaffective psychotic disorders as well as people with bipolar disorder have elevated levels of CRP,[66,67] and elevated CRP was shown to predict the development of schizophrenia in general population studies.[68] Several other acute-phase proteins show also alterations in schizophrenia, similarly to other brain diseases.[69] Of negative acute-phase proteins that decrease during inflammation, low albumin levels predicted conversion to psychosis in patients with relevant risk symptoms.[70]

Cytokines are the most widely studied innate immunity markers in psychotic disorders. The major innate immunity cytokines are IL-1α, IL-1β, IL-6, and TNF-α. According to a meta-analysis of patients with schizophrenia, IL-1β and IL-6 are elevated in acute psychosis but are normalized with antipsychotic treatment, whereas TNF-α, remains elevated even following antipsychotic treatment.[71] Elevated IL-1β may also predict transition to psychosis in young people with psychosis risk symptoms.[72] In bipolar disorder, concentrations of TNF-α, soluble tumor necrosis factor receptor type 1 (sTNFR1), and soluble IL-6 receptor (sIL-6R) were significantly higher in bipolar patients compared with healthy controls in a meta-analysis.[73] Of them, sTNFR1 and sIL-6R were higher in manic than in depressive states.[73] In addition to these innate immunity cytokines, a variety of others have been investigated. The findings from a meta-analysis for schizophrenia[71] are summarized in Table 7.1 and for bipolar disorder[73] in Table 7.2. Of note is that findings between different studies are heterogeneous, and therefore also meta-analyses have produced somewhat different results because the inclusion and exclusion criteria have

TABLE 7.1 Significant Changes in Serum Cytokines in Patients with Schizophrenia Versus Healthy Controls According to a Meta-Analysis by Miller et al.[71]

	Drug-naïve first-episode psychosis	Acutely relapsed inpatients	Changes following antipsychotic treatment
IL-1β	0.60 (0.37–0.84)*	Not available	−0.45 (−0.70 to −0.20)
IL-2	NS	NS	NS
IL-6	1.40 (1.14–1.65)	0.96 (0.74–1.18)	−0.31 (−0.54 to −0.08)
IL-8	NA	0.59 (0.18–1.00)	NA
IL-10	NA	−0.57 (−0.98 to −0.17)	NA
IL-12	0.98 (0.61–1.35)	NA	0.33 (0.06–0.60)
IL-1RA	NA	0.49 (0.07–0.90)	NA
sIL-2R	1.03 (0.55–1.52)	NS	0.30 (0.01–0.60)
IFN-γ	0.57 (0.24–0.90)	0.49 (0.18–0.80)	NS
TGF-β	0.48 (0.22–0.74)	0.53 (0.26–0.79)	−0.37 (−0.63 to −0.11)
TNF-α	0.81 (0.61–1.01)	0.73 (0.46–0.99)	NS

NS, no significant difference between cases and controls or before and after treatment; NA, not available, no studies from this patient group.
*Mean effect sizes and 95% confidence intervals are presented for statistically significant changes.

TABLE 7.2 Significant Changes in Serum Cytokines in Patients with Bipolar Disorder Versus Healthy Controls According to a Meta-Analysis by Modabbernia et al.[73]

	Total	Euthymic	Manic	Depressive
IL-1β	NS	0.37 (0.11–0.62)*	NA	NA
IL-2	NS	NS	NS	NS
IL-4	0.46 (0.12–0.80)	NS	NS	NS
IL-6	NS	NS	0.62 (0.02–1.22)	NS
IL-8	NS	NS	NA	NA
IL-10	0.28 (0.06–0.50)	NS	0.27 (0.04–0.50)	0.39 (0.13–0.65)
IL-1RA	NS	0.32 (0.05–0.60)	0.55 (0.25–0.86)	NA
sIL-2R	0.41 (0.25–0.58)	0.37 (0.18–0.55)	0.75 (0.49–1.01)	NA
sIL-6R	0.36 (0.05–0.67)	0.45 (0.07–0.84)	NS	NA
IFN-γ	NS	NS	NS	NA
TNF-α	0.60 (0.15–1.05)	NS	0.55 (0.03–1.07)	NS
sTNFR1	0.62 (0.34–0.90)	0.65 (0.43–0.88)	0.89 (0.61–1.18)	NA
CCL2	NS	NS	NA	NA

NS, no significant difference between cases and controls; NA, not available, not measured separately according to current mood state.
*Mean effect sizes and 95% confidence intervals are presented for statistically significant changes. Findings are presented for all studies and for different affective states compared to controls separately whenever information is available.

differed (e.g., Munkholm et al.[74] for bipolar disorder and Tourjman et al.[75] for the effect of antipsychotics on cytokine levels).

Many findings in acute psychosis and in prodromal stages of psychotic disorders suggest an activation of macrophages/monocytes (reviewed by Bergink et al.).[76] In line with this, a study in which whole blood samples from people with schizophrenia, bipolar disorder, and healthy controls were cultured with TLR agonists for 24 h, an exaggerated release of proinflammatory cytokines was seen in response to stimulation with TLR-2-, TLR4-, and TLR-8 agonists.[77] However, studies that have specifically focused on monocytes suggest that they may be functioning inefficiently. In one study, monocytes showed an activation of genes characterized by different sets of transcription/mitogen-activated protein kinases regulating factors in schizophrenia and bipolar disorder, although one set of genes was downregulated in schizophrenia.[78] On the other hand, in a study that compared monocytes derived from people with schizophrenia and healthy controls before and after stimulation with either LPS or polyI:C found that the intracellular IL-1β concentration was lower in monocytes from people with schizophrenia than in those from healthy controls before and after stimulation.[79] In the same study, the expression of toll-like receptors three and four was elevated in people with schizophrenia before the stimulation, but increased less after stimulation.[79] A different pattern was observed for IL-6: it was lower in people with schizophrenia before stimulation, but increased more after stimulation.[80] Together, these findings suggest that monocyte functioning is dysregulated in schizophrenia. Furthermore, this dysregulation seems to be present together with reduced numbers and reduced proliferation activity of circulating lymphocytes, in particular of T cells.[21,76] However, the findings across studies are not consistent, probably because of the clinical heterogeneity of psychotic disorders.

Oxidative stress results in the release of enzymes, "redoxkines," which amplify signals of the TNF-α-induced inflammatory response and have also other cytokine-like activities, linking oxidative stress to innate immunity.[81] Some reviews summarize considerable evidence for an association of lowered or impaired antioxidant defenses with psychotic disorder.[25,26,82] Overall, the evidence so far is moderate for a role of oxidative stress at illness onset, suggesting interesting perspectives of early intervention by redox modulation.[83,84] Some evidence for an imbalance of antioxidant defenses can be also found at later phases of the illness.[82]

One pathway from systemic innate immunity activation to psychotic disorders may be a shift in the kynurenine pathway metabolism toward formation of KYNA, an antagonist of the glutaminergic NMDA receptors. Elevated brain KYNA levels have been observed in postmortem studies of brains of patients with schizophrenia.[20] Excessive KYNA leads to reduced NMDA receptor activity, and this may be relevant, for example, to cognitive deficits in schizophrenia and major depression.[20] On the other hand, some of the metabolites of the KYNA pathway are neurotoxic, which may also be relevant for the pathophysiology of these disorders.[20] However, kynurenine has also an important anti-inflammatory role in endotoxic tolerance,[22] and therefore activation of kynurenine pathway metabolism activation might have differing tissue- and phase-dependent effects.

On the whole, elevated innate immunity markers have been associated with clinical features of psychotic disorders, although a consistent pattern has not emerged and several studies have found contradictory results. Among the confirming findings, elevated CRP and IL-6 have been associated with insidious psychosis onset, duration of illness, and chronic schizophrenia course with mental deterioration as well as poorer cognitive functioning.[85] In another study, cytokines and chemokines of the IL-17 pathway correlated with more severe positive and negative symptoms.[86] In a large clinical study sample, the CRP levels at acute stages of schizophrenia or bipolar disorder did not differ statistically, both groups having elevated CRP levels.[87] The association of CRP and IL-6 is not specific for psychosis since it is also seen in unipolar major depressive patients.[87,88] However, a gene expression study of monocytes in patients with schizophrenia, bipolar disorder, and controls showed similarities and differences in immune gene activation, suggesting that the pathology is not identical in both conditions.[78] Systemic innate immunity markers, particularly IL-6 and CRP, have been also correlated with brain structural changes in patients with first-episode psychosis and schizophrenia,[89,90] and an aggregate index of proinflammatory cytokines predicted steeper gray matter loss in frontal cortical areas in high-risk patients who transitioned to psychosis during follow-up.[38] The results suggest that an abnormal activation of innate immunity may contribute to brain structural changes in psychotic disorders.

MICROGLIA IN PSYCHOTIC DISORDERS

The microglia hypothesis of schizophrenia suggests that microglia are in a pro-inflammatory state in schizophrenia, and contribute to neuronal pathology associated with the disease.[91] Neuropathological studies have found evidence of microglial activation and proliferation particularly in the white matter, while results concerning gray matter have been inconsistent.[92] A few studies have investigated the association of inflammatory gene expression and gray and white matter pathology, and have also found associations especially with white matter pathology.[92] Furthermore, some studies have found that the number of macrophages and activated lymphocytes were increased in people who had schizophrenia with acute psychotic episode.[93,94] There is an overexpression of several immune-response-related genes and downregulation of genes related to oxidative phosphorylation in the postmortem brain of patients who had schizophrenia.[95] A study comparing gene expression in postmortem brains of patients who had schizophrenia, bipolar disorder, and controls, found an even stronger upregulation of innate immunity-related genes in bipolar disorder compared to schizophrenia.[96]

Positron emission tomography studies have investigated microglial activation *in vivo* using (^{11}C)-(R)-PK11195, a peripheral benzodiazepine receptor (TPSO) ligand. Using this method, two small studies of patients with recent onset schizophrenia or schizophrenia spectrum psychosis found evidence of microglial activation in the brain of patients with schizophrenia compared to matched controls, one study finding microglial activation in hippocampus and the other in the total gray matter.[97,98] A study using a second-generation TPSO ligand [^{18}F]-FEPPA found no evidence of microglial activation in patients with schizophrenia.[99] However, Doorduin et al.[97] and Van Berckel et al.[98] investigated young patients with recent onset psychosis or schizophrenia, whereas Kenk et al.[99] investigated older and more chronic patients. The only study conducted in bipolar disorder, using (^{11}C)-(R)-PK11195, found evidence of microglial activation in the hippocampus in patients with bipolar I disorder.[100]

Overall, not only there is support for the activation of microglia in psychotic disorders, but also some negative findings.

NEURONAL AUTOANTIBODIES AND PSYCHOSIS

Over the recent years, a number of neuropsychiatric syndromes mediated by brain-reactive antibodies have been identified.[101,102] Anti-NMDAR encephalitis was originally identified in young women with ovarian teratoma who had an encephalitis with prominent psychiatric manifestations. Later, it was noted that anti-NMDAR encephalitis can exist without an association with cancer.[102] For some time, it was believed that even 10% of schizophrenic patients could actually have such encephalitis etiology behind their symptoms based on the studies reporting mostly IgA or IgM antibodies to NMDAR in clinically schizophrenic patients.[3] However, it appeared that IgA and IgM antibodies seem to be unassociated with clinical features, rather they are equally common in controls. At the same time, most research suggests that IgG GluN1 antibodies are specific for anti-NMDAR encephalitis.[3] GluN1 is glycosylated in transfected cells and several rat brain regions. The region around the glycosylation site GluN1-N368 controls recognition by patients' antibodies, but glycosylation itself is neither necessary nor sufficient for antibody staining.[103] Other antibrain antibodies associate with encephalitis with psychotic symptoms in case reports.[76]

MICROBIOME AND INFLAMMATION IN PSYCHOTIC DISORDERS

Gut microbiome has an important role in health and disease. One of the main roles of gut microbiome in mammals is that it guides the maturation and functioning of a host immune system, tuning it toward effector or regulatory directions.[104] Furthermore, intestinal microbiota, gut, and CNS interact, forming the microbiome–gut–brain axis.[104] This occurs via afferent and efferent neural, endocrine, nutrient, and immunological signals.[104] For example, some intestinal microbes cause anxiety- and depression-like behavior as well as modulate GABA-ergic, glutaminergic NMDA, and serotonergic 5HT1A receptors in the brain,[105–108] whereas germ-free mice exhibit reduced anxiety-like behavior.[107,108]

Several studies have found evidence of gastrointestinal (GI) inflammation in schizophrenia. Antibodies to anti-*Saccharomyces cerevisiae*, a marker of GI inflammation, are elevated in people with first-episode psychosis, schizophrenia, and bipolar disorder.[109,110] Furthermore, serological surrogate markers of bacterial translocation correlated with serum CRP levels,[111] suggesting that GI inflammation may contribute to systemic low-level inflammation. A contributing factor may be increased GI permeability, which is supported by studies finding elevated antibodies against food in people with schizophrenia.[112] These findings suggest that people with psychotic disorders may suffer from GI inflammation and "leaky gut," which may contribute to immunological alterations in psychotic disorders.

AN IMMUNE-MEDIATED TWO-HIT MODEL FOR PSYCHOSIS

Animal models of psychotic conditions (maternal stress and inflammation paradigms) suggest an immune-mediated model for the etiology of psychosis.[49,76,113] According to it, in genetically susceptible individuals, environmental influences (infection or stress *in utero* or early life, representing first hits) induce excessive inflammatory activation of monocytes/microglia, resulting in changes in the HPA axis functioning. These lead to developmental brain abnormalities (a vulnerable brain) with primed microglia, for example, microglial dysfunction in supporting neuronal growth and axon guidance for important brain areas. The second hit occurs later in the form of various environmental or endogenous alterations, including microbes, stress, puberty, hormonal changes at postpartum period, or exposure to cannabinoids.[114] These lead to a further and excessive activated microglia resulting in abnormalities of the neuronal circuitry in the brain and psychosis.[76]

The theory is based on animal models where induced maternal infection or otherwise induced inflammatory response can disrupt fetal brain development via upregulation of proinflammatory cytokines within the placenta, fetal circulation, and the fetal brain.[49,76,115] A prenatal viral infection can have an effect on gene expression in the brain postnatally, with differences in the affected genes and brain areas depending on the timing of the infection.[49] Many of these genes are associated with hypoxia, inflammation, and schizophrenia. Animal models thus show that prenatal infection can lead to long-term changes in brain morphology and behavioral development, which manifest as neuropathology. In adulthood, this leads to abnormalities of behavior, psychophysiology, cognition, and neurochemistry.[115] The interaction of maternal infection and later stress leading to illness-related behavior cited earlier is seen as supporting evidence for this model.[61]

Findings in animal models are consistent and highly interesting, especially because some changes can be reversed with medication.[115] At the same time, they cannot be generalized to humans. First, the exposure to infectious and noninfectious stressors in animal models is extreme, as compared to infections and stress in humans.[49] Also, direct evidence for the model in humans is lacking. Association of prenatal infections with increased risk of psychotic disorders,[114,115] and peripheral monocyte activation,[116] altered cytokine activity, microglia activation and gene expression in the brain,[92] altered brain energy metabolism,[117] and association of microglial and astroglial pathology, and systemic level of innate immunity cytokines and chemokines, with white and gray matter pathology in patients with psychotic disorders, provide indirect evidence for the aforementioned theory.[49,92,114,117,118]

CONFOUNDERS

Several conditions associated with chronic inflammation are more common in patients with schizophrenia and other psychotic disorders than in the general population. These include obesity, metabolic syndrome, and type 2 diabetes.[119] The most common abnormality seen in patients with schizophrenia is abdominal obesity, which is over four times more common in these patients than in general population controls.[119] In visceral obesity, both macrophages of the white adipose tissue and enlarged adipocytes produce proinflammatory cytokines.[120] However, while this comorbidity has been shown to influence the levels of inflammatory markers in studies investigating patients with multiple episode psychotic disorder,[121] it is rarely present in first-episode patients[122] who nevertheless have elevations in various proinflammatory cytokines.[71]

Lifestyle-related and socioeconomic factors that could also contribute to the association between psychotic disorders and inflammation include smoking,[123] alcohol use,[124] diet,[125] poor physical condition,[126] sleep,[127] and low socioeconomic status in childhood[128] as well as in adulthood.[129] Each of these is more common in people with schizophrenia, and each have been associated with alterations of the immune system. In studies that have been adjusted for several of these factors, the association between inflammation and psychotic disorders has been attenuated.[130] Furthermore, for example, the possible role of sleep disturbance in inflammation related to psychotic disorders has not been studied.

Most importantly, antipsychotic medication affects the immune system. According to meta-analyses of patients with schizophrenia, spectrum psychoses followed up after the initiation of antipsychotic treatment, there is a significant decrease of proinflammatory cytokine levels following antipsychotic treatment, suggesting that antipsychotics have an anti-inflammatory effect.[71,75] However, these changes may also reflect indirect effects related to alleviation of psychotic symptoms, such as improved sleep and decreased agitation. Furthermore, *in vitro* studies have found that different antipsychotics have different effects on the immune system. For example, clozapine and risperidone seem to have an inhibitory effect on Th1 differentiation and cytokines, whereas the same was not observed for haloperidol.[131,132] Other medications that are commonly used in the treatment of psychotic disorders, such as antidepressants, also have anti-inflammatory properties.[133] Interestingly, some animal studies suggest that antipsychotics also affect gut microbiota, and this might contribute to weight gain associated with antipsychotic treatment.[134] Such mechanisms could also explain some of the effects of antipsychotics on inflammatory markers.

Oxidative stress is a shared factor in psychosis and metabolic disorders. Assies et al. suggested that the imbalance in oxidative stress regulation of psychotic patients is mediated by changes in lipid metabolism, as also seen in metabolic comorbidity.[26] Consistent with this, alterations in lipid metabolism associated with cognitive functioning and brain structural changes have been identified in schizophrenia.[135]

PSYCHOSIS AS COMPARED TO AUTOIMMUNE DISORDERS

Affective and nonaffective psychosis possess many clinical features shared by autoimmune diseases.[76] First, they are etiologically multifactorial, with a polygenic inheritance and requiring exposure to one or more environmental factors. Second, psychotic disorders show familial association of psychotic and autoimmune disorders in the first-degree relatives, and autoimmune and chronic inflammatory conditions are associated with increased risks of psychotic disorders.[4,5] Also, psychotic disorders have a typical course of progression from subclinical to clinical disease, and show cyclical exacerbation-remission patterns especially when affective symptomatology is present. Interestingly, this course pattern in psychotic symptoms seems to be associated with a similar pattern of inflammatory response. In schizophrenia, where the psychotic symptoms are often persistent, some cytokines are elevated only during acute episodes, while others at acute and chronic illness.[71] In bipolar disorders, interepisode partial or full remission is rather a rule and, by definition, psychotic symptoms are present only at mania or major depressive episode. Interestingly, changes in cytokine profile are clear in a manic episode, while a trait-like inflammatory response remains more disputable.[73] However, only sporadic cases of primary psychosis are reported to be etiologically autoimmune, caused by, for example, autoantibodies against neuroreceptors, which interfere with their functioning.[3] For example, in anti-NMDA receptor encephalitis, IgG antibodies to NMDA receptors induce a reversible internalization of the receptors from synaptic and extrasynaptic space, leading to increased excitability, neurological, and psychiatric symptoms.[3]

ANTI-INFLAMMATORY DRUGS AS ADJUNCTIVE MEDICATION IN PSYCHOTIC DISORDERS

An adjunctive anti-inflammatory medication especially at illness onset is theoretically interesting, for example, because of the findings linking inflammation to progressive brain structural changes. So far, no strong conclusions of potential compounds or effectiveness of specific compounds can be made since most of the study samples have been small and heterogenic in terms of symptoms or phase of the illness. Few studies used a setting of a strict intervention study. In a meta-analysis,[136] aspirin (mean weighted effect size [ES]: $0.3, n = 270, 95\%$ CI: 0.06–0.537) and n-acetyl cysteine (ES: 0.45, $n = 140$, 95% CI: 0.112–0.779) showed significant effects on symptom severity in schizophrenia. However, the dose of aspirin had been 1000 mg daily, which as a long-term medication could cause significant side effects. Celecoxib, minocycline, davunetide, and fatty acids showed no significant effect on symptoms of schizophrenia.[136] Other randomized controlled trials (RCTs) in schizophrenia suggesting some efficacy of adjunctive anti-inflammatory treatment include three pilot RCTs with pregnenolone, two RCTs with dehydroepiandrosterone and dehydroepiandrosterone-sulfate, and one with L-theanine.[137]

In patients with a clinical high risk of psychosis, one randomized controlled trial on omega-3 fatty acids suggested a beneficial effect for a 12-week course of nutritional supplementation compared with placebo.[138] However, another large randomized controlled trial with ethyl-eicosapentaenoate in people with schizophrenia spectrum psychoses found it to worsen psychotic symptoms.[139] In terms of potential side effects, omega-3 fatty acids are safe to use.[140]

Based on a recent review of anti-inflammatory treatment in bipolar disorder, evidence is strongest for an effect of n-acetyl cysteine in bipolar depression. Although several studies were available, for other compounds and interventions in mania, the evidence is insufficient to draw any conclusions.[141]

Immune-system-based interventions in psychosis have to face several challenges. First, modifying the function of immune pathways may have systemic side effects. Second, identification of patients who would benefit from such a therapy will be challenging, because the peripheral or imaging biomarkers might not be sufficiently specific and sensitive. Third, it is likely that the maximum benefit from an immune intervention would be in early life, during the initial immune system hyperactivation in genetically susceptible individuals, long before the disease is diagnosed and at a time point when a perceived risk of developing schizophrenia will hardly justify aggressive therapeutic interventions. In the future, personalized analysis may be helpful. For example, people with schizophrenia and elevated CRP had better treatment responses with adjunctive aspirin,[142] and higher baseline erythrocyte membrane concentration of α-linolenic acid, the shortest chain fatty acid in the ω-3 family, predicted better treatment response in the mentioned omega-3 fatty acid trial.[143]

Targeting inflammatory pathways opens numerous hypothetical new options of adjunctive, also nonmedical treatment. These are as diverse as glycomimetic targets aiming at reducing viral damage in the brain by reducing inflammation, promoting cell proliferation, enhancing synaptic plasticity,[144] and targeting the purinergic P2 receptors to reduce neuroinflammation.[145] Interventions also aim at reducing oxidative stress, and changing gut microbiome, including probiotic supplementation.

FUTURE DIRECTIONS

We have reviewed evidence for an imbalance in inflammatory mechanisms at perhaps all stages of inflammation in psychotic patients: an oversensitive triggering system for exogenous and endogenous danger (e.g., stress response), a modified sensor mechanism (e.g., pattern recognition receptors), imbalance of signal transmission and production of mediators in numerous innate immunity signaling pathways (e.g., lower anti-inflammatory and higher proinflammatory cytokines, the kynurenine pathway), and altered activation of cellular effectors.

It is evident that monocyte, cytokine, and T cell aberrancies are only found in subgroups of patients with psychosis and often overlap with findings in healthy control subjects. The findings are also largely shared by all major psychiatric disorders, at least schizophrenia, bipolar disorder, major depressive disorder, and partly autism, although there are also differences, for example, in immunological gene expression. Numerous possible confounders are identified and also shared by other psychiatric illnesses. Based on current evidence from human studies, there is not enough evidence to state that immune system deregulation or an immune-related trigger causes psychosis. Nevertheless, current research suggests that the immune system is involved at least in a subgroup of patients with psychosis. Immune activation could also be seen as a phenomenon secondary to the disease state. It is also possible that the activation of innate immunity response is an etiological factor behind somatic comorbidity and has no direct, independent etiological role in psychosis.

Etiological and intervention studies including patients across categorical diagnostic boundaries are needed to further evaluate the specificity of the aforementioned findings. Further clinical studies are warranted especially in high-risk patients and at early illness onset. Longitudinal studies comparing inflammatory measures at acute phase and remission at an individual level are needed to get information about the dynamic changes in inflammatory response, whereas mediating and moderating factors, such as stress and sleep, would deserve more attention. Outcome measures should also include, in addition to categorical diagnosis and symptom measures (psychosis, mania, depression), measures of cognitive impairment, and brain imaging reflecting neuroinflammatory processes and neurodegeneration. The possible role of gut microbiome in immunological alterations should be investigated. Anti-inflammatory intervention studies aiming at reducing metabolic side effects of current antipsychotics are also warranted. Any intervention study should monitor specific inflammatory markers (hCRP, oxidative stress, etc.) to identify the individuals most likely to respond and to investigate the correlation between change and treatment outcome.

A detailed understanding of the molecular mechanisms at work in virally and other induced neuroinflammation is crucial if researchers are to uncover ways to regulate aberrant cytokine-induced initiation and propagation of neuronal damage. Precise predictive models of the prodromal phase of neurodegeneration will provide guidance for designing potential intervention regimens that delay disease onset. To this end, investigation of immune alterations should be more specific, focusing on specific cell types, whose functioning should be studied more closely. Also, cerebrospinal fluid (CSF) should be investigated more often, and blood and CSF samples should be collected and analyzed from the same individuals in order to understand similarities and differences. In particular, peripheral biomarkers that would reflect central inflammation would be highly valuable. Such work could provide guidance for designing potential intervention regimens that delay psychosis onset and progression.

REFERENCES

1. Dantzer R, O'Connor JC, Freund GG, Johnson RW, Kelley KW. From inflammation to sickness and depression: when the immune system subjugates the brain. *Nat Rev Neurosci* 2008;**9**(1):46–56.
2. Raison CL, Demetrashvili M, Capuron L, Miller AH. Neuropsychiatric adverse effects of interferon-alpha: recognition and management. *CNS Drugs* 2005;**19**(2):105–23.
3. Kayser MS, Dalmau J. Anti-NMDA receptor encephalitis, autoimmunity, and psychosis. *Schizophr Res* 2014 Oct 25. pii: S0920-9964 (14)00546-5. doi:10.1016/j.schres.2014.10.007.
4. Benros ME, Waltoft BL, Nordentoft M, Ostergaard SD, Eaton WW, Krogh J, et al. Autoimmune diseases and severe infections as risk factors for mood disorders: a nationwide study. *JAMA Psychiatry* 2013;**70**(8):812–20.
5. Benros ME, Pedersen MG, Rasmussen H, Eaton WW, Nordentoft M, Mortensen PB. A nationwide study on the risk of autoimmune diseases in individuals with a personal or a family history of schizophrenia and related psychosis. *Am J Psychiatry* 2014;**171**(2):218–26.
6. Raevuori A, Haukka J, Vaarala O, Suvisaari JM, Gissler M, Grainger M, et al. The increased risk for autoimmune diseases in patients with eating disorders. *PLoS One* 2014;**9**(8):e104845.
7. Lugrin J, Rosenblatt-Velin N, Parapanov R, Liaudet L. The role of oxidative stress during inflammatory processes. *Biol Chem* 2014;**395**(2):203–30.
8. Irwin MR, Cole SW. Reciprocal regulation of the neural and innate immune systems. *Nat Rev Immunol* 2011;**11**(9):625–32.
9. Olofsson PS, Rosas-Ballina M, Levine YA, Tracey KJ. Rethinking inflammation: neural circuits in the regulation of immunity. *Immunol Rev* 2012;**248**(1):188–204.
10. Rosas-Ballina M, Olofsson PS, Ochani M, Valdés-Ferrer SI, Levine YA, Reardon C, et al. Acetylcholine-synthesizing T cells relay neural signals in a vagus nerve circuit. *Science* 2011;**334**(6052):98–101.
11. Prinz M, Priller J. Microglia and brain macrophages in the molecular age: from origin to neuropsychiatric disease. *Nat Rev Neurosci* 2014;**15**(5):300–12.
12. Graeber MB. Changing face of microglia. *Science* 2010;**330**(6005):783–8.
13. Deverman BE, Patterson PH. Cytokines and CNS development. *Neuron* 2009;**64**(1):61–78.
14. Pribiag H, Stellwagen D. Neuroimmune regulation of homeostatic synaptic plasticity. *Neuropharmacology* 2014;**78**:13–22.
15. Calabrese F, Rossetti AC, Racagni G, Gass P, Riva MA, Molteni R. Brain-derived neurotrophic factor: a bridge between inflammation and neuroplasticity. *Front Cell Neurosci* 2014;**8**:430.
16. Borsini A, Zunszain PA, Thuret S, Pariante CM. The role of inflammatory cytokines as key modulators of neurogenesis. *Trends Neurosci* 2015;**38**(3):145–57.
17. Holtzman CW, Trotman HD, Goulding SM, Ryan AT, Macdonald AN, Shapiro DI, et al. Stress and neurodevelopmental processes in the emergence of psychosis. *Neuroscience* 2013;**249**:172–91.
18. Stetler C, Miller GE. Depression and hypothalamic-pituitary-adrenal activation: a quantitative summary of four decades of research. *Psychosom Med* 2011;**73**(2):114–26.
19. Bellavance MA, Rivest S. The HPA – Immune axis and the immunomodulatory actions of glucocorticoids in the brain. *Front Immunol* 2014;**5**:136.
20. Schwarcz R, Bruno JP, Muchowski PJ, Wu HQ. Kynurenines in the mammalian brain: when physiology meets pathology. *Nat Rev Neurosci* 2012;**13**(7):465–77.
21. Najjar S, Pearlman DM, Alper K, Najjar A, Devinsky O. Neuroinflammation and psychiatric illness. *J Neuroinflammation* 2013;**10**:43.

22. Bessede A, Gargaro M, Pallotta MT, Matino D, Servillo G, Brunacci C, et al. Aryl hydrocarbon receptor control of a disease tolerance defence pathway. *Nature* 2014;**511**(7508):184–90.
23. Heneka MT, Kummer MP, Latz E. Innate immune activation in neurodegenerative disease. *Nat Rev Immunol* 2014;**14**(7):463–77.
24. Bitanihirwe BK, Woo TU. Oxidative stress in schizophrenia: an integrated approach. *Neurosci Biobehav Rev* 2011;**35**(3):878–93.
25. Yao JK1, Keshavan MS. Antioxidants, redox signaling, and pathophysiology in schizophrenia: an integrative view. *Antioxid Redox Signal* 2011;**15**(7):2011–35.
26. Assies J, Mocking RJ, Lok A, Ruhé HG, Pouwer F, Schene AH. Effects of oxidative stress on fatty acid- and one-carbon-metabolism in psychiatric and cardiovascular disease comorbidity. *Acta Psychiatr Scand* 2014;**130**(3):163–80.
27. Steullet P, Cabungcal JH, Monin A, Dwir D, O'Donnell P, Cuenod M, et al. Redox dysregulation, neuroinflammation, and NMDA receptor hypofunction: A "central hub" in schizophrenia pathophysiology? *Schizophr Res.* 2014 Jul 4. pii: S0920-9964(14)00313-2. doi: 10.1016/j. schres.2014.06.021.
28. Perälä J, Suvisaari J, Saarni SI, Kuoppasalmi K, Isometsä E, Pirkola S, et al. Lifetime prevalence of psychotic and bipolar I disorders in a general population. *Arch Gen Psychiatry* 2007;**64**(1):19–28.
29. Pedersen CB, Mors O, Bertelsen A, Waltoft BL, Agerbo E, McGrath JJ, et al. A comprehensive nationwide study of the incidence rate and lifetime risk for treated mental disorders. *JAMA Psychiatry* 2014;**71**(5):573–81.
30. Van Os J, Kapur S. Schizophrenia. *Lancet* 2009;**374**(9690):635–45.
31. Cannon TD, Kaprio J, Lönnqvist J, Huttunen M, Koskenvuo M. The genetic epidemiology of schizophrenia in a Finnish twin cohort. A population-based modeling study. *Arch Gen Psychiatry* 1998;**55**(1):67–74.
32. Kieseppä T, Partonen T, Haukka J, Kaprio J, Lönnqvist J. High concordance of bipolar I disorder in a nationwide sample of twins. *Am J Psychiatry* 2004;**161**(10):1814–21.
33. Lichtenstein P, Yip BH, Björk C, Pawitan Y, Cannon TD, Sullivan PF, et al. Common genetic determinants of schizophrenia and bipolar disorder in Swedish families: a population-based study. *Lancet* 2009;**373**(9659):234–9.
34. Rapoport JL, Giedd JN, Gogtay N. Neurodevelopmental model of schizophrenia: update 2012. *Mol Psychiatry* 2012;**17**(12):1228–38.
35. MacCabe JH, Wicks S, Löfving S, David AS, Berndtsson Å, Gustafsson JE, et al. Decline in cognitive performance between ages 13 and 18 years and the risk for psychosis in adulthood: a Swedish longitudinal cohort study in males. *JAMA Psychiatry* 2013;**70**(3):261–70.
36. Network and Pathway Analysis Subgroup of the Psychiatric Genomics Consortium, International Inflammatory Bowel Disease Genetics Consortium (IIBDGC). Psychiatric genome-wide association study analyses implicate neuronal, immune and histone pathways. *Nat Neurosci* 2015;**18**(2):199–209.
37. Fusar-Poli P, Borgwardt S, Bechdolf A, Addington J, Riecher-Rössler A, Schultze-Lutter F, et al. The psychosis high-risk state: a comprehensive state-of-the-art review. *JAMA Psychiatry* 2013;**70**(1):107–20.
38. Cannon TD, Chung Y, He G, Sun D, Jacobson A, Van Erp TG, et al. Progressive reduction in cortical thickness as psychosis develops: a multisite longitudinal neuroimaging study of youth at elevated clinical risk. *Biol Psychiatry* 2015;**77**(2):147–57.
39. Ho BC, Andreasen NC, Ziebell S, Pierson R, Magnotta V. Long-term antipsychotic treatment and brain volumes: a longitudinal study of first-episode schizophrenia. *Arch Gen Psychiatry* 2011;**68**(2):128–37.

40. Brown AS, Derkits EJ. Prenatal infection and schizophrenia: a review of epidemiologic and translational studies. *Am J Psychiatry* 2010;**167**(3):261–80.

41. Suvisaari JM, Taxell-Lassas V, Pankakoski M, Haukka JK, Lönnqvist JK, Häkkinen LT. Obstetric complications as risk factors for schizophrenia spectrum psychoses in offspring of mothers with psychotic disorder. *Schizophr Bull* 2013;**39**:1056–66.

42. Abel KM, Wicks S, Susser ES, Dalman C, Pedersen MG, Mortensen PB, Webb RT. Birth weight, schizophrenia, and adult mental disorder: is risk confined to the smallest babies? *Arch Gen Psychiatry* 2010;**67**(9):923–30.

43. St Clair D, Xu M, Wang P, Yu Y, Fang Y, Zhang F, Zheng X, Gu N, Feng G, Sham P, He L. Rates of adult schizophrenia following prenatal exposure to the Chinese famine of 1959–1961. *JAMA* 2005;**294**(5):557–62.

44. Khashan AS, Abel KM, McNamee R, Pedersen MG, Webb RT, Baker PN, Kenny LC, Mortensen PB. Higher risk of offspring schizophrenia following antenatal maternal exposure to severe adverse life events. *Arch Gen Psychiatry* 2008;**65**(2):146–52.

45. Brown AS, Hooton J, Schaefer CA, et al. Elevated maternal interleukin-8 levels and risk of schizophrenia in adult offspring. *Am J Psychiatry* 2004;**161**(5):889–95.

46. Buka SL, Tsuang MT, Torrey EF, Klebanoff MA, Wagner RL, Yolken RH. Maternal cytokine levels during pregnancy and adult psychosis. *Brain Behav Immun* 2001;**15**(4):411–20.

47. Severance EG, Gressitt KL, Buka SL, Cannon TD, Yolken RH. Maternal complement C1q and increased odds for psychosis in adult offspring. *Schizophr Res* 2014;**159**(1):14–9.

48. Canetta S, Sourander A, Surcel HM, Hinkka-Yli-Salomäki S, Leiviskä J, Kellendonk C, et al. Elevated maternal C-reactive protein and increased risk of schizophrenia in a national birth cohort. *Am J Psychiatry* 2014;**171**(9):960–8.

49. Kneeland RE, Fatemi SH. Viral infection, inflammation and schizophrenia. *Prog Neuropsychopharmacol Biol Psychiatry* 2013;**42**:35–48.

50. Gardner RM, Dalman C, Wicks S, Lee BK, Karlsson H. Neonatal levels of acute phase proteins and later risk of non-affective psychosis. *Transl Psychiatry* 2013;**3**:e228.

51. Nielsen PR, Agerbo E, Skogstrand K, Hougaard DM, Meyer U, Mortensen PB. Neonatal levels of inflammatory markers and later risk of schizophrenia. *Biol Psychiatry* 2015;**77**(6):548–55.

52. Khandaker GM, Zimbron J, Dalman C, Lewis G, Jones PB. Childhood infection and adult schizophrenia: a meta-analysis of population-based studies. *Schizophr Res* 2012;**139**(1-3): 161–8.

53. Nielsen PR, Benros ME, Mortensen PB. Hospital contacts with infection and risk of schizophrenia: a population-based cohort study with linkage of Danish national registers. *Schizophr Bull* 2014;**40**:1526–32.

54. Blomström Å, Karlsson H, Svensson A, Frisell T, Lee BK, Dal H, Magnusson C, Dalman C. Hospital admission with infection during childhood and risk for psychotic illness – a population-based cohort study. *Schizophr Bull* 2014;**40**:1518–25.

55. Khandaker GM, Pearson RM, Zammit S, Lewis G, Jones PB. Association of serum interleukin 6 and C-reactive protein in childhood with depression and psychosis in young adult life: a population-based longitudinal study. *JAMA Psychiatry* 2014;**71**(10):1121–8.

56. Crump C, Winkleby MA, Sundquist K, Sundquist J. Comorbidities and mortality in persons with schizophrenia: a Swedish national cohort study. *Am J Psychiatry* 2013;**170**(3):324–33.

57. Crump C, Sundquist K, Winkleby MA, Sundquist J. Comorbidities and mortality in bipolar disorder: a Swedish national cohort study. *JAMA Psychiatry* 2013;**70**(9):931–9.

58. Fisher HL, Jones PB, Fearon P, Craig TK, Dazzan P, Morgan K, et al. The varying impact of type, timing and frequency of exposure to childhood adversity on its association with adult psychotic disorder. *Psychol Med* 2010;**40**(12):1967–78.

59. Coelho R, Viola TW, Walss-Bass C, Brietzke E, Grassi-Oliveira R. Childhood maltreatment and inflammatory markers: a systematic review. *Acta Psychiatr Scand* 2014;**129**(3):180–92.

60. Hepgul N, Pariante CM, Dipasquale S, DiForti M, Taylor H, Marques TR, et al. Childhood maltreatment is associated with increased body mass index and increased C-reactive protein levels in first-episode psychosis patients. *Psychol Med* 2012;**42**(9):1893–901.

61. Giovanoli S, Engler H, Engler A, Richetto J, Voget M, Willi R, et al. Stress in puberty unmasks latent neuropathological consequences of prenatal immune activation in mice. *Science* 2013;**339**(6123):1095–9.

62. Schizophrenia Working Group of the Psychiatric Genomics Consortium. Biological insights from 108 schizophrenia-associated genetic loci. *Nature* 2014;**511**(7510):421–7.

63. Schneider M, Debbané M, Bassett AS, Chow EW, Fung WL, Van den Bree M, et al. Psychiatric disorders from childhood to adulthood in 22q11.2 deletion syndrome: results from the International Consortium on Brain and Behavior in 22q11. 2 Deletion Syndrome. *Am J Psychiatry* 2014;**171**(6):627–39.

64. Ferrando-Martínez S, Lorente R, Gurbindo D, De José MI, Leal M, Muñoz-Fernández MA, Correa-Rocha R. Low thymic output, peripheral homeostasis deregulation, and hastened regulatory T cells differentiation in children with 22q11.2 deletion syndrome. *J Pediatr* 2014;**164**(4):882–9.

65. Gabay C, Kushner I. Acute-phase proteins and other systemic responses to inflammation. *N Engl J Med* 1999;**340**(6):448–54.

66. Miller BJ, Culpepper N, Rapaport MH. C-reactive protein levels in schizophrenia: a review and meta-analysis. *Clin Schizophr Relat Psychoses* 2014;**7**:223–30.

67. Bai YM, Su TP, Li CT, Tsai SJ, Chen MH, Tu PC, et al. Comparison of pro-inflammatory cytokines among patients with bipolar disorder and unipolar depression and normal controls. *Bipolar Disord* 2015;**17**(3):269–77.

68. Wium-Andersen MK, Ørsted DD, Nordestgaard BG. Elevated C-reactive protein associated with late- and very-late-onset schizophrenia in the general population: a prospective study. *Schizophr Bull* 2014;**40**(5):1117–27.

69. Chiam JT, Dobson RJ, Kiddle SJ, Sattlecker M. Are blood-based protein biomarkers for Alzheimer's disease also involved in other brain disorders? A systematic review. *J Alzheimers Dis* 2015;**43**(1):303–14.

70. Labad J, Stojanovic-Pérez A, Montalvo I, Solé M, Cabezas A, Ortega L, Moreno I, Vilella E, Martorell L, Reynolds RM, Gutiérrez-Zotes A. Stress biomarkers as predictors of transition to psychosis in at-risk mental states: roles for cortisol, prolactin and albumin. *J Psychiatr Res* 2014;**60C**:163–9.

71. Miller BJ, Buckley P, Seabolt W, Mellor A, Kirkpatrick B. Meta-analysis of cytokine alterations in schizophrenia: clinical status and antipsychotic effects. *Biol Psychiatry* 2011;**70**(7):663–71.

72. Perkins DO, Jeffries CD, Addington J, Bearden CE, Cadenhead KS, Cannon TD, et al. Towards a psychosis risk blood diagnostic for persons experiencing high-risk symptoms: preliminary results from the NAPLS Project. *Schizophr Bull* 2015;**41**(2):419–28.

73. Modabbernia A, Taslimi S, Brietzke E, Ashrafi M. Cytokine alterations in bipolar disorder: a meta-analysis of 30 studies. *Biol Psychiatry* 2013;**74**(1):15–25.

74. Munkholm K, Braüner JV, Kessing LV, Vinberg M. Cytokines in bipolar disorder vs. healthy control subjects: a systematic review and meta-analysis. *J Psychiatr Res* 2013;**47**(9):1119–33.

75. Tourjman V, Kouassi É, Koué MÈ, Rocchetti M, Fortin-Fournier S, Fusar-Poli P, Potvin S. Antipsychotics' effects on blood levels of cytokines in schizophrenia: a meta-analysis. *Schizophr Res* 2013;**151**(1-3):43–7.

76. Bergink V, Gibney SM, Drexhage HA. Autoimmunity, inflammation, and psychosis: a search for peripheral markers. *Biol Psychiatry* 2014;**75**(4):324–31.
77. McKernan DP, Dennison U, Gaszner G, Cryan JF, Dinan TG. Enhanced peripheral toll-like receptor responses in psychosis: further evidence of a pro-inflammatory phenotype. *Transl Psychiatry* 2011;**1**:e36.
78. Drexhage RC, Van der Heul-Nieuwenhuijsen L, Padmos RC, Van Beveren N, Cohen D, Versnel MA, et al. Inflammatory gene expression in monocytes of patients with schizophrenia: overlap and difference with bipolar disorder. A study in naturalistically treated patients. *Int J Neuropsychopharmacol* 2010;**13**(10):1369–81.
79. Müller N, Wagner JK, Krause D, Weidinger E, Wildenauer A, Obermeier M, et al. Impaired monocyte activation in schizophrenia. *Psychiatry Res* 2012;**198**(3):341–6.
80. Krause DL, Wagner JK, Wildenauer A, Matz J, Weidinger E, Riedel M, et al. Intracellular monocytic cytokine levels in schizophrenia show an alteration of IL-6. *Eur Arch Psychiatry Clin Neurosci* 2012;**262**(5):393–401.
81. Salzano S, Checconi P, Hanschmann EM, Lillig CH, Bowler LD, Chan P, Vaudry D, Mengozzi M, Coppo L, Sacre S, Atkuri KR, Sahaf B, Herzenberg LA, Herzenberg LA, Mullen L, Ghezzi P. Linkage of inflammation and oxidative stress via release of glutathionylated peroxiredoxin-2, which acts as a danger signal. *Proc Natl Acad Sci USA* 2014;**111**(33):12157–62.
82. Flatow J, Buckley P, Miller BJ. Meta-analysis of oxidative stress in schizophrenia. *Biol Psychiatry* 2013;**74**(6):400–9.
83. Cabungcal JH, Counotte DS, Lewis EM, Tejeda HA, Piantadosi P, Pollock C, et al. Juvenile antioxidant treatment prevents adult deficits in a developmental model of schizophrenia. *Neuron* 2014;**83**(5):1073–84.
84. Emiliani FE, Sedlak TW, Sawa A. Oxidative stress and schizophrenia: recent breakthroughs from an old story. *Curr Opin Psychiatry* 2014;**27**(3):185–90.
85. Frydecka D, Misiak B, Pawlak-Adamska E, Karabon L, Tomkiewicz A, Sedlaczek P, Kiejna A, Beszłej JA. Interleukin-6: the missing element of the neurocognitive deterioration in schizophrenia? The focus on genetic underpinnings, cognitive impairment and clinical manifestation. *Eur Arch Psychiatry Clin Neurosci* 2014 Sep 12. [Epub ahead of print] PubMed PMID: 25214388.
86. Dimitrov DH, Lee S, Yantis J, Valdez C, Paredes RM, Braida N, et al. Differential correlations between inflammatory cytokines and psychopathology in veterans with schizophrenia: potential role for IL-17 pathway. *Schizophr Res* 2013;**151**(1-3):29–35.
87. Wysokiński A, Margulska A, Strzelecki D, Kłoszewska I. Levels of C-reactive protein (CRP) in patients with schizophrenia, unipolar depression and bipolar disorder. *Nord J Psychiatry* 2015;**69**(5):346–53.
88. Valkanova V, Ebmeier KP, Allan CL. CRP, IL-6 and depression: a systematic review and meta-analysis of longitudinal studies. *J Affect Disord* 2013;**150**(3):736–44.
89. Mondelli V, Cattaneo A, Belvederi Murri M, Di Forti M, Handley R, Hepgul N, et al. Stress and inflammation reduce brain-derived neurotrophic factor expression in first-episode psychosis: a pathway to smaller hippocampal volume. *J Clin Psychiatry* 2011;**72**(12):1677–84.
90. Prasad KM, Upton CH, Nimgaonkar VL, Keshavan MS. Differential susceptibility of white matter tracts to inflammatory mediators in schizophrenia: an integrated DTI study. *Schizophr Res* 2015;**161**(1):119–25.
91. Monji A, Kato T, Kanba S. Cytokines and schizophrenia: microglia hypothesis of schizophrenia. *Psychiatry Clin Neurosci* 2009;**63**(3):257–65.
92. Najjar S, Pearlman DM. Neuroinflammation and white matter pathology in schizophrenia: systematic review. *Schizophr Res* 2015;**161**(1):102–12.

93. Nikkilä HV, Müller K, Ahokas A, Miettinen K, Rimón R, Andersson LC. Accumulation of macrophages in the CSF of schizophrenic patients during acute psychotic episodes. *Am J Psychiatry* 1999;**156**(11):1725–9.

94. Nikkilä HV, Müller K, Ahokas A, Rimón R, Andersson LC. Increased frequency of activated lymphocytes in the cerebrospinal fluid of patients with acute schizophrenia. *Schizophr Res* 2001;**49**(1-2):99–105.

95. Mistry M, Gillis J, Pavlidis P. Meta-analysis of gene coexpression networks in the post-mortem prefrontal cortex of patients with schizophrenia and unaffected controls. *BMC Neurosci* 2013;**14**:105.

96. de Baumont A, Maschietto M, Lima L, Carraro DM, Olivieri EH, Fiorini A, Barreta LA, Palha JA, Belmonte-de-Abreu P, Moreira Filho CA, Brentani H. Innate immune response is differentially dysregulated between bipolar disease and schizophrenia. *Schizophr Res* 2015;**161**(2–3):215–21.

97. Doorduin J, de Vries EF, Willemsen AT, de Groot JC, Dierckx RA, Klein HC. Neuroinflammation in schizophrenia-related psychosis: a PET study. *J Nucl Med* 2009;**50**(11):1801–7.

98. Van Berckel BN, Bossong MG, Boellaard R, Kloet R, Schuitemaker A, Caspers E, et al. Microglia activation in recent-onset schizophrenia: a quantitative (R)-[^{11}C]PK11195 positron emission tomography study. *Biol Psychiatry* 2008;**64**(9):820–2.

99. Kenk M, Selvanathan T, Rao N, Suridjan I, Rusjan P, Remington G, et al. Imaging neuroinflammation in gray and white matter in schizophrenia: an *in vivo* PET study with [^{18}F]-FEPPA. *Schizophr Bull* 2015;**41**(1):85–93.

100. Haarman BC, Riemersma-Van der Lek RF, de Groot JC, Ruhé HG, Klein HC, Zandstra TE, Burger H, Schoevers RA, de Vries EF, Drexhage HA, Nolen WA, Doorduin J. Neuroinflammation in bipolar disorder - A [(11)C]-(R)-PK11195 positron emission tomography study. *Brain Behav Immun* 2014;**40**:219–25.

101. Diamond B, Honig G, Mader S, Brimberg L, Volpe BT. Brain-reactive antibodies and disease. *Annu Rev Immunol* 2013;**31**:345–85.

102. Coutinho E, Harrison P, Vincent A. Do neuronal autoantibodies cause psychosis? A neuroimmunological perspective. *Biol Psychiatry* 2014;**75**:269–75.

103. Gleichman AJ, Spruce LA, Dalmau J, Seeholzer SH, Lynch DR. Anti-NMDA receptor encephalitis antibody binding is dependent on amino acid identity of a small region within the GluN1 amino terminal domain. *J Neurosci* 2012;**32**(32):11082–94.

104. Wang Y, Kasper LH. The role of microbiome in central nervous system disorders. *Brain Behav Immun* 2014;**38**:1–12.

105. Bercik P, Verdu EF, Foster JA, Macri J, Potter M, Huang X, et al. Chronic gastrointestinal inflammation induces anxiety-like behavior and alters central nervous system biochemistry in mice. *Gastroenterology* 2010;**139**(6):2102–12.

106. Bravo JA, Forsythe P, Chew MV, Escaravage E, Savignac HM, Dinan TG, et al. Ingestion of Lactobacillus strain regulates emotional behavior and central GABA receptor expression in a mouse via the vagus nerve. *Proc Natl Acad Sci USA* 2011;**108**(38):16050–5.

107. Heijtz RD, Wang S, Anuar F, Qian Y, Björkholm B, Samuelsson A, Hibberd ML, Forssberg H, Pettersson S. Normal gut microbiota modulates brain development and behavior. *Proc Natl Acad Sci USA* 2011;**108**(7):3047–52.

108. Neufeld KM, Kang N, Bienenstock J, Foster JA. Reduced anxiety-like behavior and central neurochemical change in germ-free mice. *Neurogastroenterol Motil* 2011;**23**(3):255–64.

109. Severance EG, Alaedini A, Yang S, Halling M, Gressitt KL, Stallings CR, et al. Gastrointestinal inflammation and associated immune activation in schizophrenia. *Schizophr Res* 2012;**138**(1):48–53.

110. Severance EG, Gressitt KL, Yang S, Stallings CR, Origoni AE, Vaughan C, et al. Seroreactive marker for inflammatory bowel disease and associations with antibodies to dietary proteins in bipolar disorder. *Bipolar Disord* 2014;**16**(3):230–40.

111. Severance EG, Gressitt KL, Stallings CR, Origoni AE, Khushalani S, Leweke FM, et al. Discordant patterns of bacterial translocation markers and implications for innate immune imbalances in schizophrenia. *Schizophr Res* 2013;**148**(1-3):130–7.

112. Samaroo D, Dickerson F, Kasarda DD, Green PH, Briani C, Yolken RH, et al. Novel immune response to gluten in individuals with schizophrenia. *Schizophr Res* 2010;**118**(1-3):248–55.

113. Feigenson KA, Kusnecov AW, Silverstein SM. Inflammation and the two-hit hypothesis of schizophrenia. *Neurosci Biobehav Rev* 2014;**38**:72–93.

114. Debnath M, Venkatasubramanian G, Berk M. Fetal programming of schizophrenia: select mechanisms. *Neurosci Biobehav Rev* 2015;**49**:90–104.

115. Reisinger S, Khan D, Kong E, Berger A, Pollak A, Pollak DD. The Poly(I:C)-induced maternal immune activation model in preclinical neuropsychiatric drug discovery. *Pharmacol Ther* 2015;**149**:213–26.

116. Girgis RR, Kumar SS, Brown AS. The cytokine model of schizophrenia: emerging therapeutic strategies. *Biol Psychiatry* 2014;**75**(4):292–9.

117. Rajasekaran A, Venkatasubramanian G, Berk M, Debnath M. Mitochondrial dysfunction in schizophrenia: pathways, mechanisms and implications. *Neurosci Biobehav Rev* 2015;**48**:10–21.

118. Mäntylä T, Mantere O, Raij TT, Kieseppä T, Laitinen H, Leiviskä J, Torniainen M, Tuominen L, Vaarala O, Suvisaari J. Altered activation of innate immunity associates with white matter volume and diffusion in first-episode psychosis. *PLoS One* 2015;**10**(5):e0125112.

119. Vancampfort D, Wampers M, Mitchell AJ, Correll CU, De Herdt A, Probst M, et al. A meta-analysis of cardio-metabolic abnormalities in drug naïve, first-episode and multi-episode patients with schizophrenia versus general population controls. *World Psychiatry* 2013;**12**(3):240–50.

120. Després JP, Lemieux I. Abdominal obesity and metabolic syndrome. *Nature* 2006;**444**(7121):881–7.

121. Beumer W, Drexhage RC, De Wit H, Versnel MA, Drexhage HA, Cohen D. Increased level of serum cytokines, chemokines and adipokines in patients with schizophrenia is associated with disease and metabolic syndrome. *Psychoneuroendocrinology* 2012;**37**(12):1901–11.

122. Foley DL, Morley KI. Systematic review of early cardiometabolic outcomes of the first treated episode of psychosis. *Arch Gen Psychiatry* 2011;**68**(6):609–16.

123. Shiels MS, Katki HA, Freedman ND, Purdue MP, Wentzensen N, Trabert B, et al. Cigarette smoking and variations in systemic immune and inflammation markers. *J Natl Cancer Inst* 2014;**106**(11):1–8.

124. Afshar M, Richards S, Mann D, Cross A, Smith GB, Netzer G, et al. Acute immunomodulatory effects of binge alcohol ingestion. *Alcohol* 2015;**49**(1):57–64.

125. Dias JA, Wirfält E, Drake I, Gullberg B, Hedblad B, Persson M, et al. A high quality diet is associated with reduced systemic inflammation in middle-aged individuals. *Atherosclerosis* 2015;**238**(1):38–44.

126. Rubin DA, Hackney AC. Inflammatory cytokines and metabolic risk factors during growth and maturation: influence of physical activity. *Med Sport Sci* 2010;**55**:43–55.

127. Axelsson J, Rehman JU, Akerstedt T, Ekman R, Miller GE, Höglund CO, et al. Effects of sustained sleep restriction on mitogen-stimulated cytokines, chemokines and T helper 1/ T helper 2 balance in humans. *PLoS One* 2013;**8**(12):e82291.

128. Packard CJ, Bezlyak V, McLean JS, Batty GD, Ford I, Burns H, et al. Early life socioeconomic adversity is associated in adult life with chronic inflammation, carotid atherosclerosis, poorer lung function and decreased cognitive performance: a cross-sectional, population-based study. *BMC Public Health* 2011;**11**:42.

129. Friedman EM, Herd P. Income, education, and inflammation: differential associations in a national probability sample (The MIDUS study). *Psychosom Med* 2010;**72**: 290–300.

130. Suvisaari J, Loo BM, Saarni SE, Haukka J, Perälä J, Saarni SI, Viertiö S, Partti K, Lönnqvist J, Jula A. Inflammation in psychotic disorders: a population-based study. *Psychiatry Res* 2011;**189**(2):305–11.

131. Chen ML, Tsai TC, Wang LK, Lin YY, Tsai YM, Lee MC, Tsai FM. Risperidone modulates the cytokine and chemokine release of dendritic cells and induces TNF-α-directed cell apoptosis in neutrophils. *Int Immunopharmacol* 2012;**12**(1):197–204.

132. Chen ML, Tsai TC, Wang LK, Lin YY, Tsai YM, Lee MC, Tsai FM. Clozapine inhibits Th1 cell differentiation and causes the suppression of IFN-γ production in peripheral blood mononuclear cells. *Immunopharmacol Immunotoxicol* 2012;**34**(4):686–94.

133. Walker FR. A critical review of the mechanism of action for the selective serotonin reuptake inhibitors: do these drugs possess anti-inflammatory properties and how relevant is this in the treatment of depression? *Neuropharmacology* 2013;**67**:304–17.

134. Morgan AP, Crowley JJ, Nonneman RJ, Quackenbush CR, Miller CN, Ryan AK, Bogue MA, Paredes SH, Yourstone S, Carroll IM, Kawula TH, Bower MA, Sartor RB, Sullivan PF. The antipsychotic olanzapine interacts with the gut microbiome to cause weight gain in mouse. *PLoS One* 2014;**9**(12):e115225.

135. Orešič M, Seppänen-Laakso T, Sun D, Tang J, Therman S, Viehman R, Mustonen U, van Erp TG, Hyötyläinen T, Thompson P, Toga AW, Huttunen MO, Suvisaari J, Kaprio J, Lönnqvist J, Cannon TD. Phospholipids and insulin resistance in psychosis: a lipidomics study of twin pairs discordant for schizophrenia. *Genome Med* 2012;**4**(1):1.

136. Sommer IE, Van Westrhenen R, Begemann MJ, de Witte LD, Leucht S, Kahn RS. Efficacy of anti-inflammatory agents to improve symptoms in patients with schizophrenia: an update. *Schizophr Bull* 2014;**40**(1):181–91.

137. Suvisaari J, Mantere O. Inflammation theories in psychotic disorders: a critical review. *Infect Disord Drug Targets* 2013;**13**(1):59–70.

138. Amminger GP, Schäfer MR, Papageorgiou K, Klier CM, Cotton SM, Harrigan SM, et al. Long-chain omega-3 fatty acids for indicated prevention of psychotic disorders: a randomized, placebo-controlled trial. *Arch Gen Psychiatry* 2010;**67**(2):146–54.

139. Bentsen H, Osnes K, Refsum H, Solberg DK, Bøhmer T. A randomized placebo-controlled trial of an omega-3 fatty acid and vitamins E+C in schizophrenia. *Transl Psychiatry* 2013;**3**:e335.

140. Shlögelhofer M, Amminger GP, Schaefer MR, Fusar-Poli P, Smesny S, McGorry P, Berger G, Mossaheb N. Polyunsaturated fatty acids in emerging psychosis: a safer alternative? *Early Interv Psychiatry* 2014;**8**(3):199–208.

141. Ayorech Z, Tracy DK, Baumeister D, Giaroli G. Taking the fuel out of the fire: evidence for the use of anti-inflammatory agents in the treatment of bipolar disorders. *J Affect Disord* 2015;**174C**:467–78.

142. Laan W, Grobbee DE, Selten JP, Heijnen CJ, Kahn RS, Burger H. Adjuvant aspirin therapy reduces symptoms of schizophrenia spectrum disorders: results from a randomized, double-blind, placebo-controlled trial. *J Clin Psychiatry* 2010;**71**(5):520–7.

143. Amminger GP, Mechelli A, Rice S, Kim SW, Klier CM, McNamara RK, Berk M, McGorry PD, Schäfer MR. Predictors of treatment response in young people at ultra-high risk for psychosis who received long-chain omega-3 fatty acids. *Transl Psychiatry* 2015;**5**:e495.

144. Rowlands D, Sugahara K, Kwok JC. Glycosaminoglycans and glycomimetics in the central nervous system. *Molecules* 2015;**20**(3):3527–48.

145. Fiebich BL, Akter S, Akundi RS. The two-hit hypothesis for neuroinflammation: role of exogenous ATP in modulating inflammation in the brain. *Front Cell Neurosci* 2014;**8**:260.

Chapter 8

Modulation of the Interferon Response by Environmental, Noninfectious Stressors

Elisabetta Razzuoli,* Cinzia Zanotti,** Massimo Amadori**

*Laboratory of Diagnostics, S.S. Genova, Istituto Zooprofilattico Sperimentale del Piemonte, Liguria e Valle d'Aosta, Piazza Borgo Pila, Genova, Italy; **Laboratory of Cellular Immunology, Istituto Zooprofilattico Sperimentale della Lombardia e dell'Emilia-Romagna, Brescia, Italy

INTRODUCTION

Interferons (IFNs) are a class of proteins synthesized and secreted by most cell types that elicit pleiotropic biological effects. They are named after the ability to interfere with viral infections of animal cells. Yet, after the serendipitous discovery of their antiviral activity,[1] IFNs were shown to exert a plethora of regulatory, and effector biological functions. Thus, IFNs can affect cell proliferation, differentiation, and also play a pivotal role in the innate immune system and in the regulation of the adaptive immune response.[2] IFNs can modulate the balance between pro- and antiinflammatory mediators secreted by T lymphocytes and antigen-presenting cells, which may be associated with detrimental or beneficial effects for the host.[3] To date, three distinct categories of IFN molecules are known, that is, types I, II, and III IFNs. As for type I IFNs, a major role in the homeostatic control of the inflammatory response has been clearly demonstrated, as well.[2]

Type I IFNs include different families: IFN-α, IFN-β, IFN-ω, IFN-κ, IFN-ε, IFN-τ, IFN-ζ, and IFN-δ.[4] IFN-α represents a multigene family coding for different proteins, named subtypes.[5] In this respect, human, porcine, and mice IFN-α systems consist of a multigene family with 30, 17, and 14 intronless, functional genes, respectively.[6-8] In humans, the IFN-α gene family is located on the short arm of chromosome 9, consisting of 13 functional genes and 1 pseudogene; differently, this gene family is located in mice on chromosome 4, including 14 functional IFN-α genes and 3 pseudogenes.[9,10] The porcine IFN-α gene cluster is located in chromosome 1;[11] this gene family shares 96–99.8%

and 91.1–100% homology at the nucleotide and amino acid level, respectively;[5] yet, different IFNs-α show profound differences in their biological effects.[12]

Concerning type II IFN, there is one molecular species only (IFN-γ), produced by T lymphocytes and natural killer (NK) cells; this IFN family is located on the long arm of chromosome 12 in humans and on chromosome 10 in mice.[13] The expression and release of this protein is mediated by T helper (Th) 1 cytokines like IL-12 and it is crucial for the control of intracellular pathogens (viruses and intracellular bacteria) and tumors.

Regarding type III IFNs, these include three molecular species: IFNs λ1, λ2, and λ3, also named interleukin (IL)-29, IL-28A, and IL-28B, respectively, showing similar biological properties.[14] At the amino acid level IFN-λ2 and IFN-λ3 are highly similar with 96% of sequence identity, while IFN-λ1 shares approximately 81% of sequence identity with IFN-λ2 and IFN-λ3.[15] Phylogenetically, type III IFNs are closely related to type I IFN and IL-10 gene families,[14] showing at the amino acid level 15–19% homology with type I IFNs and 11–13% homology with IL-10. This shows that type III IFNs are more closely related to type I IFNs than IL-10,[15] and probably represent the ancestral IFN molecule that resulted into intronless type I IFNs.[4]

The biological effects of IFNs are mediated through IFN-regulated genes. Three major IFN-regulated pathways involving RNA-dependent protein kinase (PKR)/the eukaryotic initiation factor (eIF)-2a system, 2-5A synthetase/RNase L system, and Janus kinase (JAK)/signal transducer and activator of transcription (STAT) system have been identified. The PKR/eIF2a system mainly mediates type I IFN effector functions, and the protein synthesis factor eIF-2a works as target of PKR-induced effects in this pathway.[16]

The effects of IFNs are exerted after binding to specific receptors (Fig. 8.1). The type I IFN receptor (IFNAR I) belongs to the class II family of cytokine receptors and consists of two chains of transmembrane·glycoproteins, named IFNAR1 and IFNAR2, respectively;[17] the IFN-λ receptor system is composed of IL-10 receptor-β and IL-28 receptor-α. The IFN-γ receptor, consisting of the IFNγR1 and IFNγR2 subunits, is structurally and functionally different from the types I and III receptors.[18]

BIOLOGICAL FUNCTIONS

The IFN system plays a pivotal role in the innate immune system and in the regulation of the adaptive immune response. Also, recent evidence accumulated in farm animals, humans, and mice points at type I IFN as a crucial homeostatic system, aimed at avoiding unnecessary tissue damage and waste of food energy as a result of a dysregulated inflammatory response.[2] On the whole, there is strong evidence that IFN responses are displayed by the host toward successful adaptation to infectious and noninfectious stressors. As such, the IFN system is constantly operated through mechanisms of constitutive gene expression and possible low-grade protein release.[19] In this conceptual framework, constitutive

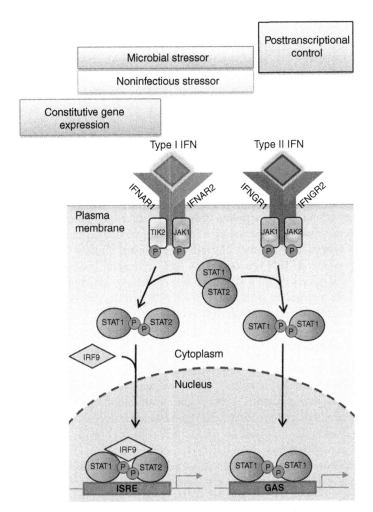

FIGURE 8.1 Activation of classic JAK–STAT pathways by interferons in response to different stimuli. IFNAR I and II, the two subunits of type I IFN receptor; JAKs, Janus activated kinases; TYK2, tyrosine kinase 2; IFNGR1 and IFNGR2, the two subunits of IFN-γ receptor; STAT 1 and 2, signal transducer and activator of transcription 1 and 2; IRF9, IFN-regulatory factor 9; ISREs, IFN-stimulated response elements; GAS, IFN-γ activated site.

production of IFN-α can be recognized in human and porcine PBMC, and protein can be either released or maintained in intracellular stores.[20,21] An overt IFN response with moderate to large protein release takes place through peculiar mechanisms after exposure to infectious and noninfectious stressors.[22] The same biological functions were not shown by type III IFNs; their functions could be partly distinct from type I IFNs because of the low-level tissue expression of the type III receptor complexes.

These findings outline a major role of type I IFNs in the process of environmental adaptation, which prompted us to analyze in this review the expression of IFNs following exposure to noninfectious stressors as diverse as weaning, transportation, pregnancy, toxins, and cancer cells.

CONSTITUTIVE EXPRESSION

The IFN system has been progressively reappraised as a fundamental physiological regulator associated with crucial homeostatic functions for the host's survival. As such, a few members of the aforementioned IFN families show low-grade constitutive expression in tissues as gene and protein in healthy subjects, not exposed to detectable, infectious or noninfectious stressors. In particular, strong evidence points at the constitutive expression of type I IFNs in different organs and tissues as a foundation of homeostatic control in the immune system, and in other physiological control circuits. The first reports about spontaneous IFN production by leukocytes and bone marrow cells of healthy individuals date back to the 1960s.[23,24] Later on, a physiological role of IFNs was postulated in the early 1980s by Velio Bocci[25] on the basis of the antiviral activity detected in uninfected tissue extracts. As indicated in a recent review,[26] IFN-β plays the most important role in constitutive expression, which has at least four aims:

1. Maintenance of hematopoietic stem cells.
2. Sustaining crucial immune cell functions: myeloid cell function and macrophage homeostasis, survival and proliferation of CD8+ blasts, maintenance of NK cell functions, and maintenance of IFNγ-dependent antiviral responses.
3. Bone remodeling.
4. General maintenance of homeostasis and priming of cells for rapid, robust, innate, and adaptive immune responses.

In particular, constitutive expression of IFN-β is induced by a peculiar occupancy profile of the positive regulatory domains of the IFN-β promoter by AP-1 and NF-κB components, which differs from acutely induced IFN expression.[26] In addition to that, IFN-β is also an immediate early IFN protein as a result of primary, IRF 3-driven stimulation, its expression being conducive to a further, wider boost of type I IFN responses.[27] The low basal expression level of type I IFNs results in weak signaling and intracellular tyrosine phosphorylation of IFNAR-1, the type I IFN receptor α-chain. The signal does not elicit the signaling cascade that leads to transcriptional activation of IFN-response genes.[28]

Strong evidence of constitutive expression has been accumulated for IFN-α in humans,[21] mice,[10] and pigs.[20–29] The evidence accumulated so far in the pig model indicates that constitutive expression can vary in terms of intensity and panel of involved IFN-α subtypes, in the framework of a constant expression of the IFN-β gene.[29] In this scenario, direct and circumstantial evidence points at an important role of IFN-α at vanishingly low concentrations in the fine tuning and control of the inflammatory responses in tissues.[2-30] Tissue concentrations are of paramount importance. The proinflammatory effector functions of high titered IFN-α are exerted in the framework of innate immune responses to microbial stressors. However, the low tissue concentrations of IFN-α (≤ 10 U/mL) in the late phases of microbial infections and under healthy conditions underlie a major shift to a potent anti-inflammatory activity, based on transcriptional and post-transcriptional control of genes coding for inflammatory cytokines, pathogen-associated molecular pattern (PAMP) receptors (e.g., CD14) and, possibly, other undetected structures.[2] This kind of regulation can be reproduced by second messengers released by lymphoid cells stimulated with very low concentrations of IFN-α, as shown in several models of low dose, oral, IFN-α treatment.[31] Most important, this assumption is in agreement with the very potent anti-inflammatory control actions exerted *in vitro* by IFN α-treated tonsil cells.[32] These activities mainly consist of a post-transcriptional regulation of inflammatory cytokines through different, nonmutually exclusive, dose-dependent pathways: mRNA stability control by tristetraprolin induction,[33] TAM receptor-mediated activation of SOCS proteins through IFNAR I signaling,[34] and downregulation of CD14 expression.[35] As expected, inability to produce IFN-α is associated with recurrent inflammatory disorders, such as chronic vestibular inflammation in women,[36] allergic asthma in children,[37] and chronic idiopathic urticaria.[38] In addition to these regulatory functions, there is also evidence that constitutively produced IFNs α/β play a preventive role in cellular transformation. The weak signal generated by these IFNs can prevent cells from transforming by hitherto-unknown pathway(s) downstream of type I IFN receptor.[19]

The aforementioned findings stress the importance of IFNs in diverse homeostatic control circuits in the host. These crucial functions imply a fine-tuning and adjustment of IFN responses following exposure to diverse environmental stimuli. Such a fine regulation is afforded by a continuous adjustment of minute gene and protein expression levels and, most importantly, by the heterogeneity of IFN families. In this respect, 16 porcine IFN-α genes expressed in mammalian cells were shown to exert significantly different antiviral, anti-inflammatory, and immunoregulatory control actions at low, autocrine/paracrine concentrations, despite limited nucleotide and amino acid divergence (C. Zanotti and M. Amadori, unpublished results). This finding underlies in the authors' opinion powerful coping responses of the host, based on continuously changing ratios among IFN-α subtypes and expression levels. Poor and/or defective regulation of these steady-state responses underlies a risk factor for the development of the aforementioned disease types.

Constitutive IFN gene expression coexists with a subsequent profile of expression induced by infectious and noninfectious stressors. This concept is of paramount importance. IFN-inducing, infectious or noninfectious stressors exert their effects in the host in the presence of an ongoing type I IFN response. In the case of IFN-α, the previous levels of IFN-α gene expression are substantially unaffected by, for example, a viral agent *in vitro*[22] and *in vivo*,[39] the difference being the production and release of IFN-α proteins at detectable levels.[22] Therefore, IFN protein expression might be the possible result of side signals leading to a higher stability of mRNAs following removal of inhibitors at their 3' untranslated regions (3' UTR). In particular, as in other cytokine gene models, AU-rich (ARE) sequences in the three' untranslated region of IFN mRNAs are probably a key target of post-transcriptional control actions,[40] and several models of gene expression support this tenet.

On the basis of the aforementioned concepts, the noninfectious stressors dealt with in this chapter should be viewed as elements modifying the profile of an ongoing IFN-α response in terms of protein expression and/or inducing *de novo* expression of further IFN families and/or types.

STRESS, TISSUE DAMAGE, AND IFN RESPONSES

Noninfectious stressors often cause inflammatory responses and tissue damage, which may be associated with detectable IFN responses. Such responses to tissue damages can be accounted for by damage-associated molecular patterns (DAMPs), released by damaged tissues, and including ATP, the cytokine IL-1β, uric acid, the calcium-binding, cytoplasmic proteins S100A8 and S100A9, and the DNA-binding, nuclear protein HMGB1.[41] DAMPs can signal through pattern-recognition receptors like toll-like receptors (TLRs).[42] It should be stressed that TLR ligands can induce the expression of all IFN-α, -β, and -λ (Type III) subtypes in plasmacytoid dendritic cells, whereas TLR-4 or TLR-3 stimulations induce only IFN-β and IFN-λ gene expression in monocyte-derived DC.[43] Interestingly, the inflammasome reaction triggered by DAMPs[41] generates IL-1β and IL-18, which can also sustain type I IFN responses.[22] In particular, a robust induction of IL-1β and IL-18 is caused by ATP through the P2X-7 receptor.[44] In this respect, IL-1β and IL-18 represent a common, final outcome of both microbial and nonmicrobial stresses involved in the generation of innate immune responses in tissues. As such, it could prove to be a unifying conceptual key of infectious and noninfectious stressors with respect to IFN responses. In addition to that, IL-18 in association with IL-12 (Th1 environment) is a very potent inducer of IFN-γ,[45] which sets another rational link between tissue damage, inflammation, and IFN responses. Another important link is the expression of stress antigens (MIC A and B, ULBP 1–3) in diverse cell types after exposure to infectious and noninfectious stressors. These antigens are recognized by $\gamma\delta$ T and NK cells in the framework of the "lymphoid stress surveillance response," that is, the network of lymphocyte populations, which recognize neoantigens like MIC on stressed cells,[7] exposed to events as diverse as heat shock, infections, DNA damage, and so on. Stress proteins are ligands for activating cell receptor NKG2D, expressed on NK cells, CD8+ αβ T cells, and γδ T cells. NKG2D ligands can give rise to IFN-γ responses,[46] being thus another fundamental link between tissue damage-related stress and IFN responses.

As already shown for microbial infections,[47] moderate IFN responses are likely to exert a favorable influence after exposure to noninfectious stressors, while the excessive ones may contribute to immunopathology. Interestingly, the expression of antiviral IFN stimulated genes (ISGs) is highly sensitive to IFN induction, whereas potentially dangerous ISGs (IL-6, CXCL11, and TRAIL) require 100-fold higher IFN concentrations.[47]

HUMAN MODELS

The occurrence of IFN responses to noninfectious stressors in humans has been reported for a long time. Thus, over 30 years ago, IFN responses were reported *in vivo* in models of human autoimmune disease like systemic lupus erythematosus, vasculitis, rheumatoid arthritis, scleroderma, and Sjogren's syndrome, often with a positive correlation between IFN response and disease activity.[48] In the same years, human B-lymphoblastoid cell lines were shown to produce IFN-α constitutively and IFN-γ after heat shock.[49] These early findings were later confirmed on PBMC of human blood donors; an IFN-γ response was observed at 39–41°C, which was inhibited by antibodies to MHC class II; this response was accompanied by enhanced proliferation of PBMC and an increased immunoglobulin production.[50] On the whole, these early data provided evidence that the IFN system could be activated also in humans by diverse noninfectious stressors and sometimes contribute to pathogenesis and disease progression.

After these early reports, other noninfectious stimuli were shown to induce diverse IFN responses, and the molecular basis of such responses was partly clarified. Among noninfectious stimuli, even fundamental physiological control mechanisms were shown to induce IFN responses. Thus, there is evidence that humans can mount antibody responses to their self IFN proteins.[51] Interestingly, such neutralizing antibodies to IFNs can cause an IFN response in human cells. This implies the activation of the transcription factor ISGF3 and the expression of IFN responsive genes.[28] The stimulatory capacity of anti-IFN-α/β antibodies was related to autocrine production of very low IFN levels, involved the type I IFN receptor, and was dependent on the Fc antibody domain.[28] These findings underlie the crucial importance of an effective, steady-state control of IFN responses by the host. The host's control strategy dictates the need for an antibody response to self IFN molecules, as previously shown in sera of human patients after viral infections, showing detectable levels of anti-IFN-γ antibodies.[52] Interestingly, low titered antibodies to IFN-γ can be also revealed in sera of healthy, uninfected subjects. These antibodies can inhibit the expression of HLA-DR antigens induced by IFN-γ, and interfere with the proliferation of lymphocytes and the generation of cytotoxic lymphocytes.[52] Apart from the serious problems posed to IFN-based therapies,[51] this kind of regulation is not surprising if one considers that natural or therapy-induced antibodies to interleukin (IL)-1, IL-2, IL-6, IL-10, granulocyte colony-stimulating factor, granulocyte–macrophage colony-stimulating factor, insulin, and recombinant factor VIII have been also reported in humans.[53] In this conceptual framework, Ab to IFNs are instrumental in controlling inflammation and tissue damage associated with high titered cytokine responses. At the same time, they can promote low titered autocrine and paracrine IFN responses probably contributing to the same control actions.

IFN responses to tissue damage can be observed in humans experiencing chronic degenerative diseases. Thus, intermittent interferonemia can be demonstrated in patients with multiple sclerosis (MS), often showing expression of IFN-α genes in brain and nonbrain tissues. Interestingly, such an expression was also detected in the same study in patients with other neural diseases, and patients with other illnesses.[54]

As for autoimmune diseases, an involvement of IFN in active Lupus patients has been known since 1979.[55] The reasons underlying IFN responses (a mixture of IFN-α subtypes or IFN-α and IFN-γ) and their role in the pathogenesis of the disease were extensively investigated in the following years. It was thus recognized that IFN-α responses are caused in these patients by apoptotic blebs incorporating nucleosomes, containing nucleic acids and other endogenous danger ligands. Therefore, such a response is associated with increased production, defective handling, and presentation of autoantigens during apoptosis. Unabated activation of DCs by IFN-α sustains the presentation of autoantigens and the production of relevant Ab.[56] As in the case of antibodies to self IFNs, an apparently harmless biological function (sensing endogenous nucleic acids during apoptosis) can turn into a dangerous inducer of dysregulated IFN responses, leading to serious clinical consequences for the host. Thus, IFN-α should be regarded as a double-edged sword. On the one hand abnormal responses in tissues can be associated with serious diseases. On the other hand, the same IFN molecules under different conditions (concentrations, subtype mixture, timing, and tissue compartment) can exert opposite, therapeutic effects. Thus, as reported in a previous review paper of ours,[2] oral, low dose IFN-α treatment proved effective in patients having active Sjogren's syndrome, that is, an autoimmune disease characterized by inflammation of the exocrine glands and secretory failure. This is the outcome of a dysregulated activation of the type I IFN system in plasmacytoid dendritic cells after exposure to RNA-containing immune complexes. Likewise, parenteral high dose IFN-α treatments exert proinflammatory control actions, which may coexist with opposite effects in the digestive tract of patients with ulcerative colitis and Crohn's disease.[2] Most important, a dysregulated type I IFN response in tissues can undermine fundamental regulatory circuits of innate immunity in macrophages, which turns IL-10 into a potent proinflammatory cytokine.[57] IL-10 and IFN-γ-associated responses may thus cause a gain of proinflammatory activity, as shown in human models of endotoxemia.[58]

ANIMAL MODELS

Weaning Stress

Weaning is a physiological event in mammals, which occurs when dam milk production is progressively reduced and the cub is able to find and utilize feed on its own. It is a stepwise process, whereby cubs get access to solid food during lactation, and gradually decrease suckling as a function of increasing age and feed availability.[59] On the contrary, weaning is usually a very stressful event for farmed piglets, which experience at 20–28 days of life a sudden separation from the sow, mixing with other litters, end of lactation immunity, a novel environment, and change of feed and gut microbiota with an alteration of intestinal barrier functions.[60] Moreover, changing the feeding regime at weaning causes histological and morphological changes in the intestine, which are detrimental to an immature digestive system. In this phase, the main metabolic responses are characterized as diet–dependent and diet–independent; in particular, McCracken et al.[61] demonstrated that major metabolic and immunological responses, that is, decreased plasma glucose, increased plasma glucagon, fibrinogen, and interleukin (IL)-1, were diet independent. In this scenario, a lot of scientific contributions highlighted an inflammatory response to the early weaning (EW) stress in pigs, characterized by increased serum level of IL-6 and TNF-α.[62,63] Moreover, Hu et al.[63] demonstrated that EW determines also an increased IFN-γ gene expression ($P < 0.05$) until day 7 after weaning, which is associated with alterations of the intestinal barrier and decreased expression of tight junction proteins.[64] This inflammatory response induces in turn a low titered IFN-α response in piglets at day 6 after weaning, which probably checks IFN-γ and other proinflammatory cytokines.[65] This assumption was confirmed in trials of oral, low dose IFN-α treatment of piglets at weaning.[62–65] The potent anti-inflammatory control actions of IFN α-treated pig tonsil lymphocytes[32] can account for these *in vivo* results.

In calves, weaning causes an immediate and short lived acute stress response modulated by gender and proximity of the dam; in particular, O'Loughlin et al.[66] demonstrated a significant increase of IFN-γ and TNF-α gene expression related to an interaction between gender and time ($P < 0.05$). IFN-γ increased over threefold ($P < 0.001$) in all calves at day 1 after weaning and remained elevated ($P < 0.01$) until day 7. Moreover, the expression of this cytokine was significantly greater ($P < 0.001$) in female, compared with male calves. Weaning can alter the homeostasis of leukocytes for at least 7 days, indicating long-term effects in cattle. Also in cattle, EW gives rise to greater serum IFN-γ concentration.[67]

Transportation Stress

Transportation represents a critical phase in the life of farm animals; it is one of the major causes of stress and may lead to negative repercussions in terms of animal health and welfare. Some factors like fatigue, handling and mixing of animals, duration of transport, stocking density, and ventilation may contribute to stress, which may be expressed by specific physiological changes.[68] This stress causes a modulation of IFN responses; in particular, transportation significantly reduces ($P < 0.05$) IFN-γ production in bulls[69] and gives rise to a low titered IFN-α response after a long distance journey (M. Amadori and E. Razzuoli, unpublished results, Fig. 8.2). The same effects on type I IFNs were observed in bulls after a short (4 h) transportation stress.[70] A type I IFN response was also shown in serum samples of healthy piglets after transportation to the fattening farms (M. Amadori and E. Razzuoli, unpublished results), in agreement with the results of a previous study.[71]

Exposure to Mycotoxins

The main biological and toxicological features of mycotoxins are illustrated in the preface to this book. The reader is referred to this introductory section for an overview of mycotoxins and their impact on humans and animals. Deoxynivalenol (DON), fumonisins (FB), and T-2 toxin are mycotoxins produced by *Fusarium* species. The gastrointestinal tract represents the first target of contaminated food/feed compounds, which also affects the immune system. In particular, the T-2 toxin affects the established levels of cytokine gene expression in porcine ileal Peyer's patches. After 42 days of exposure to T-2 (200 μg T-2 toxin kg^{-1} feed), a gradual decrease was observed in the amount of IFN-γ cytokine transcripts in the study of Obremski et al.[73] Pinton et al.[74] reported a downregulation of IFN-γ in spleen and lymph nodes of pigs fed DON (2.2–2.5 mg DON/kg

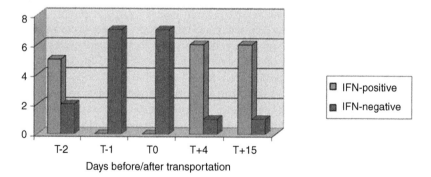

FIGURE 8.2 **IFN-α was measured in sera of calves transported from Poland to Italy by a virus inhibition assay on MDBK cells.** The y axis indicates the number of calves under study. T-2: samples collected in the Polish farm 2 days before transportation to Italy. T-1: samples collected in the Polish transit center after commingling calves from different farms on the day before transportation. T-0: arrival day in Italy. +4: 4 days after arrival. +15: 15 days after arrival. The transport conditions were described in a previous paper. *(Adapted from Ref. [72].)*

feed) for 9 weeks. The same effect was shown in the gut of broilers[75] after 5 weeks of exposure to a diet contaminated with DON (10 mg DON/kg feed). Zearalenone is a mycotoxin produced by *Fusarium* species, which can be present in feed associated with other mycotoxins or alone. The reproductive tract is the main target of this compound and its metabolites, but toxic effects are also exerted on the immune system. Chen et al.[76] evaluated the effects of diet supplementation with 1 mg DON/Kg and 250 μg ZON/Kg on 24 weaning piglets. The results showed that DON and ZON have a strong effect on pigs. Indeed, DON and ZON caused a significant ($P < 0.05$) decrease of type II IFN levels. On the contrary, DON caused an increase of serum levels of IFN-γ in mice.[77,78] Among the various mycotoxins, aflatoxin B1 (AFB1) also causes immunosuppression in domestic animals (pigs, poultry, and ruminants) and humans.[79] In a 1-day-old male broilers fed a diet supplemented with AFB1 (0.3 mg/kg AFB1) for 21 days, there was a decrease of serum levels of IFN-γ.[80] On the whole, there is strong evidence that mycotoxins induce a proinflammatory environment that causes a modulation of the IFN system.

Pregnancy

During pregnancy, maternal recognition of the conceptus results from signals exchanged between membranes associated with the embryo (trophoblast) and the mother's immune system. Some studies suggest that an important signal is generated by the IFN system,[81] which could be involved in the maintenance of structural and functional integrity of the corpus luteum (CL). Type I and/or type II IFNs are conducive to fetal implant in the mammalian uterus. In 1993, Imakawa et al.[82] determined the amino acid sequence of sheep's trophoblastin and stressed a close correlation with an IFN-α sequence and the ability to bind to the same receptor. Today this protein is known as IFN-tau (IFN-τ);[83] this compound is detectable in sheep between day 10 and 21 postinsemination, and acts as a paracrine antiluteolytic hormone on the endometrium. In particular, it causes inhibition of prostaglandin secretion and downregulation of estrogen receptor (ER) expression.[84] Albeit inessential for maternal recognition of pregnancy in primates, IFNs play a central role in these species; indeed, human placenta constitutively express IFN-α and can release IFN-β in response to virus infection. *In vitro* studies demonstrated a toxic effect of type II IFN on human trophoblast cells; moreover, high levels of proinflammatory cytokines (IL-2, TNF-α, and IFN-γ) are associated with recurrent miscarriage;[85] the same results were obtained in a murine model of pregnancy where Th1 cytokines (in particular IFN-γ) were associated with unsuccessful pregnancies. On the contrary, IFN-γ is important in pig in the maintenance of pregnancy. Indeed, trophectoderm and uterus epithelial cells interact through endocrine, paracrine, and autocrine pathways to allow for implant of the conceptus. The latter releases estrogens and IFNs.[86] In particular, between day 13 and 20 of pregnancy trophectoderm secretes IFN-γ, and IFN-δ is detectable at day 14.[87]

The role of these IFNs at embryonic level is not well understood. Some studies suggest a possible role in the modulation of the endometrium as support to implantation and development of functional placenta. There is no evidence of antiluteinic action. Yet, IFNs can induce PGE2 secretion and ISGs gene expression in the uterus lumen. Another type I IFN associated with the reproductive system is IFN-ε. Hermant et al.[88] highlighted an unusual expression pattern and restriction in the secretion of this member of the type I IFN group. As this IFN is constitutively expressed in cells of the female and male reproductive tracts, IFN-ε secretion might be regulated by a specific factor expressed in these cells. In humans, IFN-ε was identified in 1999. IFN-ε has been reported later on in other species (mice, pigs, and cattle), and recent studies demonstrated that seminal plasma can upregulate its expression in cervico-vaginal tissues. Therefore, IFN-ε may be involved in reproductive functions, in terms of either viral protection or early placental development in mammals.[89] On the whole, these findings outline the pivotal role of the IFN system in reproductive physiology.

CONCLUSIONS

The innate immune system can rapidly react to infectious and noninfectious stressors by exerting diverse effector and regulatory functions. In this scenario, the constitutive expression of some IFNs is involved in steady state physiological functions, and it is conducive to prompt and powerful reactions to infectious and noninfectious *noxae*. At the same time, the IFN system can keep safe fundamental control circuits of the inflammatory response. By a "gas and brake" adaptation strategy, IFNs can adjust regulatory actions toward either increased inflammatory and immune responses, or prevention of tissue damage. In a "one health" scenario,[90] the discovery of the fine regulatory mechanisms exerted by diverse IFNs will open new opportunities for successful prophylactic and therapeutic treatments, as well as for the definition of disease predicting and prognostic parameters in human and veterinary medicine.

REFERENCES

1. Isaacs A, Lindenman J. Virus interference. I. The interferon. *Proc R Soc London B* 1957;**147**:258–67.
2. Amadori M. The role of IFN-α as homeostatic agent in the inflammatory response: a balance between danger and response? *J Interferon Cytokine Res* 2007;**27**:181–9.
3. Touzot M, Grandclaudon M, Cappuccio A, Satoh T, Martinez-Cingolani C, Servant N, Manel N, Soumelis V. Combinatorial flexibility of cytokine function during human T helper cell differentiation. *Nat Commun* 2014;**28**(5):3987.
4. Uzé G, Monneron D. IL-28 and IL-29: newcomers to the interferon family. *Biochimie* 2007;**89**(6–7):729–34.
5. Cheng G, Chen W, Li Z, Yan W, Zhao X, Xie J, Liu M, Zhang H, Zhong Y, Zheng Z. Characterization of the porcine alpha interferon multigene family. *Gene* 2006;**382**:28–38.

6. Díaz MO, Pomykala HM, Bohlander SK, Maltepe E, Malik K, Brownstein B, Olopade OI. Structure of the human type-I interferon gene cluster determined from a YAC clone contig. *Genomics* 1994;**22**:540–52.

7. Hayday AC. γδ T cells and the lymphoid stress-surveillance response. *Immunity* 2009;**31**:184–96.

8. Sang Y, Rowland RR, Hesse RA, Blecha F. Differential expression and activity of the porcine type I interferon family. *Physiol Genomics* 2010;**42**:248–58.

9. Kelley KA, Kozak CA, Dandoy F, Sor F, Skup D, Windass JD, DeMaeyer-Guignard J, Pitha PM, DeMaeyer E. Mapping of murine interferon-alpha genes to chromosome 4. *Gene* 1983;**26**:181–8.

10. Van Pesch V, Michiels T. Characterization of interferon-α 13, a novel constitutive murine interferon-α subtype. *J Biol Chem* 2003;**47**:46321–8.

11. Yerle M, Gellin J, Echard G, Lefevre F, Gillois M. Chromosomal localization of leukocyte interferon gene in the pig (*Sus scrofa domestica* L.) by *in situ* hybridization. *Cytogenet Cell Genet* 1986;**42**:129–32.

12. Razzuoli E, Villa R, Amadori M. IPEC-J2 cells as reporter system of the anti-inflammatory control actions of interferon-α. *J Interferon Cytokine Res* 2013;**10**:597–605.

13. Schoenborn JR, Wilson CB. Regulation of interferon-γ during innate and adaptive immune responses. *Adv Immunol* 2007;**96**:41–101.

14. Donnelly RP, Kotenko SV. Interferon-λ: a new addition to an old family. *J Interferon Cytokine Res* 2010;**30**:555–64.

15. Gad HH, Dellgren C, Hamming OJ, Vends S, Paludan SR, Hartmann R. Interferon-λ is functionally an interferon but structurally related to the interleukin-10 family. *J Biol Chem* 2009;**284**:20869–75.

16. Dafny N. Is interferon-α a neuromodulator? *Brain Res Brain Res Rev* 1998;**26**:1–15.

17. Durbin RK, Kotenko SV, Durbin JE. Interferon induction and function at the mucosal surface. *Immunol Rev* 2013;**255**:25–39.

18. Zaidi MR, Merlino G. The two faces of interferon-γ in cancer. *Clin Cancer Res* 2011;**17**:6118–24.

19. Chen HM, Tanaka N, Mitani Y, Oda E, Nozawa H, Chen JZ, Yanai H, Negishi H, Choi MK, Iwasaki T, Yamamoto H, Taniguchi T, Takaoka A. Critical role for constitutive type I interferon signaling in the prevention of cellular transformation. *Cancer Sci* 2009;**100**:449–56.

20. Amadori M, Cristiano A, Ferrari M. Constitutive expression of interferons in swine leukocytes. *Res Vet Sci* 2010;**88**:64–71.

21. Greenway AL, Hertzog PJ, Devenish RJ, Linnane AW. Constitutive and virus-induced interferon production by peripheral blood leukocytes. *Exp Hematol* 1995;**23**:229–35.

22. Razzuoli E, Villa R, Sossi E, Amadori M. Characterization of the interferon-α response of pigs to the weaning stress. *J Interferon Cytokine Res* 2011;**31**:237–47.

23. Northrop RL, Deinhardt F. Production of IFN-like substances by human bone marrow tissues *in vitro*. *J Nat Cancer Inst* 1967;**39**:685–9.

24. Minnefor AB, Halsted CC, Seto DS, Glade PR, Moore GE, Carver DH. Production of interferon by long-term suspension cultures of leukocytes derived from patients with viral and nonviral diseases. *J Infect Dis* 1970;**121**:442–4.

25. Bocci V. Is interferon produced in physiological conditions? *Med Hypotheses* 1980;**6**:735–45.

26. Gough DJ, Messina NL, Clarke CJ, Johnstone RW, Levy DE. Constitutive type I interferon modulates homeostatic balance through tonic signaling. *Immunity* 2010;**36**:166–74.

27. Marie I, Durbin JE, Levy DE. Differential viral induction of distinct interferon-α genes by positive feedback through interferon regulatory factor-7. *EMBO J* 1998;**17**:6660–9.

28. Moll HP, Freudenthaler H, Zommer A, Buchberger E, Brostjan C. Neutralizing type I interferon antibodies trigger an interferon-like response in endothelial cells. *J Immunol* 2008;**180**:5250–6.

29. Razzuoli E, Villa R, Sossi E, Amadori M. Reverse transcription real-time PCR for detection of porcine interferon α and β genes. *Scand J Immunol* 2011;**74**:412–8.

30. Amadori M. Physiological response and constitutive expression of interferons: roles and functions. In: Durand M, Morel CV, editors. *New Research on Innate Immunity*. New York: Nova Science Publishers Inc; 2008. p. 1–11.

31. Tompkins W. Immunomodulation and therapeutic effect of the oral use of IFN-α: mechanism of action. *J Interferon Cytokine Res* 1999;**19**:817–28.

32. Razzuoli E, Villa R, Ferrari A, Amadori M. A pig tonsil cell culture model for evaluating oral, low-dose IFN-α treatments. *Vet Immunol Immunopathol* 2014;**160**:244–54.

33. Anderson P, Phillips K, Stoecklin G, Kedersha N. Post-transcriptional regulation of proinflammatory proteins. *J Leukoc Biol* 2004;**76**:42–7.

34. Lemke G, Rothlin CV. Immunobiology of the TAM receptors. *Nat Rev Immunol* 2008;**8**:327–36.

35. Begni B, Amadori M, Ritelli M, Podavini D. Effects of IFN-α on the inflammatory response of swine leukocytes to bacterial endotoxin. *J Interferon Cytokine Res* 2005;**25**:202–8.

36. Gerber S, Bongiovanni AM, Ledger WJ, Witkin SS. A deficiency in interferon-α production in women with vulvar vestibulitis. *Am J Obstet Gynecol* 2002;**186**:361–4.

37. Bufe A, Gehlhar K, Grage-Griebenow E, Ernst M. Atopic phenotype in children is associated with decreased virus-induced interferon-α release. *Int Arch Allergy Immunol* 2002;**127**:82–8.

38. Futata E, Azor M, Dos Santos J, Maruta C, Sotto M, Guedes F, Rivitti E, Duarte A, Sato M. Impaired IFN-α secretion by plasmacytoid dendritic cells induced by TLR9 activation in chronic idiopathic urticaria. *Brit J of Dermatol* 2011;**164**:1271–9.

39. Skovgaard K, Cirera S, Vasby D, Podolska A, Breum SO, Durrwald R, Schlegel M, Heegaard PM. Expression of innate immune genes, proteins and microRNAs in lung tissue of pigs infected experimentally with influenza virus (H1N2). *Innate Immun* 2013;**19**:531–44.

40. Khabar KS, Young HA. Post-transcriptional control of the interferon system. *Biochimie* 2007;**89**:761–9.

41. Newton K, Dixit VM. Signaling in innate immunity and inflammation. *Cold Spring Harb Perspect Biol* 2012;**4**:1–19.

42. Feldman N, Rotter-Maskowitz A, Okun E. DAMPs as mediators of sterile inflammation in aging-related pathologies. *Ageing Res Rev* 2015; doi: 10.1016/j.arr.2015.01.003; In press.

43. Coccia EM, Severa M, Giacomini E, Monneron D, Remoli ME, Julkunen I, Cella M, Lande R, Uzé G. Viral infection and Toll-like receptor agonists induce a differential expression of type I and λ interferons in human plasmacytoid and monocyte-derived dendritic cells. *Eur J Immunol* 2004;**34**:796–805.

44. Dinarello CA. Interleukin-1 family. In: Thomson AW, Lotze MT, editors. *The Cytokine Handbook*. 4th ed London: Academic Press; 2003. p. 709–33.

45. Okamura H, Lotze MT, Tsutsui H, Kashiwamura S, Ueda H, Yoshimoto T, Nakanishi K. Interleukin-18 [IL-1F4]. In: Thomson AW, Lotze MT, editors. *The Cytokine Handbook*. 4th ed. London: Academic Press; 2003. p. 709–33.

46. Guzman E, Birch JR, Ellis SA. Cattle MIC is a ligand for the activating NK cell receptor NKG2D. *Vet Immunol Immunopathol* 2010;**136**:227–34.

47. Davidson S, Maini MK, Wack A. Disease-promoting effects of type I interferons in viral, bacterial, and coinfections. *J Interferon Cytokine Res* 2015;**35**:252–64.

48. Hooks JJ, Moutsopoulos HM, Notkins AL. Circulating interferon in human autoimmune disease. Baron S, Dianzani F, Stanton GJ, editors. *The Interferon System: A Review to 1982*, 41. Texas: Reports on Biology and Medicine; 1982. p. 164–8.

49. Taylor MW, Long T, Martinez-Valdez H, Downing J, Zeige G. Induction of γ-interferon activity by elevated temperatures in human B-lymphoblastoid cell lines. *Proc Natl Acad Sci* 1984;**81**:4033–6.

50. Huang YH, Haegerstrand A, Frostegård J. Effects of *in vitro* hyperthermia on proliferative responses and lymphocyte activity. *Clin Exp Immunol* 1996;**103**:61–6.

51. Sbardella E, Tomassini V, Gasperini C, Bellomi F, Cefaro LA, Morra VB, Antonelli G, Pozzilli C. Neutralizing antibodies explain the poor clinical response to interferon beta in a small proportion of patients with multiple sclerosis: a retrospective study. *BMC Neurol* 2009;**13**:9–54.

52. Caruso A, Turano A. Natural antibodies to interferon-γ. *Biotherapy* 1997;**10**:29–37.

53. Dianzani F, Antonelli G. What is the practical significance of antibodies to interferons? *Bio Drugs* 1998;**9**:187–95.

54. Brandt ER, Mackay IR, Hertzog PJ, Cheetham BF, Sherritt M, Bernard CC. Molecular detection of interferon-α expression in multiple sclerosis brain. *J Neuroimmunol* 1993;**44**:1–5.

55. Hooks JJ, Moutsopoulos HM, Geis SA, Stahl NI, Decker JL, Notkins AL. Immune interferon in the circulation of patients with autoimmune disease. *N Engl J Med* 1979;**301**:5–8.

56. Kontaki E, Boumpas DT. Innate immunity in systemic lupus erythematosus: sensing endogenous nucleic acids. *J Autoimmun* 2010;**35**:206–11.

57. Sharif MN, Tassiulas I, Hu Y, Mecklenbrauker I, Tarakhovsky A, Ivashkiv LB. IFN-α priming results in a gain of proinflammatory function by IL-10: implications for systemic lupus erythematosus pathogenesis. *J Immunol* 2004;**172**:6476–81.

58. Lauw FN, Pajkrt D, Hack CE, Kurimoto M, van Deventer SJ, van der Poll T. Proinflammatory effects of IL-10 during human endotoxemia. *J Immunol* 2010;**165**:2783–9.

59. Manners MJ. The development of digestive function in the pig. *Proc Nutr Soc* 1976;**35**:49–55.

60. Wijtten PJ, van der Meulen J, Verstegen MW. Intestinal barrier function and absorption in pigs after weaning: a review. *Br J Nutr* 2011;**105**:967–81.

61. McCracken BA, Gaskins HR, Ruwe-Kaiser PJ, Klasing KC, Jewell DE. Diet-dependent and diet-independent metabolic responses underlie growth stasis of pigs at weaning. *J Nutr* 1995;**125**:2838–45.

62. Razzuoli E, Dotti S, Archetti IL, Amadori M. Clinical chemistry parameters of piglets at weaning are modulated by an oral, low-dose interferon-α treatment. *Vet Res Commun* 2010;**34**:S189–92.

63. Hu CH, Xiao K, Luan ZS, Song J. Early weaning increases intestinal permeability, alters expression of cytokine and tight junction proteins, and activates mitogen-activated protein kinases in pigs. *J Anim Sci* 2013;**91**:1094–101.

64. Beaurepaire C, Smyth D, McKay DM. Interferon-γ regulation of intestinal epithelial permeability. *J Interferon Cytokine Res* 2009;**29**:133–44.

65. Amadori M, Razzuoli E, Nassuato C. Issues and possible intervention strategies relating to early weaning of piglets. *CAB Rev* 2012;7–46.

66. O'Loughlin A, McGee M, Waters SM, Doyle S, Earley B. Examination of the bovine leukocyte environment using immunogenetic biomarkers to assess immunocompetence following exposure to weaning stress. *BMC Vet Res* 2011;**7**:45.

67. O'Loughlin A, Lynn DJ, McGee M, Doyle S, McCabe M, Earley B. Transcriptomic analysis of the stress response to weaning at housing in bovine leukocytes using RNA-seq technology. *BMC Genomics* 2012;**13**:250.

68. Cafazzo S, Magnani D, Calà P, Razzuoli E, Gerardi G, Bernardini D, Amadori M, Nanni Costa L. Effect of short road journeys on behaviour and some blood variables related to welfare in young bulls. *Appl Anim Behav Sci* 2012;**139**:26–34.

69. Gupta S, Earley B, Crowe MA. Effect of 12-hour road transportation on physiological, immunological and haematological parameters in bulls housed at different space allowances. *Vet J* 2007;**173**:605–16.

70. Razzuoli E, Olzi E, Cafazzo S, Magnani D, Calà P, Archetti IL, Nannicosta L, Amadori M. Valutazione di alcuni parametri di immunologia-clinica in bovini sottoposti a trasporti brevi nella filiera del centro genetico ANAFI. *Buiatria* 2011;**2**:23–30 [in Italian].

71. Artursson K, Wallgren P, Alm GV. Appearance of interferon-α in serum and signs of reduced immune function in pigs after transport and installation in a fattening farm. *Vet Immunol Immunopathol* 1989;**23**:345–53.

72. Bernardini D, Gerardi G, Peli A, Nanni Costa L, Amadori M, Segato S. The effects of different environmental conditions on thermoregulation and clinical and hematological variables in long-distance road-transported calves. *J Anim Sci* 2012;**90**(4):1183–91.

73. Obremski K, Podlasz P, Zmigrodzka M, Winnicka A, Woźny M, Brzuzan P, Jakimiuk E, Wojtacha P, Gajecka M, Zielonka Ł, Gajecki M. The effect of T-2 toxin on percentages of CD4+, CD8+, CD4+ CD8+ and CD21+ lymphocytes, and mRNA expression levels of selected cytokines in porcine ileal Peyer's patches. *Pol J Vet Sci* 2013;**16**:341–9.

74. Pinton P, Accensi F, Beauchamp E, Cossalter AM, Callu P, Grosjean F, Oswald IP. Ingestion of deoxynivalenol (DON) contaminated feed alters the pig vaccinal immune responses. *Toxicol Lett* 2008;**177**:215–22.

75. Ghareeb K, Awad WA, Soodoi C, Sasgary S, Strasser A, Böhm J. Effects of feed contaminant deoxynivalenol on plasma cytokines and mRNA expression of immune genes in the intestine of broiler chickens. *PLoS One* 2013;**8**:e71492.

76. Chen F, Ma Y, Xue C, Ma J, Xie Q, Wang G, Bi Y, Cao Y. The combination of deoxynivalenol and zearalenone at permitted feed concentrations causes serious physiological effects in young pigs. *J Vet Sci* 2008;**9**:39–44.

77. Choi BK, Jeong SH, Cho JH, Shin HS, Son SW, Yeo YK, Kang HG. Effects of oral deoxynivalenol exposure on immune-related parameters in lymphoid organs and serum of mice vaccinated with porcine parvovirus vaccine. *Mycotoxin Res* 2013;**29**:185–92.

78. Islam MR, Roh YS, Kim J, Lim CW, Kim B. Differential immune modulation by deoxynivalenol (vomitoxin) in mice. *Toxicol Lett* 2013;**221**:152–63.

79. Marin S, Ramos AJ, Cano-Sancho G, Sanchis V. Mycotoxins: occurrence, toxicology, and exposure assessment. *Food Chem Toxicol* 2013;**60**:218–37.

80. Chen K, Yuan S, Chen J, Peng X, Wang F, Cui H, Fang J. Effects of sodium selenite on the decreased percentage of T cell subsets, contents of serum IL-2 and IFN-γ induced by aflatoxin B in broilers. *Res Vet Sci* 2013;**95**:143–5.

81. Micallef A, Grech N, Farrugia F, Schembri-Wismayer P, Calleja-Agius J. The role of interferons in early pregnancy. *Gynecol Endocrinol* 2014;**30**:1–6.

82. Imakawa K, Helmer SD, Nephew KP, Meka CS, Christenson RK. A novel role for GM-CSF: enhancement of pregnancy specific interferon production, ovine trophoblast protein-1. *Endocrinology* 1993;**132**:1869–71.

83. Leaman DW, Cross JC, Roberts RM. Genes for the trophoblast interferons and their distribution among mammals. *Reprod Fertil Dev* 1992;**4**:349–53.

84. Bazer FW, Spencer TE, Ott TL. Placental interferons. *Am J Reprod Immunol* 1996;**4**:297–308.

85. Polgar K, Hill JA. Identification of the white blood cell populations responsible for Th1 immunity to trophoblast and the timing of the response in women with recurrent pregnancy loss. *Gynecol Obstet Invest* 2002;**53**:59–64.

86. Joyce MM, Burghardt RC, Geisert RD, Burghardt JR, Hooper RN, Ross JW, Ashworth MD, Johnson GA. Pig conceptuses secrete estrogen and interferons to differentially regulate uterine STAT1 in a temporal and cell type-specific manner. *Endocrinology* 2007;**148**:4420–31.

87. Bazer FW. Pregnancy recognition signaling mechanisms in ruminants and pigs. *J Anim Sci Biotechnol* 2013;**4**:23.

88. Hermant P, Francius C, Clotman F, Michiels T. IFN-ε is constitutively expressed by cells of the reproductive tract and is inefficiently secreted by fibroblasts and cell lines. *PLoS One* 2013;**8**:e713–20.

89. Fung KY, Mangan NE, Cumming H, Horvat JC, Mayall JR, Stifter SA, De Weerd N, Roisman LC, Rossjohn J, Robertson SA, Schjenken JE, Parker B, Gargett CE, Nguyen HP, Carr DJ, Hansbro PM, Hertzog PJ. Interferon-ε protects the female reproductive tract from viral and bacterial infection. *Science* 2003;**339**:1088–92.

90. Pearce N, Douwes J. Research at the interface between human and veterinary health. *Prev Vet Med* 2013;**111**:187–93.

Chapter 9

Disease-Predicting and Prognostic Potential of Innate Immune Responses to Noninfectious Stressors: Human and Animal Models

Erminio Trevisi,* Livia Moscati,** Massimo Amadori†

*Faculty of Agriculture, Food and Environmental Sciences, Istituto di Zootecnia, Università Cattolica del Sacro Cuore, Piacenza, Italy; **Laboratory of Clinical Sciences, Istituto Zooprofilattico Sperimentale Umbria e Marche, Perugia, Italy; †Laboratory of Cellular Immunology, Istituto Zooprofilattico Sperimentale della Lombardia e dell'Emilia-Romagna, Brescia, Italy

INTRODUCTION

Health and Disease

Disease is the possible state of the body and brain in relation to the effect of pathogens, parasites, tissue damage, and physical or psychological disorder. Since all of these effects can cause pathology, health refers to the state of an individual as it attempts to cope with pathogens or pathology-inducing circumstances.[1] Disease can be induced by infectious and noninfectious stressors. Stress can be defined as an environmental effect on an individual that overtaxes its control systems and reduces its fitness or seems likely to do so.[2] The immune response to a stressor is part of a global adaptive response of the host to restore homeostasis. Acute stress is usually associated with transient increase in immune activation, while chronic stress is associated with suppression of a variety of immune parameters.[3,4] The coping ability implies control over mental and body stability. Prolonged failure to cope results in growth check, failure to reproduce, disease, and sometimes death.

Innate Immunity and Inflammation

Disease causes negative experiences in man and animals, including pain, discomfort or distress,[5] as well as injuries of tissues and organs and changes in metabolism. Disease-inducing infectious and noninfectious stressors are confronted by a first barrier of defense represented by the innate immune system, ready to recognize and fight any potentially harmful invader, or environmental *noxa* affecting homeostasis. Janeway and Medzhitov[6] stressed that innate immunity is an evolutionarily ancient part of the host defense mechanisms and that the same molecular modules are found in plants and animals. Interestingly, several studies clarified that the onset of the condition of sickness is strictly preserved in living beings and it is partly independent of the inducers.[7–9] The inducers of the immune response are classified as biotic (e.g., bacteria and viruses) and abiotic (e.g., injury, trauma, and psychological burden) stressors. These inducers can derive from exogenous or endogenous sources (Fig. 9.1). The first step of the innate immune response is the recognition of particular types of molecules that are common to many pathogens and absent in the healthy host. These pathogen-associated molecules (called pathogen-associated immunostimulants) stimulate two types of innate immune responses: (1) inflammatory responses and (2) phagocytosis by neutrophils and macrophages.[10] These responses occur quickly, even if the host has never been previously exposed to a particular pathogen.

Mediators of Inflammation: Local and Systemic Effects

Medzhitov[7] classified the inflammatory mediators into seven groups, according to their biochemical properties; (1) vasoactive amines, (2) vasoactive peptides, (3) fragments of complement components, (4) lipid mediators, (5) cytokines, (6) chemokines, and (7) proteolytic enzymes (Table 9.1). The most obvious

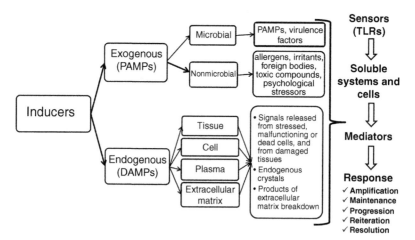

FIGURE 9.1 **The sequence of a generic inflammatory pathway in animals.** PAMPs, pathogen-associated molecular patterns; DAMPs, damage-associated molecular patterns.

TABLE 9.1 Classification of the Inflammatory Mediators According to Their Origin and Physiological Effects

	Inflammatory mediators		Source/	
	Type	Molecules	origin	Effects
1	Vasoactive amines	Histamine and serotonin	Degranulation of mast cells and platelets	Fever; increased vascular permeability, vasodilation or vasoconstriction (depending on the context). Highly detrimental in sensitized organisms, resulting in vascular and respiratory collapse during anaphylactic shock
2	Vasoactive peptides	Substance P (stored in an active form in secretory vesicles)	Released by sensory neurons (substance P causes mast-cell degranulation)	Vasodilation and increased vascular permeability (directly or indirectly inducing the release of histamine from mast cells)
		Kinins, fibrinopeptide A, fibrinopeptide B and fibrin degradation products, etc.	Generated through proteolysis of inactive precursors in the extracellular fluid by the Hageman factor, thrombin or plasmin	Hageman factor has a key role in coordinating these responses; it functions as both sensor of vascular damage and inducer of inflammation. The Hageman factor activates the kallikrein–kinin cascade, and the main product of this cascade, bradykinin, affects the vasculature and exerts a potent pro-algesic (pain-stimulating) effect. Pain sensation has an important physiological role in inflammation by alerting the organism to the abnormal state of the damaged tissue
3	Fragments of complement called anaphylatoxins	C3a, C4a, C5a etc.	Produced by distinct pathways of complement activation	C'5a (and to a lesser extent C'3a and C'4a) promote granulocyte and monocyte recruitment, induce mast cell degranulation, affect the vasculature

(Continued)

TABLE 9.1 Classification of the Inflammatory Mediators According to Their Origin and Physiological Effects *(cont.)*

	Inflammatory mediators		Source/	
	Type	Molecules	origin	Effects
4	Lipid media-tors (derived from phos-pholipids present in the inner leaflet of cellular membranes) generated by cytosolic phospholi-pase A2	Eicosanoids (prostaglan-dins = PG, thrombox-anes = TBX, leukotrienes, lipoxins)	Metabolites of arachidonic acid generated by cyclooxy-genases (COX1 and COX2): PG and TBX; or by lipoxygenases: leukotrienes and lipoxins	PGE2 and PGI2 cause vasodilation. PGE2 is hyperalgesic and a potent inducer of fever. Lipoxins inhibit inflammation (by inhibiting the recruitment of neutrophils); promote resolution of inflammation and tissue repair (by promoting the recruitment of monocytes, which remove dead cells and initiate tissue remodelling). The effects of resolvins and protectins (dietary ω3-fatty-acid-derived) are similar to those of lipoxins
		Platelet-activating factors	After acetyla-tion of lyso-phosphatidic acid	They induce an inflam-matory response (i.e. recruitment of leuko-cytes, vasodilation and vasoconstriction, increase of vascular permeability, platelet activation)
5	Inflammato-ry cytokines	Tumor-ne-crosis factor-α (TNF-α), IL-1, IL-6	Macrophages, mast cells and many other cells	Inflammatory response (i.e., activation of the endothelium and leukocytes, induction of the acute-phase response)
6	Chemokines	Four sub-families: CXC, CC, CX3C, and XC	Many cell types in response to inducers of inflammation	Modulation of leukocyte extravasation and chemotaxis toward the affected tissues
7	Proteolytic enzymes	Elastin, cathepsins, matrix metallopro-teinases	Many cell types	Inflammation (by degrading extracellular matrix and basement-membrane proteins), host defence, tissue remodelling and leukocyte migration

Adapted from Ref. [7].

effects of these mediators are exerted locally, including redness, heat, swelling, and pain. Nevertheless, many inflammatory mediators have important systemic effects[11] on the neuroendocrine system, metabolic functions, and maintenance of tissue homeostasis. Among mediators, proinflammatory cytokines (PIC) are considered the main stimulators of systemic inflammation. The responsiveness to PIC is almost ubiquitous, although with distinct effects in different tissues and cell types.[7] The main systemic effects of PIC can be summarized as follows:[12–16]

1. Exaggerated activation of the pituitary–adrenal system, resulting in a rise in body temperature, lethargy and sickness, lower bodycare activity, decreased locomotion, and social exploration.
2. Modification of the eating behavior (or overt anorexia), through an altered neurotransmitter and neuropeptide profile in the hypothalamus.
3. Modulation of gastrointestinal activities.
4. Increase of catabolic activities in adipose and muscle tissues.
5. Metabolic and endocrine modifications (i.e., increase of plasma glucose levels, probably due to increased cortisol release and insulin resistance).
6. Induction of the acute-phase reaction in the liver, with the synthesis of peculiar proteins, referred to as positive acute-phase proteins (posAPPs, i.e., haptoglobin, serum amiloyd A, C-reactive protein, ceruloplasmin, and pentraxins), and the reduced synthesis of usual hepatic proteins, as the likely outcome of competition for substrates. These are collectively named negative acute-phase proteins (negAPPs; e.g., albumins, enzymes, "carriers" of vitamins and hormones, and apolipoproteins).

Possible Causes of Dysregulated Inflammatory Response

The NF-κB complex accounts for many inflammatory effector activities. After the exposure to inflammatory stimuli, there is an accumulation of functional NF-κB dimers in the nucleus, which activate the gene transcription of proinflammatory mediators (cytokines, chemokines, adhesion molecules, and also enzymes and molecules with microbicidal activity).[17] Two distinct NF-κB activation pathways have been described[17] as canonical (classical) and noncanonical (alternative) pathways. The classical pathway is activated by a large number of stimuli as PIC, bacterial and viral products, γ-radiation, ultraviolet light, and oxidative stress. The alternative pathway occurs during the development of lymphoid organs responsible for the generation of B and T lymphocytes and produces p100/RelB complexes. The canonical pathway regulates the expression of immunoregulatory and antiapoptotic genes, and inhibits the accumulation of reactive oxygen metabolites (ROM), helping cells to survive, and eliciting a protective response to infection and injury. Trials with genetic manipulated animals confirmed that an activation of NF-κB has a strong inflammatory effect, but also that its inhibition in nonimmune cells (epithelial or parenchymal) does not attenuate inflammation-related pathologies. On the contrary, such inhibition can trigger the spontaneous development of severe inflammatory conditions.[17] These results indicate the multifaceted roles of NF-κB signaling and suggest that inhibition of NF-κB in certain tissues and cellular compartments might disrupt the physiological immune homeostasis and cause a dysregulated proinflammatory effect.

Inflammation and Disease

The systemic functions of inflammatory mediators support a role for inflammation in the control of tissue homeostasis and in adaptation to noxious conditions. These effects can help stop pathogens and favor repair of tissue damage. In fact, a good inflammatory response is essential to reduce the sensitivity to infections[18] and has a protecting role. Nevertheless, an exaggerated inflammatory response (i.e., chronic inflammation or low-grade systemic inflammatory conditions) causes potentially harmful effects in the host. These adverse properties can also affect the quality of life, due to their detrimental consequences at physical and mental levels.[19] Inflammation is common to any health disorder, and the sickness behavior is associated with the release of PIC, as recently reviewed by Bertoni et al.[20] Interestingly, some of the blood changes induced by mediators of inflammation can contribute to a correct evaluation of the host's response in terms of beginning of the stimuli, duration, and severity of *noxae* (efficacy of the defense response) in both humans[13,21,22] and livestock.[15,23,24]

To summarize, inflammation should be considered as the host's protective attempt to restore a homeostatic state. To achieve this goal, the inflammatory response must be tightly regulated in terms of timing, extent, cellular components, and tissues involved. Beyond such borders, the inflammatory response turns into the actual cause of disease. This is the conceptual framework in which the predictive and prognostic value of innate immune responses should be reasonably set and evaluated.

HUMAN MODELS

In agreement with the aforementioned tenets, several disease models in humans have revealed a significant association with diverse types of innate immune response in terms of either disease risk assessment, or prognosis of ongoing disease conditions. This was clearly shown for both infectious and noninfectious stressors.

Thus, incidence and severity of cold or flu symptoms was significantly associated with *in vitro* IL-6 and IFN-γ secretion after stimulation of PBMC with LPS and antihuman CD3, respectively. In particular, IL-6 secretion from LPS-stimulated PBMC cultures was significantly higher in subjects with self-reported cold or flu symptoms in the past month. On the contrary, IFN-γ secretion was significantly lower in the subjects experiencing more severe cases of cold and flu in the same previous period. Interestingly, these cytokine response profiles remained significantly associated with incidence of cold or flu after incorporating important dietary factors in the model.[25] On the whole, the significant association of respiratory disease with IL-6 responses confirms once again that poor homeostatic control of the inflammatory response underlies also in humans the occurrence of disease cases due to common, opportunistic, microbial agents. Lack of adequate control may be associated with genetic markers, like single-nucleotide polymorphisms of crucial genes like that coding for human IL-6[26,27] and bovine TLR-4,[28] and/or a negative imprinting caused by environmental, noninfectious stressors.[29] Also, the data about IL-6 complement previous reports about IL-6 as marker of ongoing inflammation during cold or flu infection in humans[30,31] and of bacterial burden during antibiotic therapies in pigs.[32] The emerging picture outlines a complex of pro- and anti-inflammatory activities of IL-6,[33] which need a tight regulation during exposure to infectious and noninfectious stressors. Most important, abnormal release of IL-6 and/or IL-6 responses to minor environmental stressors might predispose the host to adverse upshots later on.

IL-6 levels also have a diagnostic and prognostic value after a serious tissue damage. IL-6 and glucocorticoids induce in fact acute-phase response (APR) proteins, involved in protection of tissues and endued with potent scavenger, opsonizing, chemiotactic, and hemoglobin-binding properties.[34] Interestingly, serum IL-6 levels in burned patients are related to body temperature and APR, as shown by C-reactive protein (CRP) levels.[35] Also, IL-6 is involved in induction of ACTH and, most important, in direct glucocorticoid induction in adrenal cells,[36] as well as in inhibition of TNF-α and IL-1β expression in human macrophages.[37] By sustaining adrenal functions, the IL-6 response might thus determine an efficient control of inflammation during heat stress and high levels of immune competence, as shown in models of *Escherichia coli*, *Listeria monocytogenes*, and *Candida albicans* infection in IL-6-deficient mice.[38] IL-6 is also an emerging disease activity marker during spondyloarthritis (a group of arthritides characterized by inflammation in the joints of the axial spine), along with soluble cytotoxic T-lymphocyte-associated molecule-4.[39]

APR can be prognostic in diverse kinds of disease. Among neoplasias, CRP was shown to be an independent prognostic marker in patients with melanoma in terms of overall survival, melanoma-specific survival, and disease-free survival.[40] CRP has been also shown to be significant in the prediction of outcomes of urological cancers. The elevation of CRP levels, underlying the presence of cancer-associated systemic inflammatory response, is linked to poorer survival in patients with urological cancers, including renal cell carcinoma, upper urinary tract and bladder cancers, and prostate cancer.[41] There is also evidence that CRP can be a useful prognostic marker for a wider array of solid tumors, as well as a valuable risk assessment parameter for the same types of neoplasias in humans.[42]

Neutrophil gelatinase-associated lipocalin (NGAL) is emerging as an excellent biomarker in the urine and plasma for the early prediction of acute kidney injury (AKI), and for the prognosis of AKI in several common clinical scenarios. In particular, NGAL can enable practitioners to get early, useful diagnostic indications independent of serum creatinine concentrations, and it can provide a rational basis for a treatment for AKI based on high biomarker levels.[43]

The decrease of mean platelet volume (MPV) is an important inflammatory marker in patients with severe periodontitis. Most important, MPV increase is an accurate prognostic marker of treatment efficacy in terms of periodontal probing depth.[44,45] This may be of some importance because of the significant association between periodontitis and cardiovascular diseases.[46] These findings are in agreement with the role of MPV as an inflammatory marker in many chronic diseases like ulcerative colitis,[47] ankylosing spondylitis, and rheumatoid arthritis.[48]

Damage-associated molecular patterns (DAMPs) are usual end products of both infectious and noninfectious stressors, leading to different inflammasomes and eventual production of IL-1β.[49] The extent and timing of these early inflammatory responses can be of some importance during viral infections, too. Thus, west Nile virus (WNV) can cause asymptomatic or severe neurological disease and death, particularly in older patients. By a systems immunology approach, a reduced IL-1β induction following *ex vivo* infection of macrophages with WNV and a reduced expression of the CXCL10 gene in myeloid dendritic cells were shown to be significantly associated with severe cases of WNV infection.[50] Likewise, the combined high expression of IL-1β and IL-18 is an independent predictor for poor prognosis in patients with localized clear cell renal cell carcinoma, and the prognostic value is more pronounced in patients with low-risk disease.[44] Also, IL-1β levels were shown to be significantly associated with disease severity in methotrexate-treated psoriasis patients.[51]

Impaired immune surveillance as a result of chronic stress can be conveniently detected on the basis of the poor containment of otherwise strictly controlled viral infections. Thus, reduced immune surveillance of persistent viral infections as a result of chronic stress causes resumption of, or enhanced viral replication. In this scenario, torque teno virus (TTV) is an important, validated model in humans. It is a ubiquitous unenveloped DNA virus belonging to the Anelloviridae family, infecting humans and many animal species, like nonhuman primates, pig, cow, sheep, dog, cat, and chicken.[52] Therefore, TTV viremia could be a cross-species parameter of immunocompetence, and its scope might be widened in further studies to common environmental stressors, neoplasias, and immunosuppressive microbial agents. TTV viremia has been shown to increase in humans in many conditions of chronic immunosuppression (congenital, acquired, or iatrogenic), like congenital mannose-binding lectin deficiencies, HIV infection, cancer, heart and lung transplant, and high-dose chemotherapy for neoplasias.[53–55]

ANIMAL MODELS: THE PERIPARTURIENT DAIRY COW

Disease Occurrence in Periparturient Dairy Cows

The transition period of dairy cows represents the key phase of the whole lactation.[56] In the last part of pregnancy, the demand for nutrients gradually increases to satisfy the fetal development and, later, mammary activity, but the adaptation of the digestive system is slowed and insufficient, inducing a large mobilization of body reserves. The severe negative energy balance combined with many other adverse factors, which occur in this phase and are not always well understood,[24,56–58] account for the increased susceptibility to metabolic and infectious diseases. Several studies support this statement; in fact, LeBlanc et al.[59] reported that 75% of the metabolic and infectious diseases occur in the first month of lactation, whereas Mulligan and Doherty[60] observed that about 50% of the periparturient cows suffer at least one metabolic disease.

The situation could be more severe if the subclinical cases were to be included, for example, by the detection of plasma indices as NEFA or BHB[23,61] or APPs.[14,62,63] Among diseases that occur more frequently in the transition period and that have been related either to inflammatory conditions or to negative energy balance, the more important are retained placenta and metritis,[64–67] ketosis,[59,61] displacement of abomasum,[68,69] liver lipidosis,[70,71] mastitis,[72–74] lameness,[73] and rumen subacute acidosis.[75] Nevertheless, the incidence of many other health disturbances increases during an unsatisfactory transition period (e.g., virus infections, parasitoses, intestinal upsets), but unfortunately the registration of these problems is difficult and reports are lacking.

Causes of the Inflammatory Response in Periparturient Dairy Cows

In cattle, the most studied humoral components induced under inflammatory conditions are APPs.[14,76,77] Both posAPP and negAPP show clear changes of their concentrations after any stimulus that activates the innate immune system. In dairy cows, a typical inflammatory condition is also observed around calving[23,63] in the "transition period." This response often occurs in the absence of clinical symptoms, and several causes concur to trigger these responses:[20,24,77]

1. Mammary gland differentiation and proliferation (e.g., edema, rash).
2. Uterus/placenta interaction. In women, placenta produces continuously cytokines to improve its function; a lack of IL-10 (anti-inflammatory cytokine) seems associated with preterm parturition, and administration of anti-inflammatories decreases the incidence of preeclampsia. These facts suggest a cross-talk between placenta and body, which is largely unknown.
3. Physical effort and trauma during calving (dystocia). Strenuous exercise can determine, directly or indirectly a PIC response by increasing the

permeability of intestinal mucosa. In cows, dystocia gives rise to strenuous exercise, and is often accompanied by other typical disturbances (e.g., trauma, psychological stress), also associated with PIC release.

4. Immunosuppression, which increases frequency and severity of opportunistic infections. The ability of leukocytes to respond to an infectious challenge is impaired in the transition period and this is accompanied by dramatic changes in the endocrine, nutritional, and metabolic status.

5. Psychological burden related to the farming conditions (e.g., grouping and movement of cows, deficiency in housing, and animal–human interactions). Several studies on humans showed that chronic psychological stressors (e.g., loneliness) can lead to increased PIC levels,[78] which elicit pain, mental symptoms of sickness (fever, nausea, loss of interest in food, physical and social environment, fragmented sleep), depression, irritability, and some mild cognitive disorders.[19] In a review, Tian et al.[79] suggest a possible explanation of this phenomenon. They hypothesize that the chronic activation of the hypothalamus–pituitary–adrenal axis can induce a cortisol-resistance status, the result being an increase of PIC release in spite of the high concentrations of plasma cortisol.

6. Nutritional modifications (affecting e.g., nutrient balancing, rumen microbiota, rumen fermentations, modulation of immune pathways). In humans, particularly relevant is the link between a form of subclinical, low-grade systemic inflammation ("metaflammation," referring to metabolically triggered inflammation), obesity and chronic disease.[80] Recently, a similar condition has been also described in cattle.[24] Indeed, cows that receive over-feeding energy until calving showed a more severe inflammation until calving and an increased susceptibility to developing fatty liver syndrome (and related disorders), greater body condition score (BCS) loss, and lower fertility.

Altogether, these phenomena affect the homeostatic adaptation strategies of the cows in the transition period.

Blood Indexes to Assess the Inflammatory Response in Dairy Cows

The presented tenets outline the perspective to monitor the ongoing innate immune response to the described stressors, and to verify poor homeostasis as a foundation of later disease cases. In this respect, a crucial issue concerning the inflammation is how to evaluate the severity of this condition. To this purpose, APPs have been investigated as biomarkers of disease in ruminants for a long time.[14,76] Despite posAPP and negAPP being useful to describe the effects of inflammation, particular attention has been devoted to posAPP as a result of infection (e.g., mastitis, metritis), as reviewed by Ceciliani et al.[14]

An important role in the inflammatory response is also attributed to negAPPs, which play a role in its control and resolution. This class of APPs includes proteins with fundamental physiological functions[14,81] such as the following:

- Albumin, apolipoproteins, and transferrin, mainly involved in the blood transport of proteins, lipids, and iron, respectively;[76,81,82]
- Paraoxonase, a calcium-dependent ester hydrolase that catalyzes the hydrolysis of many xenobiotics and has anti-inflammatory activity;[63]
- Enzymes involved in bilirubin clearance;[83]
- Carriers of vitamins (e.g., retinol-binding protein for vitamin A;[84] lipoproteins for vitamin E[85]) and hormones (e.g., transcortin for cortisol,[85] thyroxine-binding-prealbumin or transthyretin for thyroxine[86]).

The functions of negAPPs are essential to maintain the metabolic integrity of the whole body; for this reason their syntheses are highly maintained. Nevertheless, in case of inflammation, negAPPs syntheses are reduced in the liver. If the reduction of negAPPs is marked, the body is exposed to severe damage. As a result, cows that show important and prolonged reduction of negAPPs or retarded increases of negAPPs after calving also show *a higher incidence of health problems and a marked reduction of performance.*[63,87] These findings support the role of negAPPs as proper markers to measure consequences of inflammatory conditions in the peripartum period[88] and predict related health disorders.

Currently, the scientific community has a great interest in identifying reliable biomarkers to be used in the field for monitoring energy balance status, liver function, inflammatory status, and depicting poor homeostasis.[24] Biomarkers should reflect various functions (i.e., digestive tract, metabolic, and immune state) in the attempt to identify animals that are at a greater risk of developing disease conditions.[89]

Aggregate Indices of the Inflammatory Response After Calving Allow Early Diagnosis and/or Prognosis of Disease Conditions

The first aggregate index developed at the Institute of Zootechnics, Piacenza, included a combination of three negAPPs, and it aimed to classify dairy cows in accordance with the physiological consequences of the inflammatory challenge occurred around calving.[88] This index was named liver activity index (LAI) and measured the changes in concentrations of albumin, cholesterol, and vitamin A (Table 9.2) during the first month of lactation. Albumin is the most important negAPP, cholesterol and vitamin A are indirect indexes of negAPP, but their changes in plasma are strictly related to lipoproteins and retinol-binding protein concentrations, respectively. By classifying cows in accordance with their LAI values and comparing classes of animals under extreme conditions (lowest vs. highest scores), we demonstrated that cows with the lowest scores showed the following:

1. A higher susceptibility to metabolic and infectious diseases; in fact these cows displayed a greater frequency of clinical symptoms (e.g., 42% vs. 5%,

TABLE 9.2 Physiological Meaning and Assessment of the LAI, LFI, and PIRI

Item	LAI	LFI	PIRI
References	[23,29,88,90–92]	[29,70,90–93]	[94]
Plasma parameters	Concentrations of albumin, lipoproteins (indirectly measured as total cholesterol), and retinol-binding protein (RBP, measured as retinol, the level of which in blood is strictly related to RBP synthesized by the liver)	Concentrations of albumin, lipoproteins (indirectly measured as total cholesterol), and bilirubin (as indirect measure of the enzymes synthesized by the liver, which also regulates bilirubin clearance)	Haptoglobin, Reactive Metabolites of Oxygen (ROMs), cholesterol and paraoxonase (PON)
Checks (days after calving)	7, 14, 28	3, 28	7
Calculation	Data of each parameter are transformed into units of standard deviation for each cow. The mean values of the herd population of each plasma parameter (albumin, total cholesterol, and RBP) are subtracted from each cow value (days 7, 14, 28 after calving) and divided by the corresponding standard deviation. The final LAI score for each cow is the arithmetical mean of the 3 partial values obtained from the 3 selected blood indices from 3 bleedings [in Ref. [15] an example is provided]	Sum of the changes in concentrations between day 3 and 28 after calving of the three plasma parameters, standardized on the basis of an optimal pattern of change for the three parameters observed in healthy cows at the same stage of lactation.[23] In Ref. [15] an example is provided	For each parameter a range of variations is defined, based on literature data [extreme values = score 10 (best) and 0 (worst)]. The score for each parameter of a cow is calculated using a linear correlation procedure. The final PIRI score for each cow is the arithmetical sum of the four partial values

TABLE 9.2 Physiological Meaning and Assessment of the LAI, LFI, and PIRI *(cont.)*

Item	LAI	LFI	PIRI
Range of score	−1/+1 (higher is better)	−15/+6 (higher is better)	0/40 (higher is better)
Diagnostic meaning	The index provides a retrospective ranking of the successful transition of a cow through the calving period (i.e., it estimates the consequence of an inflammation that occurs in the periparturient period within a defined herd)	The index measures the consequences of an inflammation occurring at or after calving. The index represents an absolute value	The index measures the consequences of the environmental challenges occurring in the periparturient period
Practical implications	Identification of cows with subclinical problems in the first month of lactation; anticipation of therapies mainly to improve the fertility	Identification of cows with subclinical problems in the first month of lactation; comparison of inflammatory profiles among herds and periods; anticipation of therapies, mainly to improve the fertility	Identification of cows with subclinical problems in the first week of lactation; comparison of the inflammatory profiles among herds and periods
Limitation	It allows a meaningful comparison only within a herd; it does not promptly identify subclinical problems	It does not identify subclinical problems promptly	It does not measure possible effects due to metabolic and infectious diseases occurred after the first week of lactation

comparing the lower and upper quartiles of LAI;[23] 60% vs. 9%, comparing the lower and upper halves of the LAI distribution[95]). Data were often referred to more than one disease case per cow.[23,90]

2. Reduction of milk yield and fertility.[23]
3. A more serious negative energy balance, as confirmed by the more marked losses of BCS and the higher levels of β-hydroxy-butyrate.[23,29] Interestingly,

the lower reduction of BCS in cows with the highest LAI value was observed also when the milk yield was higher.

4. A lower feed intake.[91,92]
5. A lower efficiency in feed energy conversion, as a consequence of the increased energy to support the activity of the immune system.[91,92]
6. Higher peaks of posAPPs; plasma haptoglobin in the days following the parturition,[23,29,63] and higher concentrations of ceruloplasmin for >1 week,[29,95] which confirms a more severe inflammatory status.

On the whole, LAI identifies subjects that need more attention by the breeder and more time (and care) to regain satisfactory conditions and reproductive efficiency. In particular, two inadequate physiological conditions will be observed in case of low LAI values:[77]

1. Subjects showing inflammatory phenomena (e.g., high plasma haptoglobin level) without clinical signs. This condition demands an accurate diagnosis, concerning organs at risk (i.e., uterus, mammary gland, and feet).
2. Subjects without acute inflammatory events, but showing poor liver functions. This condition requires some kind of support (i.e., nutraceutical, galenic, dietary) to accelerate liver recovery and onset of reproductive functions.

Despite the utility of the information inferred by LAI, this measurement is time-consuming (at least three bleedings per cow in the first month of lactation) and expensive. Moreover, LAI does not allow for a comparison with animals of other herds.

To simplify the assessment of the global effect of the transition period in terms of inflammatory response, our laboratory has proposed the liver functionality index (LFI). This index is calculated on the basis of two blood samplings, and measurement of vitamin A is replaced by a total bilirubin assay, another parameter related to negAPPs, but measurable by a quick and easy method (Table 9.2). Furthermore, the changes of the parameters are adjusted in accordance with the physiological changes observed in healthy cows, characterized by good productive performance.[15,70] LFI is well correlated with LAI ($r = 0.87$; $P < 0.001$),[92] which supports its reliability. Interestingly, cows with a high LFI score experienced lower disease prevalence[29,96] and a lower number of drug treatments over the whole transition period.[96] This implied a two- to fourfold reduction of the costs related to drug treatments, compared with cows showing low LFI scores. Nevertheless, LFI (as LAI) cannot promptly identify subclinical problems in the transition period because the final score is available only at the end of the first month of lactation, when plenty of disease cases have already occurred.

A third aggregate index was therefore developed to identify subclinical problems in the first week of lactation. The postcalving inflammatory response index (PIRI) (Table 9.2)[94] includes four assays related to inflammation (haptoglobin, posAPPs, cholesterol and paraoxonase, negAPPs) and oxidative stress (ROM).

Despite PIRI requiring a validation in the field, cows with lower scores showed greater prevalence of postcalving diseases, more severe inflammatory conditions in the early lactation period, higher lipomobilization and ketone body concentrations, and also lower milk production.[94] From these data, PIRI index is a good candidate to identify the subclinical subjects at risk very early after calving. Yet, this approach does not allow to monitor the whole transition period, thus missing the health disorders occurring after the first week of lactation.

Owing to these issues, it seems reasonable to employ both LFI and PIRI aggregate indices. In this perspective, two blood samples will be collected at 3–7 and 28–30 days from parturition. The former will be useful to calculate PIRI and promptly identify cows with subclinical problems, whereas the latter will be used to calculate LFI and identify cows with later occurring disease conditions. This should enable bovine practitioners to anticipate therapeutic treatments toward adequate health and welfare conditions.

Blood Indices in Late Pregnancy Allow to Predict Disease Occurrence After Calving

A profound impairment of innate immunity has been observed in the transition period. Kehrli et al.[97,98] reported that leukocyte activity was suppressed or impaired at least from the week before calving. In the whole transition period, neutrophils exhibit a reduced ability to ingest and kill bacteria, while lymphocytes showed a decreased ability to respond to mitogens and to produce antibodies.[72] Several authors, as reviewed by LeBlanc,[65] observed an association between (1) some of the presented changes in innate immunity some weeks before calving, and (2) postpartum uterine diseases, such as retained placenta or metritis. Hammon et al.[99] suggested that the energy status can account for changes in neutrophil functions in Holstein cows and, consequently, for the uterine disorders. The decrease of dry matter intake (DMI) or the inadequate levels of DMI prior to parturition,[100,101] are the most important causes of impaired immunity in this period. Inadequate DMI leads to a condition of negative energy balance (NEB), which might start mobilization of lipids prior to and not after calving, thus increasing nonesterified fatty acids (NEFA) concentrations and suppressing important immune functions.[102] Nevertheless, besides NEB, many other causes can negatively affect the immune system and metabolism in late pregnancy:[20,24,58,65,77] diet changes (e.g., high energy feed in the "dry," nonlactating period); drops in energy, vitamin, and mineral intake around calving; rumen adaptation; mobilization of body protein; dramatic endocrine changes such as reduction of progesterone and increase of estrogen concentrations in late gestation; massive increase in cortisol concentration at calving;[103] psychological stresses; and viral and parasitic infections. Therefore, we can postulate that during the "dry" period, the peculiar physiological conditions of dairy cows associated with suboptimal environmental conditions (mainly poor hygiene) may exert a negative imprinting on the innate immune system. As a result, commonly harmless opportunistic bacteria could pose a threat. Also, no adequate control over the inflammatory response would be exerted after calving.

In agreement with the tenets presented, recent studies confirmed that some blood indices of innate immune response can be used for disease risk assessment in late pregnancy.[29,90,104,105] As a matter of fact, the concentrations of some biomarkers were shown to change a few days or weeks before calving, in association with appearance and severity of the inflammatory response in the early lactation period. The most interesting biomarkers known to date are as follows:

1. Hemolytic complement (reduced during inflammatory responses), sialic acid (a part of the larger chemical family of glycans and generally considered as a marker of APP release), ROM (markers of oxidative stress)[90]: lower concentrations of sialic acid and ROM and higher concentration of hemolytic complement[106] were found during the last month of pregnancy in cows with the highest LAI value in comparison with cows with a low LAI value. This suggests that cows with high LAI values were not challenged by adverse events in late pregnancy and at calving time. Therefore, cows with high LAI seem to have lower inflammatory and oxidative stimuli at parturition and/or a balanced immune response in case of stimulus;

2. Total bilirubin, ceruloplasmin and lysozyme. Trevisi et al.[29] compared cows with the lowest (worst 10%) and highest LFI values (best 10%) in a population of 54 cows, and confirmed the worse performance in early lactation in cows with the lowest LFI. In addition, these cows showed higher concentrations of bilirubin and ceruloplasmin and a lower concentration of lysozyme in the 3–4 weeks preceding calving. The levels of these biomarkers suggest the presence of a persisting inflammatory condition in late gestation in cows showing low LFI later on, regardless of any acute inflammatory stimulus and/or tissue damage, as confirmed by the low concentrations of posAPPs (e.g., haptoglobin). Moreover, these data suggest a possible role of lysozyme in the homeostatic regulation of the inflammatory response, as previously indicated in other models.[77] In a survey carried out in 26 commercial herds, Amadori et al.[104] also observed that cows with abnormal serum lysozyme concentrations 1 month before calving, but not in the week before calving, showed a significantly greater prevalence of disease in the first 2 months of lactation;

3. PIC like IL1β and IL6. Dry cows showed a high variability of their plasma concentrations of IL-1β, IL-6,[29,105] and TNF-α.[87] Surprisingly, in a more recent investigation we observed that concentrations of PIC remained almost stable in the month before calving,[105] and cows with the highest PIC concentrations showed the worst health status in the early lactation period, and a lower milk yield. Indeed, the susceptibility to inflammatory challenges, measured with the release of PIC from leukocytes after lipopolysaccharides

stimulation in an *ex vivo* test,[107] proved to be substantially constant during the dry period and to increase around calving (from -3 to 3 days from parturition). Interestingly, Jahan et al.[107] reported that the increase of *in vitro* susceptibility occurs when the peripheral response to inflammation, measured by aseptic stimulation in a carrageenan skin test, showed a significant reduction. Amadori et al.[104] also observed on farm a greater prevalence of disease in the first 2 months of lactation in cows with elevated serum concentrations of IL-6, measured 4–5 weeks before calving.

On the whole, these data suggest that some crucial events in the late gestation period may determine a negative imprinting of the innate immune response to infectious and noninfectious stressors after calving, thus worsening the homeostatic response capacity of dairy cows. This conclusion is not surprising, since previous inflammatory challenges tend to depress the immune system and make the organism more susceptible to new stressors, as also confirmed in humans.[108,109]

Therefore, some humoral components of the immune response of dairy cows (i.e., hemolytic complement, lysozyme, PIC, and some acute-phase proteins) can be considered as biomarkers to be used in late gestation for disease risk assessment in the following phases (parturition and lactation). This implies that the negative imprinting occurring in late pregnancy can exert effects over a few weeks, as a possible outcome of the peculiar physiological conditions of pregnant cows, and/or of a specific genetic background.

ANIMAL MODELS: THE FARMED PIG

Disease Occurrence in Farmed Pigs

In swine intensive farms there are critical points that have to be controlled to prevent the onset of diseases sustained by opportunistic pathogens. These are present in the herds, but do not cause disease without critical environmental conditions, as shown, for example, around early weaning at 3–4 weeks of age. A substantial immunosuppression is often observed in this period, because piglets are deprived of the sow's milk (containing protective IgA antibody[110]), and they are moved, mixed, and consequently stressed. Under these conditions, disease occurrence results from an interaction between pathogens and the environment, in which early weaning undoubtedly plays an important role. The most frequent opportunistic infections observed in the 1970s and 1980s, such as swine dysentery, pleuropneumonia (*Actinobacillus pleuropneumoniae*), atrophic rhinitis, and *Mycoplasma* (enzootic) pneumonia, have greatly subsided, being then replaced by other diseases such as porcine reproductive and respiratory syndrome (sustained by a porcine *Arterivirus*, PRRSV), postweaning multysistemic wasting syndrome (PMWS, sustained by porcine circovirus 2), swine influenza, and enteritis.[110]

The efficient production of healthy growers and finishing pigs depends on management, feed, type of housing, and genetic potential of the animals. The main opportunistic infections that affect growers and finishing pigs are PMWS,[111] swine dysentery (SD), PRRSV, lameness, and stomach ulcers. In this phase, poor growth is often a sign of subclinical infections.

Lean Type Pig: Borderline Animal

Various noninfectious stressors may adversely bear on the welfare of farmed pigs under intensive farming conditions, and may cause chronic stress as a long-term effect of modern husbandry techniques. Moreover, genetic selection for lean pigs has caused the appearance of some undesirable traits, which are likely to worsen the adaptation process to modern husbandry techniques. Genetic improvements in pig production have been concentrated on increasing lean tissue deposition in the carcass at the expense of fat, with lean growth rates up to 1000 g/day.[112] The underlying metabolic effort can cause a conflict between immune response and performance under conditions of chronic stress and suboptimal environmental conditions, which is likely to overtax the animals' coping ability and force them to long-lasting homeostatic control actions.

Also, as illustrated in the preface to this book, the genetic selection for lean, large muscle blocks and fast growth is associated with cardiovascular inadequacy and tissue hypoxia. The hypoxia is linked to the production of free radicals/reactive oxygen species (ROS) that are naturally produced reactive compounds. The apparent paradox of an ROS response under conditions of low oxygen pressure was solved some years ago, when it was demonstrated that the electron transport chain in mitochondria is actually an oxygen sensor, which releases ROS under hypoxia conditions.[113] In this scenario, an imbalance between free radical production and antioxidant defense leads to an oxidative stress state, which may be involved in serious clinical conditions like Mulberry Heart Disease, Porcine Stress Syndrome, and Osteochondrosis.[114]

The lean type pig has often to cope with an unfavorable environment in terms of housing, feeding management, mutilations, early weaning, commingling of groups, and high infectious pressure due to poor hygiene conditions. In this context, clinical immunology assays can reveal innate immune responses to these environmental stressors and signal a disease risk.[115] In the authors' experience, assays of cytokines, APPs, serum lysozyme, complement, and bactericidal activity can provide a useful disease risk assessment. Also, these parameters can help identify the environmental fitness of pigs after introducing improved environmental conditions.

A few field cases reported hereunder depict the critical association between innate immune responses to environmental stressors and subsequent decrease of disease resistance, in the context of defective immunocompetence for environmental, opportunistic microbial agents.

Case 1: Innate Immunity Parameters as Prognostic and Diagnostic Tools

This field case was described in detail in a previous paper.[116] Hemolytic complement activity,[117] serum lysozyme,[118] and serum bactericidal activity[119] were investigated in different age groups to get an insight into innate immune responses in a farrow-to-finish pig operation with a breeding unit of 250 sows. This was affected by disease problems in the prefattening sector (reduction of the growth rate, respiratory symptoms, paleness, and weakness). Disease onset was clearly correlated with abnormal values of the innate immunity parameters under study in the age group at risk (70-day old pigs). This could be traced back in turn to a high microbial load in the environment. After the adoption of an effective cleaning protocol, a parallel improvement of clinical conditions and innate immunity parameters was demonstrated 8 months later in pigs of the same age group.

Case 2: Human–Animal Relationship in Pig Production: Influence on Innate Immunity

Under intensive farming conditions, the animals' fear related to livestock people can cause chronic stress, which can progressively limit animal growth and reproductive performance. Therefore, when evaluating causes of low production or reproduction figures, the animals' psychological status should be carefully investigated. This assumption was verified in a modern pig production farm with 400 breeding sows, where wrong handling and behavior of the personnel were clearly recorded.

To characterize the animals' response to such unfavorable conditions, the reactivity test described by Hemsworth et al.[120] was applied to 60 sows between 30 and 90 days of gestation. Three categories of sows were defined and classified on the basis of the test results: fearful, timorous, and trustful. The following data were also collected:

- Total number of piglets and number of piglets born alive.
- P2 thickness (internationally recognized anatomic point, 6.5 cm from the back bone, behind the last rib) at the time of delivery.
- Serum lysozyme,[118] serum bactericidal activity,[119] and total hemolytic complement.[117]

Data obtained from laboratory analyses were processed by analysis of variance. Fearful sows showed a significant alteration of serum bactericidal activity, a lesser back-fat depth and a productive performance far below that of the other two groups (Table 9.3).

These findings confirm the role of human–animal interactions in predisposing animals to disease under intensive farming conditions.

TABLE 9.3 Innate Immunity Parameters, Fat Depth (P2) and Productive Performance of Sows

	Bactericidal activity (%)	Lysozyme (μg/mL)	Complement C'H$_{50}$ (U/mL)	P2 (mm)	Total piglets (born/ litter)	Born piglets (alive/ litter)
Fearful sows	17.77^A	3.37	41.34^a	15.45^a	9.36^A	11.05
Timorous sows	30.58^B	3.44	57.87^b	17.20^b	9.09^A	11
Trustful sows	36.32^B	3.09	64.50^b	18.56^b	12.22^B	11.78

Results are shown as group averages. Different superscripts indicate significant differences. ^{a,b}, $P < 0.05$; ^{A,B}, $P < 0.001$.

Case 3: Innate Immune Response to Thermal Stress

One of the most significant stressors for a newborn piglet is the challenge to adapt to the thermal environment. Thermal stress has complex interactions with diverse homeostatic circuits, including innate immunity (see Preface). Therefore, the aim of this work was the evaluation of some innate immunity parameters in piglets kept in a cold environment. The details of this study were reported in a previous paper.[116] Briefly, the owner of a pig breeding unit with 200 sows, reported high newborn mortality (>20%), mostly in 24–72 h old piglets, in traditional farrowing rooms with slatted floor crates lifted from the ground. The values recorded by max and min thermometers at different levels in the crates revealed temperatures by far below the thermoneutrality value (34°C) of newborn piglets.[121]

On visiting the farm, sows presented BCS values below the expected range. Newborn piglets showed wide weight differences and clear signs of sickness like diarrhea. After ruling out the presence of the usual environmental pathogens, innate immunity tests (C', lysozyme, serum bactericidal activity) were shown to be affected by the thermal discomfort and sickness conditions recorded on farm. On the basis of these results, corrective measures were adopted for a better piglet thermal comfort. Two months later, four sows and their progeny (five piglets per each) were checked in the same pen, and a significant improvement of the aforementioned parameters of innate immunity was recorded in the framework of satisfactory animal health conditions.[116]

On the whole, the reported field cases indicate that timely assays of innate immunity can contribute to an objective evaluation of animal welfare on farm. They can also provide useful diagnostic and prognostic data toward improved disease control. Finally, as shown in dairy cattle farms,[96] such a timely recognition of disease-prone pigs could contribute to reduced usage of antibiotics on farm, with very favorable repercussions in terms of food safety and public health at large.

ACKNOWLEDGMENTS

We thank Dr P. Grossi and Dr A. Ferrari (Università Cattolica, Piacenza, Italy) for their skillful technical assistance.

REFERENCES

1. Broom DM, Johnson KG. *Stress and Animal Welfare*. Londra, UK: Chapman and Hall; 1993.
2. Broom DM. The stress concept and ways of assessing the effects of stress in farm animals. *Appl Anim Ethol* 1983;**11**(1):79.
3. Yu S-F, Jiang K-Y, Zhou W-H, Wang S. Relationship between occupational stress and salivary siga and lysozyme in assembly line workers. *Chin Med J (Engl)* 2008;**121**(17):1741–3.
4. Dhabhar FS, Viswanathan K. Short-term stress experienced at time of immunization induces a long-lasting increase in immunologic memory. *Am J Physiol Regul Integr Comp Physiol* 2005;**289**(3):R738–44.
5. Fregonesi JA, Leaver JD. Behaviour, performance and health indicators of welfare for dairy cows housed in strawyard or cubicle systems. *Livest Prod Sci* 2001;**68**(2–3):205–16.
6. Janeway CA, Medzhitov R. Innate immune recognition. *Annu Rev Immunol* 2002;**20**:197–216.
7. Medzhitov R. Origin and physiological roles of inflammation. *Nature* 2008;**454**(7203):428–35.
8. Mills KHG. TLR-dependent T cell activation in autoimmunity. *Nat Rev Immunol* 2011;**11**(12):807–22.
9. Segerstrom SC, Miller GE. Psychological stress and the human immune system: a meta-analytic study of 30 years of inquiry. *Psychol Bull* 2004;**130**(4):601–30.
10. Alberts B, Johnson A, Lewis J, Raff M, Roberts K, Walter P. *Innate immunity. Molecular biology of the cell*. 4th ed New York: Garland Science; 2002.
11. Turnbull AV, Rivier CL. Regulation of the hypothalamic-pituitary-adrenal axis by cytokines: actions and mechanisms of action. *Physiol Rev* 1999;**79**(1):1–71.
12. Plata-Salamán CR. Cytokine-induced anorexia. behavioral, cellular, and molecular mechanisms. *Ann NY Acad Sci* 1998;**856**:160–70.
13. Bottazzi B, Doni A, Garlanda C, Mantovani A. An integrated view of humoral innate immunity: pentraxins as a paradigm. *Annu Rev Immunol* 2010;**28**:157–83.
14. Ceciliani F, Ceron JJ, Eckersall PD, Sauerwein H. Acute phase proteins in ruminants. *J Proteomics* 2012;**75**(14):4207–31.
15. Bertoni G, Trevisi E. Use of the liver activity index and other metabolic variables in the assessment of metabolic health in dairy herds. *Vet Clin North Am Food Anim Pract* 2013;**29**(2):413–31.
16. Petersen HH, Nielsen JP, Heegaard PMH. Application of acute phase protein measurements in veterinary clinical chemistry. *Vet Res* 2004;**35**(2):163–87.
17. Pasparakis M. Regulation of tissue homeostasis by NF-κB signalling: implications for inflammatory diseases. *Nat Rev Immunol* 2009;**9**(11):778–88.
18. Sorci G, Faivre B. Inflammation and oxidative stress in vertebrate host-parasite systems. *Philos Trans R Soc Lond B Biol Sci* 2009;**364**(1513):71–83.

19. Dantzer R, O'Connor JC, Freund GG, Johnson RW, Kelley KW. From inflammation to sickness and depression: when the immune system subjugates the brain. *Nat Rev Neurosci* 2008;**9**(1):46–56.

20. Bertoni G, Minuti A, Trevisi E. Immune system, inflammation and nutrition. *Anim Prod Sci* 2015;**55**(6):354–60.

21. Frossard JL, Hadengue A, Pastor CM. New serum markers for the detection of severe acute pancreatitis in humans. *Am J Respir Crit Care Med* 2001;**164**(1):162–70.

22. Vermeire S, Van Assche G, Rutgeerts P. C-reactive protein as a marker for inflammatory bowel disease. *Inflamm Bowel Dis* 2004;**10**(5):661–5.

23. Bertoni G, Trevisi E, Han X, Bionaz M. Effects of inflammatory conditions on liver activity in puerperium period and consequences for performance in dairy cows. *J Dairy Sci* 2008;**91**(9):3300–10.

24. Loor JJ, Bertoni G, Hosseini A, Roche JR, Trevisi E. Functional welfare – using biochemical and molecular technologies to understand better the welfare state of peripartal dairy cattle. *Anim Prod Sci* 2013;**53**(9):931–53.

25. Meng H, Lee Y, Ba Z, Fleming JA, Furumoto EJ, Roberts RF, et al. *In vitro* production of IL-6 and IFN-γ is influenced by dietary variables and predicts upper respiratory tract infection incidence and severity respectively in young adults. *Front Immunol* 2015;**6**:94.

26. Fishman D, Faulds G, Jeffery R, Mohamed-Ali V, Yudkin JS, Humphries S, et al. The effect of novel polymorphisms in the interleukin-6 (IL-6) gene on IL-6 transcription and plasma IL-6 levels, and an association with systemic-onset juvenile chronic arthritis. *J Clin Invest* 1998;**102**(7):1369–76.

27. Nieters A, Brems S, Becker N. Cross-sectional study on cytokine polymorphisms, cytokine production after T-cell stimulation and clinical parameters in a random sample of a German population. *Hum Genet* 2001;**108**(3):241–8.

28. Catalani E, Amadori M, Vitali A, Lacetera N. Short communication: lymphoproliferative response to lipopolysaccharide and incidence of infections in periparturient dairy cows. *J Dairy Sci* 2013;**96**(11):7077–81.

29. Trevisi E, Amadori M, Cogrossi S, Razzuoli E, Bertoni G. Metabolic stress and inflammatory response in high-yielding, periparturient dairy cows. *Res Vet Sci* 2012;**93**(2):695–704.

30. Kishimoto T. Il-6: from its discovery to clinical applications. *Int Immunol* 2010;**22**(5):347–52.

31. Hussell T, Goulding J. Structured regulation of inflammation during respiratory viral infection. *Lancet Infect Dis* 2010;**10**(5):360–6.

32. Fossum C, Wattrang E, Fuxler L, Jensen KT, Wallgren P. Evaluation of various cytokines (IL-6, IFN-alpha, IFN-gamma, TNF-alpha) as markers for acute bacterial infection in swine – a possible role for serum interleukin-6. *Vet Immunol Immunopathol* 1998;**64**(2):161–72.

33. Scheller J, Chalaris A, Schmidt-Arras D, Rose-John S. The pro- and anti-inflammatory properties of the cytokine interleukin-6. *Biochim Biophys Acta* 2011;**1813**(5):878–88.

34. Baumann H, Gauldie J. The acute phase response. *Immunol Today* 1994;**15**(2):74–80.

35. Nijsten MWN, De Groot ER, Ten Duis HJ, Klasen HJ, Hack CE, Aarden LA. Serum levels of interleukin-6 and acute phase responses. *Lancet* 1987;**330**(8564):921.

36. Päth G, Scherbaum WA, Bornstein SR. The role of interleukin-6 in the human adrenal gland. *Eur J Clin Invest* 2000;**30**(Suppl 3):91–5.

37. Aderka D, Le JM, Vilcek J. IL-6 inhibits lipopolysaccharide-induced tumor necrosis factor production in cultured human monocytes, U937 cells, and in mice. *J Immunol* 1989;**143**(11):3517–23.

38. Kishimoto T. Interleukin-6 (IL-6). In: Thomson AG, Lotze MT, editors. *The cytokine handbook*. 4th ed London: Academic Press; 2003. p. 281–304.

39. Maksymowych WP. Biomarkers in spondyloarthritis. *Curr Rheumatol Rep* 2010;**12**(5):318–24.

40. Fang S, Wang Y, Sui D, Liu H, Ross MI, Gershenwald JE, et al. C-reactive protein as a marker of melanoma progression. *J Clin Oncol* 2015;**33**(12):1389–96.

41. Saito K, Kihara K. Role of C-reactive protein in urological cancers: a useful biomarker for predicting outcomes. *Int J Urol* 2013;**20**(2):161–71.

42. Allin KH, Nordestgaard BG. Elevated C-reactive protein in the diagnosis, prognosis, and cause of cancer. *Crit Rev Clin Lab Sci* 2011;**48**(4):155–70.

43. Devarajan P. Biomarkers for the early detection of acute kidney injury. *Curr Opin Pediatr* 2011;**23**(2):194–200.

44. Xu L, Zhu Y, An H, Liu Y, Lin Z, Wang G, et al. Clinical significance of tumor-derived IL-1β and IL-18 in localized renal cell carcinoma: associations with recurrence and survival. *Urol Oncol* 2015;**33**(2):68e9–68e16.

45. Wang X, Meng H, Xu L, Chen Z, Shi D, Lv D. Mean platelet volume as an inflammatory marker in patients with severe periodontitis. *Platelets* 2015;**26**(1):67–71.

46. Beck J, Garcia R, Heiss G, Vokonas PS, Offenbacher S. Periodontal disease and cardiovascular disease. *J Periodontol* 1996;**67**(10 Suppl):1123–37.

47. Kapsoritakis AN, Koukourakis MI, Sfiridaki A, Potamianos SP, Kosmadaki MG, Koutrouba-kis IE, et al. Mean platelet volume: a useful marker of inflammatory bowel disease activity. *Am J Gastroenterol* 2001;**96**(3):776–81.

48. Kisacik B, Tufan A, Kalyoncu U, Karadag O, Akdogan A, Ozturk Mehmet A, et al. Mean platelet volume (MPV) as an inflammatory marker in ankylosing spondylitis and rheumatoid arthritis. *Joint Bone Spine* 2008;**75**(3):291–4.

49. Martinon F, Mayor A, Tschopp J. The inflammasomes: guardians of the body. *Annu Rev Immunol* 2009;**27**:229–65.

50. Qian F, Goel G, Meng H, Wang X, You F, Devine L, et al. Systems immunology reveals markers of susceptibility to West Nile Virus infection. *Clin Vaccine Immunol* 2015;**22**(1):6–16.

51. Tamilselvi E, Haripriya D, Hemamalini M, Pushpa G, Swapna S. Association of disease severity with IL-1 levels in methotrexate-treated psoriasis patients. *Scand J Immunol* 2013;**78**(6):545–53.

52. Okamoto H. TT viruses in animals. De Villiers E-M, Zur Hausen H, editors. *TT viruses – the still elusive human pathogens. Current topics in microbiology and immunology*, 331. Heidelberg: Springer; 2009. p. 35–52.

53. Focosi D, Maggi F, Albani M, Macera L, Ricci V, Gragnani S, et al. Torque teno virus viremia kinetics after autologous stem cell transplantation are predictable and may serve as a surrogate marker of functional immune reconstitution. *J Clin Virol* 2010;**47**(2):189–92.

54. Maggi F, Pifferi M, Michelucci A, Albani M, Sbranti S, Lanini L, et al. Torque teno virus viremia load size in patients with selected congenital defects of innate immunity. *Clin Vaccine Immunol* 2011;**18**(4):692–4.

55. Focosi D, Macera L, Pistello M, Maggi F. Torque teno virus viremia correlates with intensity of maintenance immunosuppression in adult orthotopic liver transplant. *J Infect Dis* 2014;**210**(4):667–8.

56. Drackley JK. ADSA Foundation Scholar Award. Biology of dairy cows during the transition period: the final frontier? *J Dairy Sci* 1999;**82**(11):2259–73.

57. Sordillo LM, Raphael W. Significance of metabolic stress, lipid mobilization, and inflammation on transition cow disorders. *Vet Clin North Am Food Anim Pract* 2013;**29**(2):267–78.

58. Van-Knegsel ATM, Hammon HM, Bernabucci U, Bertoni G, Bruckmaier RM, Goselink RMA, et al. Metabolic adaptation during early lactation: key to cow health, longevity and a sustainable dairy production chain. *CAB Rev Perspect Agric Vet Sci Nutr Nat Resour* 2014;**9**:15.

59. LeBlanc SJ, Lissemore KD, Kelton DF, Duffield TF, Leslie KE. Major advances in disease prevention in dairy cattle. *J Dairy Sci* 2006;**89**(4):1267–79.

60. Mulligan FJ, Doherty ML. Production diseases of the transition cow. *Vet J* 2008;**176**(1):3–9.

61. Walsh RB, Walton JS, Kelton DF, LeBlanc SJ, Leslie KE, Duffield TF. The effect of subclinical ketosis in early lactation on reproductive performance of postpartum dairy cows. *J Dairy Sci* 2007;**90**(6):2788–96.

62. Murata H, Shimada N, Yoshioka M. Current research on acute phase proteins in veterinary diagnosis: an overview. *Vet J* 2004;**168**(1):28–40.

63. Bionaz M, Trevisi E, Calamari L, Librandi F, Ferrari A, Bertoni G. Plasma paraoxonase, health, inflammatory conditions, and liver function in transition dairy cows. *J Dairy Sci* 2007;**90**(4):1740–50.

64. Cai TQ, Weston PG, Lund LA, Brodie B, McKenna DJ, Wagner WC. Association between neutrophil functions and periparturient disorders in cows. *Am J Vet Res* 1994;**55**(7):934–43.

65. LeBlanc SJ. Postpartum uterine disease and dairy herd reproductive performance: a review. *Vet J* 2008;**176**(1):102–14.

66. Trevisi E, Ferrari AR, Bertoni G. Productive and metabolic consequences induced by the retained placenta in dairy cows. *Vet Res Commun* 2008;**32**(Suppl 1):S363–6.

67. Moretti P, Probo M, Morandi N, Trevisi E, Ferrari A, Minuti A, et al. Early post-partum hematological changes in Holstein dairy cows with retained placenta. *Anim Reprod Sci* 2015;**152**:17–25.

68. Trevisi E, Ferrari A, Piccioli Cappelli F, Bertoni G. Blood changes occurring before and after abomasum displacement in dairy cows. In: XXIV *World Buiatrics Congress*. Nice; 2006, p. 869

69. Grosche A, Fürll M, Wittek T. Peritoneal fluid analysis in dairy cows with left displaced abomasum and abomasal volvulus. *Vet Rec* 2012;**170**(16):413.

70. Bertoni G, Trevisi E, Ferrari A, Gubbiotti A. The dairy cow performances can be affected by inflammations occurring around calving. In: *57th EAAP Meeting*. Antalya; 2006, p. 325.

71. Imhasly S, Naegeli H, Baumann S, von Bergen M, Luch A, Jungnickel H, et al. Metabolomic biomarkers correlating with hepatic lipidosis in dairy cows. *BMC Vet Res* 2014;**10**(1):122.

72. Goff JP, Horst RL. Physiological changes at parturition and their relationship to metabolic disorders. *J Dairy Sci* 1997;**80**(7):1260–8.

73. Beaudeau F, Seegers H, Ducrocq V, Fourichon C, Bareille N. Effect of health disorders on culling in dairy cows: a review and a critical discussion. *Ann Zootech* 2000;**49**(4):293–311.

74. Hoeben D, Burvenich C, Trevisi E, Bertoni G, Hamann J, Bruckmaier RM, et al. Role of endotoxin and TNF-alpha in the pathogenesis of experimentally induced coliform mastitis in periparturient cows. *J Dairy Res* 2000;**67**(4):503–14.

75. Khafipour E, Krause DO, Plaizier JC. A grain-based subacute ruminal acidosis challenge causes translocation of lipopolysaccharide and triggers inflammation. *J Dairy Sci* 2009;**92**(3):1060–70.

76. Gruys E, Toussaint MJM, Landman WJ, Tivapasi M, Chamanza R, VanVeen L. Infection, inflammation and stress inhibit growth. Mechanisms and non-specific assessment of the processes by acute phase proteins. In: Wensing T, editor. *Production diseases in farm animals*. The Netherland: Wageningen Press; 1998. p. 72–87.

77. Trevisi E, Amadori M, Archetti I, Lacetera N, Bertoni G. Inflammatory response and acute phase proteins in the transition period of high-yielding dairy cows. In: Veas F, editor. *Acute Phase Protein*. Rijeka: InTech; 2011. p. 355–80.

78. Leonard BE, Song C. Stress, depression, and the role of cytokines. In: Dantzer R, Wollman EE, Yirmiya R, editors. *Cytokines, stress, and depression*. New York: Kluwer Academic Publishers; 1999. p. 251.

79. Tian R, Hou G, Li D, Yuan TF. A possible change process of inflammatory cytokines in the prolonged chronic stress and its ultimate implications for health. *Sci World J* 2014; ID 780616, 8 pages.
80. Hotamisligil GS. Inflammation and metabolic disorders. *Nature* 2006;**444**(7121):860–7.
81. Gruys E, Toussaint MJM, Niewold TA, Koopmans SJ. Acute phase reaction and acute phase proteins. *J Zhejiang Univ Sci B* 2005;**6**(11):1045–56.
82. Ritchie RF, Palomaki GE, Neveux LM, Navolotskaia O, Ledue TB, Craig WY. Reference distributions for the negative acute-phase serum proteins, albumin, transferrin and trans-thyret: a practical, simple and clinically relevant approach in a large cohort. *J Clin Lab Anal* 1999;**13**(6):273–9.
83. Assenat E, Gerbal-Chaloin S, Larrey D, Saric J, Fabre JM, Maurel P, et al. Interleukin 1beta inhibits car-induced expression of hepatic genes involved in drug and bilirubin clearance. *Hepatology* 2004;**40**(4):951–60.
84. Rosales FJ, Ritter SJ, ZolFaghari R, Smith JE, Ross AC. Effects of acute inflammation on plasma retinol, retinol-binding protein, and its mRNA in the liver and kidneys of vitamin A-sufficient rats. *J Lipid Res* 1996;**37**:962–71.
85. Trevisi E, Bertoni G, Lombardelli R, Minuti A. Relation of inflammation and liver function with the plasma cortisol response to adrenocorticotropin in early lactating dairy cows. *J Dairy Sci* 2013;**96**(9):5712–22.
86. Ingenbleek Y, Young V. Transthyretin (prealbumin) in health and disease: nutritional implications. *Annu Rev Nutr* 1994;**14**(1):495–533.
87. Trevisi E, Amadori M, Bakudila AM, Bertoni G. Metabolic changes in dairy cows induced by oral, low-dose interferon-alpha treatment. *J Anim Sci* 2009;**87**(9):3020–9.
88. Trevisi E, Calamari L, Bertoni G. Definition of a liver activity index in the transition dairy cow and its relationship with the reproductive performance. *X Int Symp Vet Lab Diagnost, Salsomaggiore* 2001;118–9.
89. Bjerre-Harpøth V, Friggens NC, Thorup VM, Larsen T, Damgaard BM, Ingvartsen KL, et al. Metabolic and production profiles of dairy cows in response to decreased nutrient density to increase physiological imbalance at different stages of lactation. *J Dairy Sci* 2012;**95**(5):2362–80.
90. Trevisi E, Zecconi A, Bertoni G, Piccinini R. Blood and milk immune and inflammatory profiles in periparturient dairy cows showing a different liver activity index. *J Dairy Res* 2010;**77**(03):310–7.
91. Trevisi E, Gubbiotti A, Bertoni G. Effects of inflammation in peripartum dairy cows on milk yield, energy balance and efficiency. In: Ortigues-Marty I, Miraux N, Brand-Williams W, editors. *2nd International Symposium on Energy and Protein Metabolism and Nutrition*. Vichy: Wageningen Academic Publishers; 2007. p. 395–6.
92. Trevisi E, Ferrari A, Piccioli-Cappelli F, Grossi P, Bertoni G. *An additional study on the relationship between the inflammatory condition at calving time and net energy efficiency in dairy cows. 3rd EAAP International Symposium Energy and Protein Metabolism and Nutrition*. The Netherland: Wageningen Academic Publishers; 2010 489–490.
93. Soriani N, Trevisi E, Calamari L. Relationships between rumination time, metabolic conditions and health status in dairy cows during the transition period. *J Anim Sci* 2012;**90**:4544–54.
94. Grossi P, Bertoni G, Piccioli-Cappelli F, Trevisi E. Effects of the precalving administration of omega-3 fatty acids alone or in combination with acetylsalicylic acid in periparturient dairy cows. *J Anim Sci* 2013;**91**(6):2657–66.
95. Bossaert P, Trevisi E, Opsomer G, Bertoni G, De Vliegher S, Leroy JLMR. The association between indicators of inflammation and liver variables during the transition period in high-yielding dairy cows: an observational study. *Vet J* 2012;**192**(2):222–5.

96. Trevisi E, Zecconi A, Cogrossi S, Razzuoli E, Grossi P, Amadori M. Strategies for reduced antibiotic usage in dairy cattle farms. *Res Vet Sci* 2014;**96**(2):229–33.

97. Kehrli ME, Nonnecke BJ, Roth JA. Alterations in bovine neutrophil function during the periparturient period. *Am J Vet Res* 1989;**50**(2):207–14.

98. Kehrli ME, Nonnecke BJ, Roth JA. Alterations in bovine lymphocyte function during the periparturient period. *Am J Vet Res* 1989;**50**(2):215–20.

99. Hammon DS, Evjen IM, Dhiman TR, Goff JP, Walters JL. Neutrophil function and energy status in Holstein cows with uterine health disorders. *Vet Immunol Immunopathol* 2006;**113**(1–2):21–9.

100. Trevisi E, Han XT, Piccioli-Cappelli F, Bertoni G. Intake reduction before calving affects milk yield and metabolism in dairy cows. In: *53rd Annual Meeting EAAP*. Cairo; 2002, p. 54.

101. Grummer RR, Mashek DG, Hayirli A. Dry matter intake and energy balance in the transition period. *Vet Clin North Am Food Anim Pract* 2004;**20**(3):447–70.

102. Rukkwamsuk T, Kruip TAM, Wensing T. Relationship between overfeeding and overconditioning in the dry period and the problems of high producing dairy cows during the postparturient period. *Vet Q* 1999;**21**(3):71–7.

103. Henricks DM, Dickey JF, Hill JR, Johnston WE. Plasma estrogen and progesterone levels after mating, and during late pregnancy and postpartum in cows. *Endocrinology* 1972;**90**(5):1336–42.

104 Amadori M, Fusi F, Bilato D, Archetti IL, Lorenzi V, Bertocchi L. Disease risk assessment by clinical immunology analyses in periparturient dairy cows. *Research in Veterinary Science* 2015;102:25–26.

105. Trevisi E, Jahan N, Ferrari A, Minuti A. Pro-inflammatory cytokine profile in dairy cows: consequences for new lactation. *Ital J Anim Sci* 2015;**14**:285–292.

106. Barta V, Barta O. Testing of hemolytic complement and its components. In: Barta O, editor. *Veterinary clinical immunology laboratory*. Blacksburg: BAR-LAB; 1993. p. C6.1–C6.40.

107. Jahan N, Minuti A, Trevisi E. Assessment of immune response in periparturient dairy cows using *ex vivo* whole blood stimulation assay with lipopolysaccharides and carrageenan skin test. *Vet Immunol Immunopathol* 2015;**165**(3-4):119–26.

108. Karin M, Lawrence T, Nizet V. Innate immunity gone awry: linking microbial infections to chronic inflammation and cancer. *Cell* 2006;**124**(4):823–35.

109. Lucas SM, Rothwell NJ, Gibson RM. The role of inflammation in CNS injury and disease. *Br J Pharmacol* 2006;**147 Suppl**:S232–40.

110. Muirhead MR, Alexander TJL. *Managing pig health: a reference for the farm*. 2nd ed. Sheffield, UK: 5M Enterprises Ltd.; 2013.

111. Madec F, Rose N, Grasland B, Cariolet R, Jestin A. Post-weaning multisystemic wasting syndrome and other PCV2-related problems in pigs: a 12-year experience. *Transbound Emerg Dis* 2008;**55**(7):273–83.

112. Lawlor P, Lynch B, Kerry J, Allen P. Effect of sex, castration and slaughter weight on pig performance and carcass. In: *Proceedings of American Society of Animal Science Annual Meeting*. 2003, p. 201.

113. Guzy RD, Schumacker PT. Oxygen sensing by mitochondria at complex III: the paradox of increased reactive oxygen species during hypoxia. *Exp Physiol* 2006;**91**(5):807–19.

114. Brambilla G, Civitareale C, Ballerini A, Fiori M, Amadori M, Archetti LI, et al. Response to oxidative stress as a welfare parameter in swine. *Redox Rep* 2002;**7**(3):159–63.

115. Amadori M, Archetti IL, Frasnelli M, Bagni M, Olzi E, Caronna G, et al. An immunological approach to the evaluation of welfare in Holstein Frisian cattle. *Zentralbl Veterinarmed B* 1997;**44**(6):321–7.

116. Moscati L, Sensi M, Battistacci L, Archetti IL, Amadori M. Evaluation of innate immunity in pigs under field conditions. *Vet Scan On Line Vet J* 2011;**6**(2) Article 90.
117. Seyfarth M. Komplementtitration. In: Fiemel H, editor. *Immunologische arbeirsmethoden.* 1st ed. Jena, Germany: VEB Gustav Fischer Verlag; 1976. p. 145–8.
118. Osserman EF, Lawlor DP. Serum and urinary lysozyme (muramidase) in monocytic and monomyelocytic leukemia. *J Exp Med* 1966;**124**(5):921–52.
119. Dorn W, Mehlhorn G, Klemm C. Blood bactericidal activity in calves. *Arch Exp Veterinarmed* 1980;**34**(5):635–50.
120. Hemsworth PH, Barnett JL, Coleman GJ, Hansen C. A study of the relationships between the attitudinal and behavioural profiles of stockpersons and the level of fear of humans and reproductive performance of commercial pigs. *Appl Anim Behav Sci* 1989;**23**(4):301–14.
121. Berthon D, Herpin P, Bertin R, De Marco F, le Dividich J. Metabolic changes associated with sustained 48-hr shivering thermogenesis in the newborn pig. *Comp Biochem Physiol B Biochem Mol Biol* 1996;**114**(4):327–35.

Subject Index

Printed in the United States
By Bookmasters